CHRONIC PAIN

PAIN MANAGEMENT

Advisory Board

Walter L. Nieves, M.D.
Tallman Medical Center
Suffern, New York, U.S.A.

Sunil Panchal, M.D.
President of COPE
(Coalition for Pain Education)
Tampa, Florida, U.S.A.

William K. Schmidt, Ph.D.
Consultant
Davis, California, U.S.A.

Marsha Stanton, M.S., R.N.
Consultant
Seal Beach, California, U.S.A.

CHRONIC PAIN

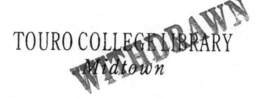

GARY W. JAY

Schwarz Biosciences, Inc.
Raleigh, North Carolina, USA

informa
healthcare

New York   London

MT

Informa Healthcare USA, Inc.
52 Vanderbilt Avenue
New York, NY 10017

© 2007 by Informa Healthcare USA, Inc.
Informa Healthcare is an Informa business

No claim to original U.S. Government works
Printed in the United States of America on acid-free paper
10 9 8 7 6 5 4 3 2 1

International Standard Book Number-10: 0-8493-3046-7 (Hardcover)
International Standard Book Number-13: 978-0-8493-3046-9 (Hardcover)

Library of Congress Cataloging-in-Publication Data

Jay, Gary W.
   Chronic pain / Gary W. Jay.
      p. ; cm. -- (Pain management ; 2)
   Includes bibliographical references and index.
   ISBN-13: 978-0-8493-3046-9 (hardcover : alk. paper)
   ISBN-10: 0-8493-3046-7 (hardcover : alk. paper)
   1. Chronic pain. 2. Chronic pain--Treatment.
   I. Title. II. Series.
   [DNLM: 1. Pain. 2. Chronic Disease. WL 704 J42c 2007]

   RB127.J38 2007
   616'.0472--dc22   2007000686

Visit the Informa Web site at
www.informa.com

and the Informa Healthcare Web site at
www.informahealthcare.com

08/01/08

As always, this book is dedicated to my wife Suzanne and daughter Samantha, for their constant love and encouragement, not to mention tolerance of my work. To my friends, old and new, who taught me and helped me along the way: Dr. David Longmire, Jim Kapp, Dr. Scott Denny, Dr. Byron Scott, Dr. Barry Cole, Dr. Mark Boswell, Dr. Richard Cox, Dr. Tim Sullivan, and Rick Johns and Jennifer Bolen, esquires both. Special thanks to Dr. Kenneth Sommerville, for teaching and leading and helping me to navigate through new, sometimes choppy, waters. To Dr. David Rudd, for putting up with my questions and being an inspiration. And Last, but certainly not least, to my patients, past and present, who have been my best teachers.

—Gary W. Jay

Preface

When I began to practice pain medicine there were no national clinical pain societies and a distinct paucity of books on pain management.

Other doctors didn't even know what I did.

Since those early years, the subspecialty has grown and evolved into something we could not have foreseen: "We" were the original thirty docs who got together in Washington, D.C., at the behest of neurosurgeon Ben Crue in 1983, to start the American Academy of Algology (later known as the American Academy of Pain Medicine).

In the beginning, there was an amorphous group of doctors with multiple specialties, all interested in treating pain patients. Now, the multiple types of physician specialties treating pain only barely exist. The way the first generation of pain specialists treated pain—using a conservative, frequently interdisciplinary medical model—has changed dramatically for many reasons, some good (to accommodate new technology) and some bad (what the insurance companies, HMOs, and PPOs deign to cover).

In the quarter century that I've specialized in the treatment of chronic headache and pain of all etiologies, I've had the good fortune to be asked to write for and lecture to my colleagues around the country and overseas literally hundreds of times. I've found great interest and need for headache and pain-related information from physicians in all specialties and have gladly acted as a resource for these physicians. I've endeavored to explain to them what I do. Because as times have changed, too many patients have not been permitted to see a pain specialist or visit a tertiary-care specialty interdisciplinary pain management clinic such as those I've run for over twenty-five years.

No one person, physician or not, is smart enough to treat a chronic pain patient by themselves. Unfortunately, the medical community's understanding of this fact, which was so marked when pain management/medicine became a specialty, has dramatically changed. Today, some believe that they can, individually and independently of anyone else, "cure" chronic pain patients. This makes little sense when the patients, as a group, carry the wrong diagnosis 65 percent of the time; have to be weaned off of inappropriate and unnecessary medications 85 percent of the time; and have seen an average of 5.6 physicians and endured an average of 1.6 surgeries prior to reaching the pain specialist (my statistically typical patient over the last several decades).

In spite of new technology, it still doesn't work that way: it takes more than one person to help identify and deal with the biological/psychological/sociological aspects that make up, in good part, the complexity of the chronic non-cancer pain patient.

Chronic non-cancer pain is a disease like diabetes and hypertension, in that for the most part it cannot be cured. It can, however, be successfully treated and controlled. Patients can lead exceptional, full lives, with their pain under significant or even excellent control.

Chronic Pain is written for all of the physicians in all of the specialties (and hopefully medical students, interns, and residents) who need to know about pain to help their patients. After all, chronic non-cancer pain is one of the top two reasons patients seek medical care. The book was written to be assessable; that is, it is not a dry encyclopedia only to be used for researching "mysterious esoteric diagnoses" in the fleeting moments between patients. The information is presented so clinicians will not find it burdensome to read right through a chapter and be able to understand the diagnosis, assessment, and treatment of the most common chronic non-cancer pain entities.

Chronic Pain starts with the anatomy and physiology and some of the molecular bases of pain, which give the basis for the pathophysiology of common chronic non-cancer pain entities, such as neuropathic pain, myofascial pain syndromes, fibromyalgia, and chronic tension-type headache. The book also delves into various treatment modalities using evidence-based medicine principles, teaching the reader about opioid and adjunctive pain medications, psychological care, interventional pain medicine, and interdisciplinary pain management treatment, among others. Other key features of the book include patient case studies, principles for pertinent examination techniques, and treatment techniques such as trigger-point injections.

Chronic Pain can be read on multiple levels—it includes the basics needed by all physicians to understand chronic non-cancer pain, while providing information meant specifically for pain specialists. I have tried to give the book an ease of understanding for physicians of all specialties who may run into the medical problems dealt with in this book—the pain specialists to whom patients are sent when their primary physician can't go any further in their treatment; the students who need to learn about pain (to get more information than the typical 3–5 hours offered in medical school regarding), and even for patients.

Gary W. Jay

Contents

Anatomy and Physiology of Pain: The Central and Peripheral Nervous Systems

DEFINING PAIN

The International Association for the Study of Pain (1) describes pain as "an unpleasant sensory and emotional experience arising from the actual or potential tissue damage or described in terms of such damage." The importance of this definition is simple—it gives a tremendous amount of latitude in the determination of the etiology of all types of pain. Clinically, pain is defined as "what the patient states it is"; it is then up to the clinician to determine exactly what the patient means.

Pain is not a simple phenomenon. Whether acute or chronic, it is a complex of biological, psychological, and sociological phenomena. The emotional and affective aspects of pain may be learned, at least in part, but are also initiated as a neurophysiological/limbic response to physical stimuli.

The central nervous system (CNS) is the site of the reception, processing, interpretation, determination, and reaction to specific stimuli—nociceptive (painful) stimuli. The closest analogy to the way pain works in the CNS appears to be the workings of a computer: the CNS has the "hard wiring" of the actual nerves, nerve pathways, and interconnections, as well as the "software," the neurotransmitters that enable the hardware to function. There is a major caveat to this analogy, however. Many cells, such as those in the spinal cord dorsal horn, appear to show a great deal of neuroplasticity; so, while they are "hard wired," the "chip type," or neurons, can change in both form and function.

Why bother with such an analogy at all? The clinical evaluation and treatment of patients with chronic noncancer pain (referred to in this book as chronic pain—CP) depends on understanding the most basic clinical physiology and pathophysiology. This understanding allows us to make clinical determinations and prescribe appropriate treatments, which can then help to relieve pain on both the "hardware" and "software" levels. That is, we can find ways to change the neurochemical milieu itself (the software) and how it affects the "hard wiring" of the CNS and the peripheral sites of nociception.

PERIPHERAL PAIN PATHWAYS

All tissues other than the CNS itself contain nociceptors, especially the skin, which is heavily innervated. The sensation of pain usually occurs when the peripheral nervous system's sensory neurons are activated by noxious stimulation to the free nerve endings of primary afferent neurons. They may be stimulated by mechanical, thermal, or chemical stimuli.

The peripheral nerves contain sensory, motor, and autonomic fibers. They are classified by their size, conduction velocity, and the absence or presence of a myelin sheath. The initial stimulation of the peripheral afferents feeds the peripheral nerves information that can change the perception of the painful stimulation. In other words, the "additive" nature of continuous stimulation, if it occurs, indicates that the sensory stimulus was intense enough to cause pain. When the nociceptors are stimulated repeatedly, typically after tissue damage, the pain threshold is decreased, so that less stimulation can induce pain. These changes in perception of peripheral painful stimulation occur in the spinal cord, as will be discussed later. Clinical manifestations include hyperalgesia, an increased subjective perception of pain, hyperpathia, a very exaggerated response to noxious stimuli, and allodynia, the perception of pain from simple, non-noxious stimuli.

Myelinated A fibers are large and have the fastest nerve impulse conduction. The A group of neurons have three subtypes, alpha (α), beta (β), and delta (δ). The Aδ fibers are small and poorly myelinated. They are the only A fibers that transmit pain impulses, particularly the pain information immediately following injury. The Aβ fibers are larger and more myelinated. They transmit pressure, touch, and vibration. They do not transmit pain impulses, but work in the spinal cord to modulate painful stimuli. The C fibers are unmyelinated. They slowly conduct pain impulses that are dull, poorly localized, and prolonged. These impulses are noted some time after injury. The Aα and A-gamma (γ) neurons are both efferent and do not transmit sensory impulses. Nevertheless, they are involved in pain, because they activate muscle fibers, inducing muscle spasms. B fibers are preganglionic fibers that are involved in the sympathetic aspects of pain.

There are three major forms of peripheral nociceptors: (*i*) the Aδ high-threshold mechanoreceptors that respond to noxious pressure, (*ii*) Aδ mechano-thermal receptors that respond to noxious thermal and mechanical stimuli, and (*iii*) the polymodal C-fiber nociceptors that respond to noxious mechanical, thermal, and chemical stimuli. After stimulation of the free nerve endings (the primary afferents), pain impulses and other sensory information travel up the peripheral nerves via the dorsal root ganglia to the spinal cord and then to the brain. The dorsal root ganglia are located outside of the spinal cord and contain the cell bodies of sensory nerves.

Nociceptors, which are part of the somatic nervous system, typically have a close correlation to specific physical areas via somatotopic representation (direct correlations between the physical area and the determination of the site, through small nociceptive fields, via the CNS) in the spinal cord and brain. The autonomic nervous system, which has a significant influence on visceral pain, sympathetic pain (e.g., complex regional pain syndrome and sympathetically mediated pain), and muscular pain, has large nociceptive fields, decreasing the specificity by which the CNS can identify exactly the area of nociception or afferent stimulation. The autonomic nervous system works to increase acetylcholine at the neuromuscular junction when the somatic nervous system, via thought or reflex, causes muscle movement. The somatic nervous system is most typically thought of as "voluntary," in that it enables us to perform specific determined tasks.

THE DORSAL HORN

From the dorsal root ganglia, pain information travels to the dorsal horn of the spinal cord, where it is processed and modulated. Modulation of painful stimuli can occur anywhere in the CNS, but it happens first in the dorsal horn. Pain information is augmented or inhibited along both ascending and descending pain pathways via neurochemical modulators, substances that can increase or inhibit algetic sensory information.

The dorsal horn is a major center for the afferent sensory information from nociceptors. This is where pain impulses are modulated by excitation, inhibition, and the integration of nociception, affecting various aspects of the expression or perception of pain. The substantia gelatinosa is an important modulation center for painful stimuli. It acts primarily to facilitate inhibition of painful stimuli. The substantia gelatinosa is stimulated by large fibers, enhancing its inhibitory effects, while small fibers inhibit this structure, thereby decreasing its inhibitory effects on fibers that stimulate its intrinsic target cells, causing pain to continue.

The dorsal horn consists of Rexed laminae I through VI. Laminae VII through X have less apparent dealings with painful stimuli. They comprise the intermediate and ventral horns of the spinal cord. Afferents from the dorsal roots enter the spinal cord with fibers traversing through Lissauer's tract and end in the dorsal horn. Lissauer's tract is a bundle of primary afferent fibers (Aδ, C, and propriospinal axons) that travels between the dorsal horn and other areas of the spinal cord. Aδ fibers terminate in laminae I, II, V, and X. C fibers end in laminae I, II, and V. Aβ fibers terminate in laminae III and IV.

There are two types of nociceptive neurons in the dorsal horn. One is the pain, or nociceptive-specific neurons, which respond to various pain-inducing stimuli, have small receptive fields, and are somatotopically organized. They are mostly found in lamina I. The others are called wide-dynamic-range neurons and respond to a wide variety of stimuli. They have larger receptive fields and are the neurons most commonly found in the dorsal horn. The wide-dynamic-range neurons are "on-off" cells that will transmit pain information and then "shut off" until stimulated again. When these cells are subjected to constant C-fiber stimulation, they are turned "on" and, via the phenomenon of "windup," do not shut off, becoming important in the genesis of central sensitization and continuation of sympathetically mediated pain syndromes.

Besides pain-specific and wide-dynamic-range neurons, the marginal layer of the dorsal horn, lamina I, includes projection cells. These cells make up projection pathways and synapse with interneurons, which are numerous in number throughout the spinal cord, and which interconnect with anterior motor neurons and are therefore responsible for most of the integrative functions of the spinal cord. Lamina II is called the substantia gelatinosa and contains both types of nociceptive neurons. The nucleus proprius consists of laminae III, IV, and V. Myelinated axons and dendrites from deeper laminae are found in lamina III. In lamina IV, low-threshold mechanoreceptors, which respond to both tactile and thermal stimuli from the skin, are the most numerous cells. Lamina V is mainly made up of wide-dynamic-range neurons and axons that are part of the ascending nociceptive systems.

Melzack and Wall's gate control theory of pain, first published in 1965 (2), described the dorsal horn's functioning as a gate that can allow painful stimuli to pass higher into the CNS or can deny passage. This theory has been modified since it was initially espoused, but it remains one of the high points of pain research.

ASCENDING PATHWAYS

Simply, there are two types of pain pathways. The oligosynaptic pathways have few synapses, long intersynaptic distances, and are rapidly conducting and topographically (somatotopically) assigned. They include the lateral spinothalamic tract (STT) with segmental crossing and nonproprioceptive parts of the dorsal columns, which cross in the medullary region. They also map somatotopically onto the posteroven-tral thalamic nuclei and the postcentral cortex. There are branches to the brain stem reticular formation.

The polysynaptic pathways have many synapses, with short intersynaptic distances and no somatotopic organization. They are relatively slow. They form part of the ascending reticular formation, and travel from the reticular activating system to the medial and intralaminar nuclei of the thalamus. Then they go to the basal ganglia, limbic system, and cerebral cortex as well as to the hypothalamus.

The STT consists of neurons that mostly originate in laminae I, II, and V, cross the midline of the spinal cord, and ascend in the anterolateral portion of the spinal cord, terminating on thalamic nuclei. The STT has both a medial and lateral system. The neospinothalamic tract (the lateral system) directly connects the dorsal horn and the thalamus. It is fast conducting and transmits initial sharp, localized pain immediately upon injury. This part of the STT consists of neurons from laminae I, II, and V, which project to the lateral thalamus and synapse with fibers that project to the somatosensory cortex, involving both the sensory and discriminatory aspects of pain. The paleospinothalamic tract (the medial system) connects to various brain stem and midbrain structures including the reticular formation, the periaqueductal gray, limbic system, and hypothalamus, before it reaches the thalamus. It is a more slowly conducting system and transmits the longer-lasting, dull, poorly localized pain experienced after injury. These neurons, which project into the medial thala-mus, come from the deeper dorsal horn laminae VI through IX. This system also activates the brain stem and midbrain structures, inducing arousal and sympathetic responses. Some of the more affective responses to pain are attributed to this system, including depression and anxiety.

The spinoreticular tract and the spinomesencephalic tract are also found in the anterolateral quadrant of the spinal cord, along with the STT. Both tracts are involved with the autonomic reflex responses to pain as well as the behavioral and motivational aspects of pain.

The dorsal column system appears to play a role in the afferent transmission of visceral pain information, as well as having a role in proprioception and possibly the inhibition of pain information. It may also provide pain-localizing information. Neurons from this system decussate, or cross, in the brain stem and terminate in the posterolateral thalamus.

Multisynaptic spinal cord interneurons make up the propriospinal tract. This system may have a role in maintaining chronic pain. It receives input from visceral and deep structures and projects to the medial thalamus and the reticular formation.

The ascending spinohypothalamic tract may play a role in the affective and motivational aspects of pain.

SUPRASPINAL SYSTEMS

Above the spinal cord, multiple CNS systems interact with the ascending nocicep-tive and descending antinociceptive pathways via multiple communicating projections.

The reticular formation, which extends throughout the brain stem, receives input from the spinoreticular tract as well as other structures in the supraspinal systems. Receptive fields are very large and come from information brought by both ipsilateral and contralateral parts of the body. The receptive field can be very precise and somatotopically indicated in the CNS, or, as described, without somato-topic functions, large and very imprecise. The reticular formation controls arousal, autonomic reflex responses, and the motivational and affective aspects of pain.

The thalamus is the major relay station in the brain for incoming nociceptive input. The paleothalamus, composed of medial and intralaminar nuclei, obtains input from the STT and the reticular formation. Its receptive fields are large and it is involved with both motor reflexes and affective aspects of pain. The paleothala-mus connects extensively with the cerebral cortex. There is no somatotopic organi-zation in this system.

The neothalamus is somatotopically organized and consists of the ventral pos-terolateral nucleus (VPL) and the ventral posteromedial nucleus (VPM). The VPL receives input from the neospinothalamic tract as well as the dorsal column tract system and the somatosensory cortex. The VPM receives input from the trigemino-thalamic tract, which carries nociceptive input from the head and face and projects to the somatosensory cortex. The neothalamus is involved in the localization of pain and its sensory and discriminative aspects.

The posterior thalamus lacks somatotopic organization. It receives input from the STT, the spinomesencephalic tract, and the dorsal column system. It projects to the somatosensory cortex and appears to be involved with the sensory expression or "texture" of pain.

The limbic system receives input from the thalamus, reticular formation, and other areas of the CNS. It has a close anatomical correlation to the "hardwired" central pain pathways; it gives and receives projections from the frontal and tempo-ral cortex. The limbic system is important in the motivational and emotional aspects of pain, especially mood and affect.

Both noxious and non-noxious stimuli from the entire body are handled by the hypothalamus. Hypothalamic neurons are not somatotopically organized. The hypothalamic nuclei send projections to the pituitary gland through the hypophy-seal stalk. The hypothalamic nuclei regulate the autonomic and neuroendocrine responses to pain and stress. The full role of the hypothalamus in pain modulation is still unknown.

The somatosensory cortex is important in sensory and discriminative aspects of pain perception, including localization. It receives input from the VPL, VPM, and posterior thalamic nuclei. Efferents from the somatosensory cortex travel back to the thalamus and mingle with the descending pathways. The limbic system receives information from the somatosensory cortex. The frontal lobe receives input from the thalamus and the limbic system, and has an effect on the behavioral and motivational aspects of pain.

DESCENDING MODULATING SYSTEMS

After the ascending nociceptive pathways have brought pain-related information to the CNS, the descending systems are primed for the modulation and inhibition or suppression of such information.

A large number of structures appear to be part of the descending pathways, including the cortex, the subcortical centers, basal ganglia, the thalamic-hypothalamic system, the midbrain, pons, and medulla, and the dorsal horn of the spinal cord.

Although there is less specific knowledge of the descending pathways/systems than we have for the ascending pathways, a great deal of information shows the importance of the pathways between the midbrain and the dorsal horn. There appear to be three pathways from the brain stem: one arises from the nucleus raphe magnus and releases serotonin (5-HT) when activated (see following text); another arises from the locus ceruleus of the pons and releases norepinephrine (see following text). The third pathway arises from the Edinger-Westphal nucleus and releases cholecystokinin (see following text). These pathways inhibit pain-responsive neurons in the dorsal horn. The periaqueductal gray (PAG) connects to all three pathways. The PAG is extremely rich in opiate receptors, and when activated, it activates the three pathways noted to modulate or inhibit pain impulses entering the dorsal horn. The spinal cord dorsal horn is also rich in opiate receptors, particularly in the substantia gelatinosa (lamina II). When stimulated, it significantly suppresses incoming C-fiber nociceptive activity.

It is also recognized that regions of the frontal lobe and the amygdala project to the PAG, inducing pain modulation. The PAG, in turn, controls spinal nociceptive neurons through relays in the rostral ventromedial medulla (RVM) and the dorsolateral pontine tegmentum (DLPT). The RVM projects directly and via the DLPT to the dorsal horn of the spinal cord through the dorsolateral funiculus (DLF). It exerts bidirectional control over pain transmission. RVM and DLPT control involves both inhibitory and excitatory interneurons in the spinal cord.

Stimulation of the somatosensory cortex appears to inhibit wide-dynamic-range neurons of the STT. Inhibition may also be mediated through the corticospinal tract, a primary motor system pathway that descends to and crosses, or decussates, in the midbrain and partially terminates in the dorsal horn.

Other supraspinal structures are also involved in descending inhibition. Limbic system structures, including the insular cortex and amygdala, appear to exert modulatory effects through input to the PAG. The paraventricular nucleus of the hypothalamus sends inputs to the PAG and is thought to be involved in the modulation of pain. The DLF is the primary descending modulatory pathway from the supraspinal regions to the dorsal horn. It carries descending modulatory processes from the cortex, limbic system, hypothalamus, and the brain stem structures, such as the PAG noted earlier.

THE "NEUROMATRIX"

Physical, behavioral, emotional, associative, and motor areas of the brain are all involved in the perception and recognition of a painful stimulus and the reaction to it.

The perceptual "mix" that takes place between painful stimuli and CNS reception and recognition of the stimuli is extremely complex. There is much more going on than what has been discussed. The idea that the brain is a passive receptacle of stimulus and response does not account for phenomena such as phantom limb pain, for example: How can the brain perceive neural information from nerves that are not there?

Melzack (3,4) hypothesized that "the brain can generate every quality of experience which is normally triggered by sensory input." He goes further to postulate that patterns (pain) are present in the brain *substrate* with genetic specifications *modified by experience.* The neuromatrix, thought to be composed of a widespread network of neurons between the thalamus and the cortex, creates a *neurosignature,* formed from repeated cyclic processing and central synthesis of the impulses within the neuromatrix. These neurosignatures are then converted into *awareness,* which initiates an action neuromatrix, a pattern of movements influenced by the awareness of pain.

The patterns "built" by the neuromatrix would incorporate physical reaction to a painful stimulus, and the recollection of similar stimuli, learned responses, and emotions. Black (5) and Melzack both hypothesize that the human body as a whole is encoded in molecular structures within the CNS that are constantly modified by external stimuli or impulses.

More recently, using functional imaging techniques such as positron emission tomography (PET), which localizes precise areas of cerebral blood flow after a painful stimulus (6), Derbyshire (7) noted that the current neuromatrix incorporates sensory, affective, and motoric processing areas of the brain, including the thalamus, anterior cingulate and primary (S1) and secondary (S2) somatosensory cortices, the midbrain region of the PAG, the lenticular complex, the insula, and cortical areas including the orbitofrontal area [Brodmann's areas (BA) 11, 47], prefrontal (BA 9,10, 44–46), motor (BA 6, supplementary motor area, and the primary motor cortex (M1), inferior parietal lobe (BA 39, 40), and anterior cingulate (BA 24, 25) cortices (ACCs).

NEUROTRANSMITTERS AND NEUROPEPTIDES

In general, the concepts of trans-synaptic facilitation of an action potential secondary to the depolarization of the postsynaptic neuron remain fairly solid: that is, messages between neurons are transduced electrically, when chemical messages are promoted to electrical or metabolic information prior to reverting to electrical impulses. The messengers are intrinsic chemicals known as neurotransmitters.

At the synapse, the postsynaptic neuron receives thousands of parcels of specific neurotransmitters and becomes depolarized. An action potential is then generated and travels via the axon to the next neuron(s). This theory essentially holds a one-to-one correspondence between presynaptic and postsynaptic neurotransmission. While this continues to hold true, it has been expanded by the postulation of indirect activity via diffusion of electrochemical or neurotransmitter signals through the extracellular medium through the interstitial spaces. Thus the neurotransmitter would diffuse in both afferent and efferent directions (8–10) This diffusion is termed volume transmission, while the former system is termed wiring transmission.

Our knowledge of the intrinsic neurochemical "software" of the nociceptive and antinociceptive systems has been enlarging, but it is certainly not total. Some of our previous conceptions have been found to be incorrect. Just a few of the neurotransmitters, which are of growing importance, include the following:

■ Calcitonin gene-related peptide (CGRP) provides antinociceptive activity that is not naloxone reversible after intracerebroventricular (ICV) injection of CGRP. (Naloxone antagonizes opiate analgesics at their receptors. Simply, if an opiate receptor is being utilized, naloxone will replace it physically and end the effective antinociception. If a neurotransmitter produces an antinociceptive effect that is not naloxone reversible, it does not work via the opiate receptors). As with many neurotransmitters, CGRP also produces contrary effects and is involved in nociception in visceral pain (11) and mediation of tolerance to opiates (12), induces slow depolarization and prolonged excitation of dorsal horn cells (12), can produce behavioral signs of mechanical hyperalgesia and sensitization of wide dynamic range neurons in the spinal cord dorsal horn of rats (13), is very active in migraine, as CGRP is one of the most potent vasodilators known (12), and when it is released from activated trigeminal sensory nerves, will dilate intra-cranial blood vessels and enhance transmission of vascular nociception (14).

- Somatostatin, distributed widely in the CNS, depresses dorsal horn neurons, and is activated by noxious stimuli.
- Cholecystokinin-8 (CCK-8), the most abundant CNS peptide, is found in the dorsal root ganglia, the substantia gelatinosa, and the PAG. It is a potent analgesic if injected into the PAG in mice, and is naloxone reversible; it has neuromodulatory behavior opposing endogenous opiates; some receptor types may be coupled on the same molecules as opiates. Caerulein, an analogue of CCK-8, is a very potent analgesic.
- Substance P (SP), if used ICV, provides naloxone-reversible antinociception, probably mediated indirectly through met-enkephalin release. Substantial support exists for SP as a mediator of nociceptive input in some primary afferents, where it appears to coexist with either 5-HT or with 5-HT and TRH (thyroid-releasing hormone).
- Endogenous opiates: Enkephalins have a more significant role in endogenous analgesia than beta-endorphin; beta-endorphin may act, as in the hippocampus, by inhibiting inhibitory interneurons, therefore disinhibiting the effect of these neurons in the analgesia-producing regions of the CNS.
- Monoamine neurotransmitters include 5-HT, norepinephrine (NEP), and dopa-mine (DA). NEP can antagonize or enhance morphine analgesia, depending on specific levels; it is possible to separate descending NEP and 5-HT pathways from the brain stem to the spinal cord via the DLF; neurons in the RVM are found that contain 5-HT, SP, enkephalin, TRH, or any combination of the four.

NEUROCHEMICAL–ANATOMICAL CORRELATES

Neurochemical–anatomical correlates exist in the peripheral nervous system, spinal cord, and supraspinal pathways.

The Peripheral Nervous System

SP, angiotensin II, and somatostatin are found in separate cell bodies of small-diameter DRG cells with projections to the substantia gelatinosa in the dorsal horn.

Spinal Cord

Primary afferents with SP, angiotensin II, and somatostatin travel to the substantia gelatinosa and the trigeminal nucleus caudalis. CCK-8, neurotensin, enkephalins, and dynorphin are found in the same regions. 5-HT and NEP are found in all Rexed laminae. Dopamine is not found in the spinal cord.

The Supraspinal Pathways

All of the neuropeptides and neuroamines just mentioned, and dopamine, are found in the supraspinal regions. High concentrations of SP, 5-HT, dynorphins, and enkephalins are found in the classic antinociceptive sites—the raphe nuclei, the PAG, and amygdala. Beta-endorphin cell bodies are found only in the basal tuberal hypothalamus with limited axonal distribution to the anterior pituitary, PAG, and limbic system. Angiotensin II cell bodies are confined to the hypothalamus but have wide distribution, especially to the amygdala, and a high density of enkephalins, dynorphins, and neurotensin are found in the amygdala and the thalamus. Neurotensin and dynorphin also are found in the pituitary. Fibers from the monoamine neurotransmitter systems arise from a small number of nuclei within the brain stem and are distributed widely, but not uniformly, to the spinal cord and brain.

NEUROCHEMICAL SYSTEMS

Three neurochemical systems are worth reviewing: the monoamine system, substance P system, and endogenous opiate system.

The Monoamine System

The mechanisms of the monoamine system (MAS) are initiated in the brain but carry out their antinociceptive action at the spinal cord level via descending pathways. Serotonergic cell bodies in the nucleus raphe magnus descend via the DLF to end in the 5-HT fields of the Rexed laminae. The release of 5-HT inhibits neurons specifically excited by nociceptive inputs. The spinal effects of a similar system involving NEP are dose dependent, alpha-receptor mediated, and separate from opioid mechanisms or vasoconstrictive effects.

Stimulation-produced analgesia (SPA) in the nucleus raphe magnus or local CNS opioid injections can activate the MAS. The interaction with the opioid system occurs both supraspinally and in the dorsal horn of the spinal cord. SPA, as the words indicate, occurs when a specific part of the CNS is electrically stimulated.

A positive correlation exists between brain dopamine and SPA from the periaqueductal gray region. 5-HT has a similar correlation. With norepinephrine, spinal, and supraspinal mechanisms appear to have opposite effects.

The Substance P System

SP terminals are involved in neurotransmission in sympathetic ganglia, its action opposed by opiates. In rats, SP-containing primary afferents are involved in pain from pressure and chemical, but not thermal, pain stimulation. Clinical correlations associated with increased levels of SP include familial dysautonomia, with decreased pain and temperature sensitivity, arachnoiditis, and dorsal rhizotomy.

The Endogenous Opiate System

There are three families of endogenous opiate peptides: (*i*) the beta-endorphin/corticotrophin family, with proopiomelanocortin as its precursor and (*ii*) the enkephalin family, with proenkephalin as the precursor. The enkephalins have seven sequences each: six met- and one leu-enkephalin; (*iii*) dynorphin/neodynorphin, with three opioid peptide sequences and a leu-enkephalin core.

Generally, dynorphin and enkephalin occur in many of the same areas including the caudate nucleus, amygdala, PAG, locus coeruleus, and the spinal cord. Dynorphin is a relatively poor analgesic.

Three of four subtypes of opiate receptors are important in this discussion: the mu (μ) receptors are possibly the most potent in inducing analgesia and the most abundant. Classic opioid agonists and antagonists have a preference for μ receptors. The kappa (κ) receptors are found predominantly in the spinal cord. The delta (δ) receptors are predominantly supraspinal and are far outnumbered by the μ receptors in CNS areas associated with nociception/antinociception—the thalamus, PAG, and raphe nuclei.

Beta-endorphin appears least likely to be primarily concerned with endogenous analgesia. ACTH and beta-endorphin together have modulatory roles that cannot function if exogenous opiates are given chronically. This, via a negative, or inhibitory feedback loop, is one mechanism for continuation of various types of chronic pain.

PHARMACOLOGY OF THE PRIMARY AFFERENT NEURONAL SYSTEMS

The pharmacology of the primary afferent neuronal systems is of great importance because it models, in some ways, the afferent changes found in muscle pain states.

C fibers, found in the skin, are very susceptible to the release of local, endogenous chemicals after local tissue damage. These chemicals both activate and sensitize the primary afferent C fibers. After a local insult, or injury, the C fibers are stimulated via an axonal, afferent reflex arc, which heralds the release of SP and CGRP from the peripheral neuronal axonal terminals. This helps sensitize the C fibers, making them more likely to fire by decreasing the threshold to sensory input. Mast cells release histamine and platelets release 5-HT. These chemicals help activate C fibers. A neurochemical cascade continues, with kinins (bradykinin) released by the local tissue injury. Kinins are very strong activators of the C fibers. Prostaglandins, leukotrienes, and potassium are released from damaged cells. Arachidonic acid, which is released from the cell membranes by phospholipase A, is synthesized by cyclo-oxygenase from lipo-oxygenase. Leukotrienes and prostoglandins continue to sensitize the end terminals on the C fibers. Potassium directly activates these terminals. Macrophages, secondary to inflammatory reactions, release cytokines, including the interleukins, which also work to sensitize end terminals of C fibers. Thus, after injury, C-fiber activation and sensitization are the result of a neurochemical cascade. The end result is hyperalgesia of the affected area. The sensitized and activated C fibers send pain information to the dorsal root ganglia and the nociception process begins. Other fibers, including Aδ fibers, also respond to this neurochemical cascade, as does muscle.

Another aspect of this cascade, which also affects muscle, is extravasation of algetic substances from local blood vessels. The vasochemical sequelae of trauma includes, after even microhemorrhage, the release of 5-HT from platelets, which induces vasoconstriction and the release of mast cells. Granules from the mast cells release histamine that causes vasodilatation and, as a result, local edema forms.

Neurotransmitters are involved in stress reactions, but so too are hormones. Structurally, hormones are proteins or polypeptides, and they are ubiquitous throughout the body. Common examples include adrenocoritcosteroids such as adrenocorticotropic hormone, thyroxin, estrogen, and the various steroids.

These compounds have various tonic effects over long periods of time. Some are phasic, with increases and decreases secondary to circadian rhythms, which are determined by the supraoptic nucleus of the hypothalamus (15).

The hormonal milieu changes in response to both physical and psychic stressors (16,17) The neuroanatomic sites of action of hormones are found, in large part, in the limbic midbrain and the ascending reticular activating system.

RECOMMENDED READING

Gilman S, Newman SW. Manter and Gatz's Essentials of Clinical Neuroanatomy and Neurophysiology. 9th ed. Philadelphia, PA: F.A. Davis, 1996.

REFERENCES

1. Mersky H. Classification of chronic pain: Description of chronic pain syndromes and definitions. Pain 1986; 16(suppl 3):S1–S225.
2. Melzack R, Wall PD. Pain Mechanisms. A new theory. Science 1965 Nov 19; 150(699): 971–979.
3. Melzack R. Phantom limbs, the self and the brain: The D. O. Hebb Memorial Lecture. Canad Psychol 1989; 30:1–16.
4. Melzack R. Central pain syndromes and theories of pain. In Casey KL, ed. Pain and Central Nervous System Disease. New York, NY: Raven Press, 1991:59–75.
5. Black IB. Information in the Brain: A Molecular Perspective. A Bradford Book, Cambridge, Mass: MIT Press, 1991.
6. Friston KJ, Frackowiak RSJ. Imaging functional anatomy. In: Lassen NA et al., eds. Brain Work and Mental Activity (Alfred Benzon Symposium 31). Copenhagen: Munksgaard, 1991:267–277.
7. Derbyshire SWG. Exploring the pain "neuromatrix". Current Rev Pain 2000; 4:467–477.
8. Agnati LF, Zoli M, Merlo Pich E, et al. NPY receptors and their interactions with other transmitter systems. In Mutt V, Fuxe K, Hokfelt T, Lundberg JM, eds. Neuropeptide Y, New York, NY: Raven Press, 1989:103–114.
9. Agnati LF, Zoli M, Merlo Pich E, et al. Aspects of neural plasticity in the central nervous system. VIII Theoretical aspects of brain communication and computation. Neurochem Int 1990; 16:479–500.
10. Swartz TW, Fuhlendorff J, Langeland N, et al. Y1 and Y2 receptors for NPY. The evolution of PP-fold peptides and their receptors. In: Mutt V, Fuxe K, Hokfelt T, Lundberg JM, eds. Neuropeptide Y, New York, NY: Raven Press, 1989:115–121.
11. Wick EC, Pikios S, Grady EF, Kirkwood KS. Calcitonin gene-related peptide partially mediates nociception in acute experimental pancreatitis. Surgery 2006; 139(2):197–201.
12. Prado MA, Evans-Bain B, Dickerson IM. Receptor component protein (RCP): a member of a multi-protein complex required for G-protein-coupled signal transduction. Biochem Soc Transact 2002; 30(4):460–464.
13. Sun RQ, Tu YJ, Lawand NB, et al. Calcitonin gene-related peptide receptor activation produces PKA- and PKC-dependent mechanical hyperalgesia and central sensitization. J Neurophysiol 2004; 92:2859–2866.
14. Arulmani U, Maassenvandenbrink A, Villalon CM, Saxena PR. Calcitonin gene-related peptide and its role in migraine pathophysiology. Eur J Pharmacol 2004; 500(1–3):15–30.
15. Moore RY. The suprachiasmic nucleus and the organization of a circadian system. Trends Neurosci 1982; 5:404.
16. Ganong W: The stress response: A dynamic overview. Hosp Prac 1988; 23(6):155–190.
17. Kalin NH, Dawson G. Neuroendocrine dysfunction in depression: Hypothalamic-anterior pituitary systems. Trends Neurosci 1986; 9:261–266.

2 Molecular Mechanisms of Nociception

It is difficult to determine the physiological substrates of nociception solely on an anatomic basis. Over the past several decades, large amounts of new information have been ascertained, much of it using multiple aspects of molecular genetics. This chapter does not focus on this specific aspect, but on the new receptor/agonist–antagonist information that is enabling us to more fully understand both the patho-physiology of pain and the mechanisms of specific drugs.

N-METHYL-D-ASPARTATE RECEPTORS

It is known that the spinal delivery of N-methyl-D-aspartate receptor (NMDAR) antagonists inhibits the hyperexcitability of spinal cord nociceptive neurons induced by C-fiber stimulation.

Activation of NMDARs after tissue injury and inflammation enables facili-tated processing in the spinal cord (1,2).

Ionotropic receptors directly gate ion channels and have three major sub-classes: AMPA (alpha-amino-3-hydroxy-5-methyl-4-isoxasolepropionic acid), kainite (kainite), and NMDA. NMDARs have crucial roles in excitatory synaptic trans-mission, plasticity, and neurodegeneration in the CNS (1).

NMDARs are different from other ligand-gated ion channels. The NMDAR controls a cation channel that is highly permeable to monovalent ions and calcium.

Simultaneous binding of glutamate and glycine, its coagonist, is required for efficient activation of NMDAR. At resting membrane potentials, the NMDAR channels are blocked by extracellular magnesium and open only on simultaneous depolarization and agonist binding.

NMDARs are composed of NR1, NR2 (A, B, C, and D), and NR3 (A and B) subunits (3).

Co-expression studies have demonstrated that formation and function of functional NMDAR channels requires a combination of NR1, an essential channel-forming subunit, and at least one of the NR2 subunits: glutamate and glycine-binding sites that have been demonstrated to be located on the homologous regions of the NR2 and NR1 subunits respectively (4,5).

The type of NR2 subunit in the heteromeric complex involves: sensitivity to magnesium block, kinetics of desensitization and offset decay, susceptibility to modulation by glycine, reducing agents, polyamines and phosphorylation, and affinity for agonists and antagonists. Subunit-dependent properties of NMDARs include their single-channel conductance and sensitivity to magnesium block (6,7).

NR2A- or NR2B-subunits-containing NMDARs generate high-conductance channel openings with a high sensitivity for blocking by magnesium, whereas NR2C or NR2C-containing receptors give rise to low-conductance openings with lower sensitivity to magnesium (7).

There is a significant contribution of NR2B subunits to nociception.

Pain associated with peripheral tissue or nerve injury involves NMDAR activation (8).

NDMAR antagonists have been shown to effectively alleviate pain-related behavior in animal models as well as in clinical situations (9,10).

NMDARs are important for normal CNS functioning; so the use of NMDAR antagonists can often be limited by serious side effects, such as memory impairment, psychotomimetic effects, ataxia, and motor incoordination (11).

A reduced side effect profile and an improved efficacy of NR2B-selective antagonists would be useful.

NMDARs located in peripheral somatic tissues and visceral pain pathways also play an important role in nociception.

NMDAR activation occurs in all aspects of the neural axis. NMDARs are found on unmyelinated and myelinated axons in peripheral somatic tissues.

Associated with NMDARs in the periphery, local injections of glutamate or NMDA result in pain behaviors that can be attenuated by peripheral administration of NMDAR antagonists (12,13). Peripheral administration of MK-801 (dizocilpine), a noncompetitive NMDAR antagonist, produces local anesthetic-like effects (14). The number of NMDARs on peripheral nerve fibers increases during inflammation, and this may contribute to peripheral sensitization in inflammation (15).

In humans, the peripheral administration of ketamine enhanced the local anesthetic and analgesic actions of bupivacaine used for infiltration anesthesia and inhibited the development of primary and secondary hyperalgesia after an experimental burn injury (16,17).

Another study found a dose-dependent antihyperalgesic effect for IV ketamine in patients with neuropathic pain, with only minimal CNS side effects encountered (18).

Topical application of ketamine ointment has been reported to reduce pain intensity and to attenuate allodynia in patients with an acute early dystrophic state of complex regional pain syndrome (CRPS) (19).

Local administration of ketamine appears to be beneficial for some patients with chronic pain.

NR2B-selective antagonists potentiate NMDAR inhibition by endogenous protons. This mode of action may be beneficial under conditions of tissue injury, ischemia, or inflammation (presumably accompanied by acidosis) when a greater degree of inhibition of NMDARs can be expected in the affected tissues than normal (11,20).

Changes in the periphery after trauma lead to the phenomenon of peripheral sensitization and primary hyperalgesia—these have a central component (8).

Central sensitization is the state where dorsal horn excitability is increased and, secondary to this, its response to sensory input is facilitated. A low-intensity stimulus acting via low-threshold afferents then generates pain (allodynia), and noxious input results in a pain response that is augmented in amplitude and duration, yielding hyperalgesia.

Evidence exists that development of spinal hyperexcitability and persistent pain involves activation of NMDARs (1). Increased NMDAR function is expressed as an increase in channel openings and may involve transcriptional, translational, and post-translational modulation.

Role of NMDARs in Central Sensitization

NMDARs do not participate in normal synaptic transmission because of their voltage-dependent block by extracellular magnesium. Postsynaptic depolarization and removal of the magnesium block of NMDARs will occur. A constant drive of noxious afferent input after tissue damage depolarizes the membrane enough to permit participation of NMDARs in synaptic transmission. Nociceptive input to the dorsal horn is further increased via positive feedback through presynaptic NMDARs. Post-translational changes of NMDARs—calcium entry—causes activation of protein kinases and results in phosphorylation of NMDARs. As a consequence, the magnesium block at resting membrane potentials is decreased and channel opening time is prolonged (1).

Observed changes in the NR subunit expression may represent an adaptive response aimed to reduce excessive neuronal excitability resulting from tissue injury. The dose–response curve of NMDAR currents were consistent with a relative increase in NR2B expression, which is important in neuropathic pain (21). Peripheral inflammation may alter the properties of NMDARs in the spinal dorsal horn (22). After Complete Freund's Adjuvant treatment, the magnesium blockade of NMDARs was reduced and the current–voltage relationship of NMDA channels was shifted in the hyperpolarized direction (22).

These changes were mediated by protein kinase C (PKC) and induced enhanced NMDA responses at negative potentials that would lead to an increase in synaptic transmission in the dorsal horn and contribute to the development of pathological nociceptive responses associated with tissue injury.

Protein phosphorylation is a major mechanism for the regulation of NMDAR function—one mechanism by which PKC regulates the function of NMDARs (23). PKC also potentiates NMDA responses indirectly by activation of the tyrosine kinase signaling cascade (24).

PKC also modulates the function of NMDARs by participating in their interactions with postsynaptic density and cytoskeletal proteins (25).

Protein phosphorylation is important for the upregulation of NMDAR function. Another protein that helps mediate many aspects of postsynaptic signaling by NMDAR is calcium–calmodulin-dependent protein kinase II (CaMKII). It is persistently activated after NMDAR stimulation (26).

Recently, evidence points to a key role for CaMKII in nociceptive transmission. A major isoform, CaMKII-alpha is preferentially localized in pain-processing regions in the CNS such as lamina II of the spinal cord dorsal horn and the dorsal root ganglion (DRG) (27).

CaMKII is upregulated in the superficial laminae of the dorsal horn and the DRG cells after inflammation or injuries to peripheral tissues: NR2 subunits in the spinal cord—NR2A and NR2B (28).

Central sensitization in the spinal cord dorsal horn is mediated via activation of postsynaptic NMDARs.

One of the features unique to the spinal cord is the presence of presynaptic NMDARs.

Many small-diameter primary afferent fibers terminating in the dorsal horn express NMDARs, and activation of presynaptic NMDARs causes the release of substance P (SP) from primary afferents (29).

Because SP, calcitonin gene-related peptide (CGRP), and glutamate cooccur in small-diameter primary afferent terminals, presynaptic NR2B-containing NMDARs can facilitate and prolong the transmission of nociceptive messages through the release of these neurotransmitters. Efficacy of NR2B-selective NMDAR antagonists is noted (30).

Drugs directed against NR2B-containing NMDARs would appear to be promising analgesics.

NMDAR activation underlies inflammation-induced neuronal hyperexcitability of brain stem circuitry (31). There is also an upregulation of NR1, NR2A, and NR2B mRNA subunits gene expression in the brain stem after inflammation (32).

Disinhibition may be caused by many factors such as a reduction in inhibitory transmitters [gamma-aminobutyric acid (GABA)] or its receptors, or losses of inhibitory neurons (33,34). Irrespective of the cause of disinhibition, the unopposed activation of NMDARs is the underlying mechanism.

In the normal state, the participation of NMDARs in synaptic transmission is prevented by $GABA_A$ receptor-mediated currents, which restore the depolarized membrane potential to a resting level and prevent the release of the magnesium block of the NMDAR. Only C-fiber input can reliably trigger central sensitization (35,36).

As NMDARs are located on both excitatory and inhibitory neurons, a drug-potentiating NMDAR function is not necessarily pain producing. Gabapentin may exert its antinociceptive effects by increasing the activity of inhibitory neurons in the dorsal horn by NMDAR activation (37). The activation of extrasynaptic NMDARs in the spinal dorsal horn (presumably containing NR2B subunits) may contribute to the antinociceptive action of gabapentin (38).

NMDARs are found on peripheral terminals of primary afferent nerves innervating the colon (39).

In visceral pain pathways, NMDARs may also be involved under inflammatory conditions (40). NMDAR antagonists may be useful analgesics for the treatment of visceral pain [including irritable bowel syndrome (IBS)].

NMDARs are critically involved in the induction and maintenance of neuronal hyperexcitability after noxious events. There are central, peripheral, somatic, and visceral NMDARs.

Accumulating evidence shows that the NR2B subunit of NMDAR is particularly important for pain perception. With a minimal side effect profile and good efficacy of NR2B-selective compounds, NR2B-selective blockade may be a variable strategy for the pharmacological treatment of pain.

As indicated earlier, windup, development of central sensitization from continuous C-fiber stimulation, results from activation of the NMDARs. Corresponding increases in dorsal horn neuronal responsiveness create rapid central hypersensitivity.

Currently, the NMDA antagonists include ketamine, dextromethorphan, and memantine, as well as, to a partial degree, methadone. Animal models and human research has demonstrated that NMDARs are, at least in part, responsible for hyperalgesia and allodynia seen most frequently in patient with postoperative, inflammatory, and neuropathic pain (41). NMDAR antagonists may have a role in the prevention of morphine tolerance. Finally, the use of oral ketamine with an opiate has been found to decrease spontaneous pain and wind-up-like pain in patients with neuropathic pain (42).

TRANSIENT RECEPTOR POTENTIAL CHANNEL RECEPTORS

Mounting evidence exists that the vanilloid (capsaicin) receptor; also known as the transient receptor potential channel, vanilloid subfamily member 1 (TRPV1) has multiple interacting levels of control. The first is secondary to reversible phosphorylation catalyzed by intrinsic kinases and phosphatases, which play an important role in receptor sensitization versus tachyphylaxis. Other levels of control involve

TRPV1 heteromers associated with suggested regulatory proteins; subcellular compartmentalization (the membranous form of TRPV1 appears to function as a nonselective cation channel); and regulation via gene expression (43).

Of equal interest is the fact that TRPV1 receptors appear to be upregulated during inflammatory processes. The TRPV1 is present on neurons that normally do not express them in the presence of experimental models of nerve injury and diabetic neuropathy (43).

These findings appear to imply that aberrant TRPV1 expression is found in neuropathic pain and hyperalgesia (43).

The TRPV1 receptors are activated by protons and significant temperature changes and capsaicin, which induces the release of the proinflammatory neuro-peptides SP, Neuropeptide A, and CGRP, all part of the "inflammatory soup" found in the presence of inflammation.

Agonists of the TRPV1, such as capsaicin, will also induce an analgesic effect after an initial excitatory response. The vanilloid system plays in important role in inflammatory hyperalgesia. TRPV1 antagonists such as capsazepine can prevent thermal hyperalgesia in animal carrageenan or Complete Fruend's Adjuvant models in mice. The analgesic effects of capsaicin appear to be enhanced during inflammation (44). It is felt that capsaicin induces desensitization by stimulating the TRPV1 receptors, which would induce the output of algetic chemicals such as SP and CGRP. When this has been done repeatedly, the amount of colocalized and other algetic chemicals induced by capsaicin from the free C-fiber nerve endings decreases and desensitization occurs (44).

When activated, the vanilloid receptor has commonly been used to facilitate neurogenic inflammation and plasma exudation, the model of which mirrors the pathogenesis of migraine (45).

The TRPV1 does appear to contribute to both acute and chronic pain. The TRP channels of the vanilloid family (TRPV1, TRPV2, TRPV3, and TRPV4) undergo stimulation by heat stimuli, although TRPV8 and ANKTM1 (a TRP-like channel expressed in nociceptive neurons activated by cold temperatures) are responsive to cold. Both TRPV1 and ANKTM1 mediate the pungency of nociceptor-specific chemicals including capsaicin and mustard oil. The resulting sensitization of TRPV1 is an important mechanism for heat hyperalgesia and enables the symptoms of chronic pain (46).

Small molecule agonists of TRPV1 [capsaicin and resiniferatoxin (RTX)] are used for a number of clinical syndromes in animal studies, including intractable neuropathic pain, spinal detrusor hyperreflexia, and bladder hypersensitivity. Vanilloid receptor 1 (VR1) antagonists have yet to reach the clinic. Capsazepine is the classic TRPV1 antagonist but it demonstrates poor pharmacokinetics and significant species selectivity issues in the laboratory (47).

The VR1 antagonist capsazepine, along with cannabinoid (CB1 and CB2) receptor antagonists, inhibit VR1 responses (48).

It is also notable that capsazepine may be mildly cytotoxic (49).

Other research indicates that TRPV1 is expressed in peripheral nociceptive neurons, and polymodal activation can occur via various agents including low extracellular pH (protons), noxious heat, capsaicin, and direct phosphorylation by PKC (50,51).

Infection, inflammation, or ischemia can produce an array of chemical media-tors, which would activate or even sensitize nociceptor terminals; adenosine triphosphate (ATP) is a part of this proalgetic response. In the presence of ATP, the temperature threshold for TRPV1 activation is reduced from 42°C to 35°C, so that normal body temperature may activate the TRPV1 (52).

A study has demonstrated morphological evidence for the distribution of TRPV1 along unmyelinated axons in peripheral nerve—giving the first view of vesicular neuropeptide exocytosis along unmyelinated axons in peripheral nerve (53).

Endogenous cannabinoid receptors are found to be distributed in the CNS and multiple peripheral tissues including the leukocytes, spleen, urinary, gastrointestinal, and reproductive systems, the endocrine glands, arteries, and heart. Anandamide is one of the five endogenous cannabinoids detected so far and is the best characterized. There are two cannabinoid receptor subtypes (CB1 and CB2) cloned so far. It is felt that additional cannabinoid receptor subtypes and vanilloid receptors (TRPV1) are involved in the very complex functions of the cannabinoid system, including memory processes, motor coordination, appetite control, neuroprotection, and pain modulation (54).

CB2 receptors, found in the periphery, with no attendant CNS effects, does appear to inhibit nociception when activated in preclinical trials (55). Human trials with CB2 receptor agonists have begun.

Endovanilloids are endogenous ligands of the TRPV1 protein, the nonselective cation channel that is part of the family of TRP ion channels and is activated by capsaicin, the pungent ingredient of hot chili peppers. TRPV1 is expressed in some nociceptor efferent neurons, which, as already noted , senses noxious heat and low pH. The fact that these channels are found in many regions of the CNS where they would not be directly exposed to these types of noxious stimuli implies the existence of endovanilloids. Three classes of endogenous lipids have been found that can activate TRPV1: unsaturated N-acyldopamines, lipoxygenase products of arachidonic acid and the endocannabinoid anandamide, and some of its cogeners. To classify a molecule as an endovanilloid, it must be formed or released in an activity-dependent manner in large enough amounts to induce a TRPV1-mediated response by direct activation of the channel (56).

The neurons located in the paraventricular nucleus (PVN) help regulate autonomic function via projections to the brain stem and spinal cord. Activation of TRPV1 receptors found in the PVN excites preautonomic PVN neurons through selective potentiation of glutamatergic synaptic inputs. Such presynaptic TRPV1 receptors and endogenous capsaicin-like substances found in the PVN may indicate a new mechanism in hypothalamic regulation of the autonomic nervous system (57).

Also of interest is a recent study showing that the TRPV1 receptor has an active role in the brain microvasculature and has a permeability-increasing effect secondary to SP. It also plays a role in the immediate blood–brain barrier disruption following ischemia and reperfusion (58). This would also presumably have an effect in the blood-brain barrier disruption post mild traumatic brain injury (59).

ACID-SENSING ION CHANNELS

The mammalian acid-sensing ion channels (ASICs) are highly expressed in sensory neurons (60). Protons are the confirmed activators of these channels, and it is felt that these channels may function in mechanotransduction (61) as the ASIC subunits are found at sites that would be appropriate to contribute to mechanosensation. Histopathological studies show that the ASIC subunits are found along the length of nerve fibers, not specifically at the end terminals. It is hypothesized that ASICs may exist in a multiple protein transduction complex that somehow masks the proton sensitivity of these channels (62). Knockout mice studies do not support a role for ASICs as mechanotransducers in mammals (63).

That sensory neurons can be directly responsive to protons or acid has engendered great clinical interest in pain research (64). Subsets of sensory neurons can express different acid-sensing ion channels (65). The two major classes of ASICs expressed on nociceptors are TRPV1 (66) and ASIC3 (67,68). Both forms of channels are excited by and sensitized by decreases in pH.

As already noted, there are currently no TRPV1 antagonists in clinical use. The TRPV1 agonist, capsaicin, is used transcutaneously.

VOLTAGE-GATED CHANNELS

Changed expression of the calcium, sodium, and potassium voltage-gated channels has been associated with neuropathic pain (69).

Calcium Channels

There is good evidence for the importance of calcium channels in the pathogenesis of neuropathic pain (70,71). The voltage-gated calcium channels involve a single α subunit and structural homology with sodium channels; accessory subunits to these channels are complex, with functional calcium channel complexes involving five proteins: α_1, α_2, β, δ, and γ (70).

The two "gabapentinoids," gabapentin and pregabalin, bind selectively to the $\alpha_2\delta$ subunit protein of the voltage-gated Ca^{2+} channels in the superficial dorsal horn of the spinal cord and different regions in the brain. These two drugs work as presynaptic inhibitors of the release of algetic or excitatory neurotransmitters in appropriately stimulated neurons. Upregulation of the $\alpha_2\delta$ subunits in the presence of neuropathic pain appears to be correlated with gabapentin sensitivity and its antiallodynic effects (72).

Further, there appears to be an increased level of calcium channel excitability in the presence of tissue damage, nerve damage, and cancer, which is felt to be indicative of increased neurotransmitter release from afferent activity; this would be expected to diminish by activation of the $\alpha_2\delta$ subunits, which should diminish both transmitter release and neuronal activity (73).

It should be noted that gabapentin and pregabalin are GABA analogues, but they have no effect at the $GABA_A$ or $GABA_B$ receptors, nor at the benzodiazepine receptors; they do not change GABA metabolism.

Conotoxin analogue ziconotide is a peptide derived from snail venom that blocks the entry of calcium into the neuronal voltage-gated calcium channels, which stops the conduction of nerve signals. These N-type voltage-gated calcium channels are found in the spinal cord dorsal horn. This drug is given intrathecally, for intractable pain (74,75).

Sodium Channels

It is felt that subtypes of tetrodotoxin-resistant voltage-gated sodium channels are also involved in the development of some forms of neuropathic pain. Sodium channels do appear to upregulate in the presence of injury, and help induce hyperexcitability. Sodium channels (particularly the $Na_V1.3$ form) also appear to be found both in the adult CNS as well as the adult peripheral nerves and they can be blocked while in a resting state (76,77).

Na$_V$1.3 is upregulated in the dorsal horn after experimental spinal cord injury, which is associated with hyperexcitability of these nociceptive neurons and associated pain (77).

Both experimental and clinical data show that changes in voltage-gated sodium channels have an important role in the pathogenesis of neuropathic pain and inflammatory pain. Drugs that block these sodium channels are potentially therapeutic (78,79).

A number of sodium channel blockers act as analgesics. Amitriptyline and other tricyclic antidepressants block these channels, along with other modes of anti-nociceptive activity. Most of the anticonvulsants used to block neuropathic pain are also sodium channel blockers.

Most drugs that block voltage-gated sodium channels do so at a site in the sodium channel pore, which is the local anesthetic receptor site. Local anesthetics block these channels when they are inactivated after prolonged depolarization. Lidocaine is effective in peripheral neuropathic pain. Mexiletine, an oral anesthetic sodium channel blocker, is also effective in some forms of neuropathic pain.

Modulation or blockade of the voltage-gated sodium channels are achieved by carbamazepine, oxcarbazepine, phenytoin, lamotrigine, valproic acid, and topiramate.

Potassium Channels

Potassium channels appear to play an important role in the development of neuronal excitability. There are four families of potassium channels that have different structures, neuropharmacological sensitivities, and functional characteristics: the voltage-gated (K$_V$), calcium activated [K (Ca)], inward rectifier [K (ir)], and the two-pore channels [K (2P)] K (+) (80). Antinociception has been associated with the opening of some forms of these K (+) channels induced by agonists of multiple G-protein coupled receptors, including alpha(2)-adrenoceptors, opioid, GABA(B), muscarinic, serotonin 5HT-1A, nonsteroidal anti inflammatory drugs (NSAIDs), tricyclic antidepressants, and cannabinoid receptors (80). New research indicates that drugs that directly open K (+) channels produce antinociceptive effects in various models of acute and chronic pain (80).

The neuropathic pain/nerve injury rat model by Chung (ligation of L5 and L6 segmental spinal nerves) (81) causes marked reductions in the K$_V$ channel subunits in the neurons of the dorsal root ganglia (82).

The specific K$_V$1.4 subunit is expressed in the smaller diameter neurons, predominating in A$_\delta$ and C fibers. It is felt that these neurons are nociceptors as they also express the TRPV1 capsaicin receptor, CGRP, and/or an Na$^+$ channel (82).

Other research has shown that the K$_V$1.2, K$_V$1.3, and K$_V$1.5 mRNA has been found in the peripheral first-order sensory neurons in the rat dorsal root ganglia; expressions of the first two potassium channels have been noted in the thalamus, the cerebral cortex, and the dorsal and ventral spinal cord (83).

REFERENCES

1. Petrenko AB, Yamakura T, Baba H, Shimoji K. The role of N-methyl-D-aspartate (NMDA) receptors in pain: a review. Anesth Analg 2003; 97:1108–1116.
2. Dickenson AH, Sullivan AF. Evidence for a role of the NMDA receptor in the frequency dependent potentiation of deep rat dorsal horn nociceptive neurones following C fibre stimulation. Neuropharmacology 1987; 26:1235–1238.

3. Mori H, Mishina M. Structure and function of the NMDA receptor channel. Neuropharmacology 1995; 34:1219–1237.
4. Hirai H, Kirsch J, Laube B, et al. The glycine binding site of the N-methyl-D-aspartate receptor subunit NR1: identification of novel determinants of co-agonist potentiation in the extracellular M3-M4 loop region. Proc Natl Acad Sci USA 1996; 93:6031–6036.
5. Laube B, Hirai H, Sturgess M, et al. Molecular determinants of agonist discrimination by NMDA receptor subunits: analysis of the glutamate binding site on the NR2B subunit. Neuron 1997; 18:493–503.
6. Cull-Candy S, Brickley S, Farrant M. NMDA receptor subunits: diversity, development and disease. Curr Opin Neurobiol 2001; 11:327–335.
7. Williams K. Ifenprodil discriminates subtypes of N-methyl-D-aspartate receptor: selectivity and mechanisms at recombinant heteromeric receptors. Mol Pharmacol 1993; 44:851–859.
8. Doubell TP, Mannion RJ, Woolf CJ. The dorsal horn: state-dependent sensory processing, plasticity and the generation of pain. In: Wall PD, Melzack R, eds. Textbook of Pain. London, UK: Churchill Livingstone, 1999:165–181.
9. Fisher K, Coderre TJ, Hagen NA. Targeting N-methyl-D-aspartate receptor for chronic pain management: preclinical animal studies, recent clinical experience and future research directions. J Pain Symptom Manage 2000; 20:358–373.
10. Hewitt DJ. The use of NMDA-receptor antagonists in the treatment of chronic pain. Clin J Pain 2000; 16:574–579.
11. Chizh BA, Headley PM, Tzschentke TM. NMDA receptor antagonists as analgesics: focus on the NR2B subtype. Trends Pharmacol Sci 2001; 22:636–642.
12. Jackson DL, Graff CB, Richardson JD, Hargreaves KM. Glutamate participates in the peripheral modulation of thermal hyperalgesia in rats. Eur J Pharmacol 1995; 284: 321–325.
13. Lawand NB, Willis WD, Westlund KN. Excitatory amino acid receptor involvement in peripheral nociceptive transmission in rats. Eur J Pharmacol 1997; 324:169–177.
14. Ushida T, Tani T, Kawasaki M, et al. Peripheral administration of an N-methyl-D-aspartate receptor antagonist (MK-801) changes dorsal horn neuronal responses in rats. Neurosci Lett 1999; 260:89–92.
15. Carlton SM, Coggeshall RE. Inflammation-induced changes in peripheral glutamate receptor populations. Brain Res 1999; 820:63–70.
16. Tverskoy M, Oren M, Vaskovich M, et al. Ketamine enhances local anesthetic and analgesic effects of bupivacaine by peripheral mechanism: a study in postoperative patients. Neurosci Lett 1996; 215:5–8.
17. Warncke T, Jorum E, Stubhaug A. Local treatment with the N-methyl-D-aspartate receptor antagonist ketamine, inhibits development of secondary hyperalgesia in man by a peripheral action. Neurosci Lett 1997; 227:1–4.
18. Leung A, Wallace MS, Ridgeway B, Yaksh T. Concentration-effect relationship of intravenous alfentanil and ketamine on peripheral neurosensory thresholds, allodynia and hyperalgesia of neuropathic pain. Pain 2001; 91:177–187.
19. Ushida T, Tani T, Kanbara T, et al. Analgesic effects of ketamine ointment in patients with complex regional pain syndrome type 1. Reg Anesth Pain Med 2002; 27:524–528.
20. Mott DD, Doherty JJ, Zhang S, et al. Phenylethanolamines inhibit NMDA receptors by enhancing proton inhibition. Nat Neurosci 1998; 1:659–667.
21. Karlsson U, Sjodin J, Angeby Moller K, et al. Glutamate-induced currents reveal three functionally distinct NMDA receptor populations in rat dorsal horn: effects of peripheral nerve lesion and inflammation. Neuroscience 2002; 112:861–868.
22. Guo H, Huang LY. Alteration in the voltage dependence of NMDA receptor channels in rat dorsal horn neurones following peripheral inflammation. J Physiol 2001; 527: 115–123.
23. Liao GY, Wagner DA, Shu MH, Leonard JP. Evidence of direct protein kinase-C mediated modulation of N-methyl-D-aspartate receptor current. Mol Pharmacol 2001; 59:960–964.
24. Lu WY, Xiong ZG, Lei S, et al. G-protein-coupled receptors act via protein kinase C and Src to regulate NMDA receptors. Nat Neurosci 1999; 2:331–338.
25. Sheng M, Pak DT. Ligand-gated ion channel interactions with cytoskeletal and signaling proteins. Annu Rev Physiol 2000; 62:755–778.

26. Bayer KU, De Koninck P, Leonard AS, et al. Interaction with the NMDA receptor locks CaMKII in an active conformation. Nature 2001; 411:801–805.
27. Bruggemann I, Schulz SK, Wiborny D, Hollt V. Colocalization of the mu-opioid receptor and calcium/calmodulin-dependent kinase II in distinct pain-processing brain regions. Brain Res Mol Brain Res 2000; 85:239-250.
28. Carlton SM. Localization of CaMKII alpha in rat primary sensory neurons: increase in inflammation. Brain Res 2002; 22:4196–4204.
29. Liu H, Mantyh PW, Basbaum AI. NMDA receptor regulation of Substance P release from primary afferent nociceptors. Nature 1997; 386:721–724.
30. Ma QP, Hargreaves RJ. Localization of N-Methyl-D-aspartate NR2B subunits on primary sensory neurons that give rise to small-caliber sciatic nerve fibers in rats. Neuroscience 2000; 101:699–707.
31. Terayama R, Guan Y, Dubner R, Ren K. Activity-induced plasticity in brain stem pain modulatory circuitry after inflammation. Neuroreport 2000; 11:1915–1919.
32. Miki K, Zhou QQ, Guo W, et al. Changes in gene expression and neuronal phenotype in brain stem pain modulatory circuitry after inflammation. J Neurophysiol 2002; 87:750–760.
33. Castro-Lopes JM, Tavares I, Coimbra A. GABA decreases in the spinal cord dorsal horn after peripheral neurectomy. Brain Res 1993; 620:287–291.
34. Azkue JJ, Zimmermann M, Hsieh TF, Herdegen T. Peripheral nerve insult induces NMDA receptor-mediated delayed degeneration in spinal neurons. Eur J Neurosci 1998; 10:2204–2206.
35. Yoshimura M, Nishi S. Primary afferent-evoked glycine- and GABA-mediated IPSPs in substantia gelatinosa neurones in the rat spinal cord in vitro. J Physiol 1995; 482:29–38.
36. Woolf CJ, Wall PD. Relative effectiveness of C primary afferent fibers of different origins in evoking a prolonged facilitation of the flexor reflex in the rat. J Neurosci 1986; 6:1433–1442.
37. Gu Y, Huang LY. Gabapentin potentiates N-methyl-D-aspartate receptor mediated currents in rat GABAergic dorsal horn neurons. Neurosci Lett 2002; 234:177–180.
38. Moore KA, Baba H, Woolf CJ. Gabapentin-actions on adult superficial dorsal horn neurons. Neuropharmacology 2002; 43:1077–1081.
39. McRoberts JA, Coutinho SV, Marvizon JC, et al. Role of peripheral N-methyl-D-aspartate (NMDA) receptors in visceral nociception in rats. Gastroenterology 2001; 120:1737–1748.
40. Meen M, Coudore-Civiale MA, Parry L, et al. Involvement of N-methyl-D-aspartate receptors in nociception in the cyclophosphamide-induced vesical pain model in the conscious rat. Eur J Pain 2002; 6:307–314.
41. Trujillo KA, Akil H. Inhibition of morphine tolerance and dependence by the NMDA-receptor antagonist MK-801. Science 1991; 251:85–87.
42. Jorem E, Warncke T, Stubhaug A. Cold allodynia and hyperalgesia in neuropathic pain: the effect of N-methyl-D-aspartate (NMDA) receptor antagonist ketamine- a double-blind cross-over comparison with alfentanil and placebo. Pain 2003; 101:229–235.
43. Cortright DN, Szallasi A. Biochemical pharmacology of the vanilloid receptor TRPV1. An update. Eur J Biochem 2004; 271(10):1814–1819.
44. Menendez L, Lastra A, Hidalgo A, Baamonde A. The analgesic effect induced by capsaicin is enhanced in inflammatory states. Life Sci 2004; 74(26):3235–3244.
45. Cheng FH, Andrews PL, Moreaux B, et al. Evaluation of the anti-emetic potential of anti-migraine drugs to prevent resiniferatoxin-induced emesis in Suncus murinus (house musk shrew). Eur J Pharmacol 2005; 508(1–3):231–238.
46. Koltzenburg M. The role of TRP channels in sensory neurons. Novartis Found Symp 2004; 260:206–213.
47. Valenzano KJ, Sun Q. Current perspectives on the therapeutic utility of VR1 antagonists. Curr Med Chem 2004; 11(24):3185–3202.
48. Golech SA, McCarron RM, Chen Y, et al. Human brain endothelium: co-expression and function of vanilloid and endocannabinoid receptors. Brain Res Mol Brain Res 2004; 132(1):87–92.
49. Teng HP, Huaung CJ, Yeh JH, et al. Capsazepine elevates intracellular Ca2+ in human osteosarcoma cells, questioning its selectivity as a vanilloid receptor antagonist. Life Sci 2004; 75(21):2515–2526.
50. Correll CC, Phelps PT, Anthes JC, et al. Cloning and pharmacological characterization of mouse TRPV1. Neurosci Lett 2004; 370(1):55–60.

51. Wang Y, Kedei N, Want M, et al. Interaction between protein kinase Cmu and the vanilloid receptor type 1. J Biol Chem 2004; 279(51):53674–53682.
52. Tominaga M, Numazaki M, Iida T, et al. Regulation mechanisms of vanilloid receptors. Novartis Found Symp 2004; 261:4–12.
53. Bernardini N, Neuhuber W, Reeh PW, Sauer SK. Morphological evidence of functional capsaicin receptor expression and calcitonin gene-related peptide exocytosis in isolated peripheral nerve axons of the mouse. Neuroscience 2004; 126(3):585–590.
54. Grotenhermen F. Pharmacology of cannabinoids. Neuro Endocrinol Lett 2004; 25(1–2):14–23.
55. Ibrahim MM, Rude ML, Stagg NJ, et al. CB2 cannabinoid receptor mediation of antinociception. Pain 2006; 122:36–42.
56. Van Der Stelt M, Di Marzo V. Endovanilloids. Putative endogenous ligands of transient receptor potential vanilloid 1 channels. Eur J Biochem 2004; 271(10):1827–1834.
57. Li DP, Chen SR, Pan HL. VR1 receptor activation induces glutamate release and postsynaptic firing in the paraventricular nucleus. J Neurophysiol 2004; 92(3):1807–1816.
58. Hu DE, Easton AS, Fraser PA. TRPV1 activation results in disruption of the blood-brain barrier in the rat. Br J Pharmacol 2005; 146:576–584.
59. Jay GW. Minor Traumatic Brain injury Handbook: Diagnosis and Treatment. Boca Raton, Fla.: CRC Press, 2000:38.
60. Waldmann R, Lazdunski M. H(+)-gated cation channels: neuronal acid sensors in the NaC/DEG family of ion channels. Curr Opin Neurobiol 1998; l8(3):418–424.
61. Lewin G, Stucky C. In: Wood JN, ed. Molecular Basis of Pain Induction. New York, NY: Wiley, 2000.
62. Welsh MJ, Price MP, Xie J. Biochemical basis of touch perception: mechanosensory function of degenerin/epithelial Na+ channels. J Biol Chem 2002; 277(4):2369–2372.
63. Drew LJ, Rohrer DK, Price MP, et al. Acid-sensing ion channels ASIC 2 and ASIC3 do not contribute to mechanically activated currents in mammalian sensory neurons. J Physiol 2004l 556(Pt 3):691–710.
64. Woolf CJ, American College of Physicians, American Physiological Society. Pain: moving from symptom control toward mechanism-specific pharmacologic management. Ann Int Med 2004; 140:441–451.
65. Julius D, Basbaum AI. Molecular mechanisms of nociception. Nature 2001; 413:203–210.
66. Tominaga M, Catarina MJ, Malmberg AB, et al. The cloned capsaicin receptor integrates multiple pain-producing stimuli. Neuron 1998; 21:531–543.
67. Bassilana F, Champigny G, Waldmann R, et al. The acid-sensitive ionic channel subunit ASIC and the mammalian degenerin MDEG form a heteromultimeric H+-gated Na+ channel with novel properties. J Biol Chem 1997; 272:28819–28822.
68. Sutherland S, Cook S, Ew M. Chemical mediators or pain due to tissue damage and ischemia. Prog Brain Res 2000; 129:21–38.
69. Wood JN, Abrahamsen B, Baker MD, et al. Ion channel activities implicated in pathological pain. Novartis Found Symp 2004; 261:32–40.
70. Wood JN. Molecular mechanisms of nociception and pain. In: Justins DM, ed. Pain 2005- An Updated Review: Refresher Course Syllabus. Seattle, Wash: IASP Press, 2005:179–186.
71. Yaksh TL. Calcium channels as therapeutic targets in neuropathic pain. J Pain 2006; 7(suppl 1):S13–S30.
72. Luo AD, Calcutt NA, Higuera ES, et al. Injury type-specific calcium channel alpha 2 delta-1 subunit up-regulation in rat neuropathic pain models correlates with antiallodynic effects of gabapentin. J Pharmacol Exp Ther 2002; 303(3):1199–1205.
73. Dickenson AH. Preclinical mechanisms related to the clinical pharmacology of analgesic therapy. Justins DM, ed. Pain 2005- An Updated Review: Refresher Course Syllabus. Seattle, Wash: IASP Press, 2005:13–18.
74. Wermeling DP. Ziconotide, an intrathecally administered N-type calcium channel antagonist for the treatment of chronic pain. Pharmacotherapy 2005; 25(8):1084–1094.
75. Prommer EE. Ziconotide: can we use it in palliative care? Am J Hosp Palliat Care 2005; 22(5):369–374.
76. Nassar MA, Stirling LC, Forlani G, et al. Nociceptor-specific gene deletion reveals a major role for NaV1.7 (PN1) in acute and inflammatory pain. Proc Natl Acad Sci USA 2004; 101:12706–12711.

77. Hains BC, Klein JP, Saab CY, et al. Upregulation of NaV1.3 and functional involvement in neuronal hyperexcitability associated with neuropathic pain after spinal cord injury. J Neurosci 2003; 26:8881–8892.

78. Amir R, Argoff CE, Bennett GJ, et al. The roll of sodium channels in chronic inflammatory and neuropathic pain. J Pain 2006; 7(suppl 3):S1–S29.

79. Devor M. Sodium channels and mechanisms of neuropathic pain. J Pain 2006; 7(suppl 1): S3–S12.

80. Ocana M, Cendan CM, Cobos EJ, Entrena JM, Baeyens JM. Potassium channels and pain: present realities and future opportunities. Eur J Pharmacol 2004; 1500(1–3):203–219.

81. Choi Y, Yoon YW, Na HS, Kim SH, Chung JM. Behavior signs of ongoing pain and cold allodynia in a rat model of neuropathic pain. Pain 1994; 59(3):369–376.

82. Rasband MN, Park EW, Vanderah TW, et al. Distinct potassium channels on pain-sensing neurons. Proc Natl Acad Sci USA 2001; 98(23):13373–13378.

83. Wichenden AD, Roeloffs R, McNaughton-Smith G, Rigdon GC. KCNQ potassium channels: drug targets for the treatment of epilepsy and pain. Expert Opin Ther Patents 2004; 14(4):1–13.

Peripheral Mechanisms of Chronic Non-Cancer Pain

MUSCLE PAIN ATTRIBUTES

Muscle pain is subjectively and objectively different from cutaneous and visceral pain. Muscle pain is most commonly described as aching and cramping. It may also be difficult to localize. Pain from cutaneous nociceptors has different attributes—sharp and pricking—and it is easily localized, while the attributes of neuropathic pain are burning and lancinating. Visceral pain is similar to muscle pain, as it is difficult to localize. It is often referred to the skin, whereas muscle pain is mostly referred to other muscles, joints, tendons, and fascia.

Objective differences, which will be dealt with in detail in the following text, also exist. Starting with the processing of the nociceptive information at the level of the spinal cord, the nociceptive impulses continue to the brain stem, where they diverge and the muscle and skin nociception terminates in different regions of the periaqueductal gray (PAG) and, more rostrally, in the thalamus.

Muscle pain frequently becomes chronic if it is not clinically attended to in an appropriate fashion within several days or weeks of its inception. Chronic non-cancer pain is typically defined clinically as non–cancer-related pain that has persisted for at least three months (1). This definition is considered by some to be arbitrary, but it is generally accepted. It is felt that after inception, via trauma, surgery, and so forth, the initial injury should be physiologically healed within three months, particularly if appropriate treatment has been utilized. Pain that exists after treatment and healing, and therefore after its initiating focus has been dealt with, is thought to be associated with different pathophysiological processes.

There are several possible mechanisms for the change from acute muscle pain to chronic.

LOCALIZED MUSCLE PAIN

Muscle nociceptors are free nerve endings that are sensitive to strong mechanical stimuli and endogenous algetic (pain-producing) substances such as bradykinin (BK), which are released from muscle at the onset of a pain-inducing event such as trauma. Prostoglandin E_2 and serotonin (5-HT) are among other algetic substances, which act as sensitizing agents that increase the sensitivity of muscle nociceptors to such chemical and mechanical stimuli. The primary etiology of local muscle tenderness is felt to be this process of sensitization of muscle nociceptors. *Sensitization is not the same as excitation.* Trauma and inflammation can be initiating events. Inflammation, even after the release of BK or 5-HT or the prostaglandins (PGs), appears to cause dysesthesias and even subjective feelings of weakness secondary to the sensitization of muscle nociceptors.

NEUROCHEMICAL MILIEU OF MUSCLE NOCICEPTORS
OR AFFERENT UNITS

No specific neurotransmitter or neuropeptide has been found to be specific for afferent muscle fibers. Similar to cutaneous nerves, dorsal root ganglion cells that project to muscle contain substance P (SP), calcitonin gene-related peptide (CGRP), and somatostatin (SOM) (2). These same neuropeptides are present in group IV muscle afferents. After activation, SP and CGRP, both of which have, in the periphery, strong vascular and other actions, influence the biochemical milieu of the receptors.

SP, produced in the dorsal root ganglia, is transported to the peripheral nerve endings (3). When released from nociceptive endings, SP triggers a cascade of events that induce neurogenic inflammation (also called a "sterile inflammatory response"), secondary to antidromic neuronal activity in sensory nerve fibers from the release of endogenous substances with both vascular and cellular actions (4,5). A nociceptor therefore acts both as a passive sensor of painful stimuli and it is also capable of inducing a change in the chemical milieu around the afferent unit as part of its reaction to noxious stimuli (6).

CGRP, considered one of the most potent cerebral vasodilitors during migraine, along with SP, is effective both in inducing vasodilation and plasma extravasation peripherally. SP also causes its vascular effects via degranulation of mast cells to liberate histamine, which is also a vasodilator. These vasoactive substances also diffuse to contiguous free nerve endings, inducing an enlargement of the area initially affected by a localized stimulus.

Small blood vessels in the regions afferent fibers are located, are also affected. Their permeability is increased and plasma extravasation occurs, shifting fluid-containing vasoneuroactive substances from the intravascular area to the interstitial space around the vessels. The most common vasoneuroactive substances may include BK (broken down from the plasma protein kallidin), 5-HT, released from platelets and PGs, particularly PGE_2 released from endothelial and other cells. All of these substances increase sensitization of nociceptors in a local area, which is also edematous.

As is commonly seen, SP appears to coexist in primary thin myelinated and unmyelinated muscle afferent units with CGRP (7,8). [Beta-endorphin also resides in hypothalamic neurons along with adrenocorticotropic hormone (ACTH)] These peptides are interactive, in that CGRP, in the spinal cord, prolongs the activity of SP by inhibiting its breakdown (9).

SP also is very capable of modulating pain sensations, particularly when found centrally (10,11).

As already noted, the algetic substances BK and 5-HT are powerful stimulants of free muscle nerve endings. High concentrations of potassium ions also act algetically (12–17). All three vasoneuroactive substances mentioned have strong abilities to sensitize muscle afferents (18).

Other algetic substance interactions exist with regard to their ability to stimulate muscle afferents. PGE_2 and 5-HT have been shown to incrementally increase the excitatory activity of BK (19). BK is known to increase both synthesis and release of PGE_2 (20).

Leukotrienes (LTs), under pathological conditions, are released from tissue, and several have been shown to promote inflammatory processes and induce, during behavioral research, hyperalgesia (LT B_4, D_4) (21–25).

OTHER MECHANISMS OF CHRONIC MUSCLE PAIN STATES

The pain-spasm-pain cycle written about by many authors may, in fact, not be physiologically accurate. This concept involves a reflex arc originating in muscle nociceptors and terminating in the neuromuscular end plates of the same muscle. This reflex circuit is felt to be triggered by a painful muscular lesion. The lesion activates muscle nociceptors that synapse with alpha and gamma motor neurons. Increased activity in these neurons induces a contraction of the muscle, via the alpha motor neurons or indirectly via the gamma loop (a neuronal circuit that leads from gamma motor neurons via muscle spindles to alpha motor neurons—the gamma motor neurons activate the muscle spindles, which then can excite alpha motor neurons monosynaptically). If there is significant force generated by the contracting muscle, it may compress blood vessels and lead to ischemia; ischemic contractions are painful and would further excite nociceptors, leading to a "vicious cycle." However, an acute painful stimulus to a muscle is likely to inhibit rather than excite homonymous motor neurons if the muscle is an extensor. If the muscle is a flexor, motor neurons typically show only short-lasting excitation, if any. Further, painful muscle frequently shows no resting electrical activity. The postulated reflex would not be functional in every muscle and could not explain long-lasting spasms (26).

Significant *hypoxia* will depress or terminate muscle spindle discharges. This will reduce the excitatory drive on homonymous alpha-motor neurons and induce relaxation of the muscle; it will also impair motor co-ordination, as during depression of spindle discharges, motor centers do not receive the information on muscle length that they need to co-ordinate movement (27).

"Psychophysiological interactions" is the term preferred by this author to use in place of "psychosomatic," as the latter term has been a possible cause of a great deal of clinical mislabeling of patients. Psychosomatic means to many clinicians that a patient's complaints of pain are entirely falsely generated by patients who essentially "believe" that they have pain, possibly for reasons of secondary gain. A patient with a preinjury history of depression, for example, can certainly sustain a painful muscular injury. Also, central pain perception relies on 5-HT, and chronic pain appears to diminish tonus of the serotonergic system. A decrement of 5-HT will lead to increased pain perception, sleep disorder, depression, and abnormalities in hypothalamic hormonal release. After the onset of pain, at least a subclinical neurochemical "set up" for depression exists. Other affective difficulties such as anxiety will also frequently begin. In these patients, chronic pain is not psychosomatic, but aggravated and perpetuated by physiological problems and affective input. Stress, as noted earlier, has physiological and neurochemical manifestations. Psychophysiological aspects can change physiological parameters in muscle-related pain, such as those found in active myofascial trigger points. The psychophysiological aspects of pain must be actively evaluated and teased apart, so that appropriate treatment can be rendered to the various physical and affective problems a chronic muscle pain patient may manifest.

MYOFASCIAL TRIGGER POINTS

Trigger points associated with myofascial pain syndrome are discussed in detail in Chapter 4.

REFERRED PAIN

One of the major clinical characteristics of myofascial trigger points is referred pain. There are four postulated neurophysiological mechanisms of sensitization that may mediate referred pain from trigger points. They are:

1. *Convergence–projection*: Pain may be initiated by muscle nociceptors but then referred to another area served by other somatic receptors that converge on the same region of the spinothalamic tract.
2. *Convergence–facilitation*: Impulses from one somatic zone are facilitated or amplified in the spinal cord by other activity originating in nociceptors from a trigger point in another area of the body.
3. *Peripheral branching of primary afferent nociceptors*: The brain may misinterpret activity from nociceptors in one part of the body as originating from nerves coming from another part of the body (28).
4. *Sympathetic modulation of peripheral nociceptors*: Induction of increased sympathetic activity causes an increase in substances that sensitize primary afferent nerve receptors in the area of referred pain (29).

These hypotheses take much into account that has already been discussed. Central nervous system (CNS) plasticity plays a role, along with dorsal horn neuronal plasticity and sensitization. Clinically, these factors need to be taken into account when examining a patient—treating the area of referred pain is obviously not helpful. One must recognize the area of primary pain that induces the referred pain.

"UPREGULATION" OF NOCICEPTIVE AFFERENTS

Central neurotransmitter receptor sites, during pathological conditions, upregulate, increasing their individual effectiveness and their density. Similarly, Reinert and Mense (30) have shown experimentally that muscle inflammation in rats lasting 12 days was associated with a marked increase in the innervation density of thin neuropeptide-containing fibers, which could be visualized with antibodies to SP. The increased nociceptive fiber density, it was felt, would cause noxious stimuli to excite more nociceptive endings and thus increase pain, or chronic hyperalgesia in the affected muscle.

PERIPHERAL AND CENTRAL NERVOUS SYSTEM ASPECTS OF NON-CANCER PAIN

Pain can be generated from the peripheral nervous system (PNS) and CNS, including the autonomic aspects of the CNS. The attributes of these forms of pain are different from those seen in myofascial pain. They can be seen in addition to myofascial pain. The diagnosis of neuropathic, or nerve–related, pain is made via both history and examination.

Neuropathic Pain Manifestations

Different pain attributes are important to note and should be used in conducting an appropriate history.

- *Spontaneous pain* is paroxysmal or constant—burning, shooting, and/or lancinating.

- *Paresthesias* are abnormal nonpainful sensations that may be spontaneous or evoked—tingling.
- *Dysesthesias* are unpleasant, abnormal pain sensations, spontaneous, or evoked—unpleasant tingling.
- *Hyperalgesia/hyperesthesia* is an increased response to a stimulus that is normally painful.
- *Allodynia* is pain from stimuli that do not normally provoke pain—burning from light touch.

Peripheral Mechanisms of Chronic Pain

Various changes in the physiology of the peripheral nerves can induce pain. These changes include:

- continued discharges unprovoked by peripheral afferents,
- demyelination secondary to chronic irritation leading to the production of spontaneous action potentials that may travel in two directions—dromically and antidromically,
- peripheral nerve lesions inducing pathological changes in the dorsal root ganglia, causing spontaneous discharge of neurons without reception of peripheral stimulation,
- spontaneous activity of axonal sprouts during regeneration, which may lead to neuroma formation, and
- increased sensitivity in a neuroma, which may be secondary to chemical or mechanical stimuli leading to excitation continued between bare sections of neurons—ephaptic transmission, or "cross talk."

Neuroma Formation

Sensory nerve axons have three functions: encoding, conduction, and relaying sensory information from the periphery to the CNS for processing. If any of these aspects does not function properly, the CNS may have difficulties determining the meaning of the projected information.

Pain that occurs after termination of the initial noxious stimuli may be secondary to:

- sensitization, or increased sensitivity of peripheral nociceptors, causing previously innocuous stimuli to elicit pain from otherwise normal CNS pathways,
- abnormal ectopic impulses produced from new sites (previously injured) in peripheral nerve axons,
- abnormal neuronal discharges from within the CNS, and
- the inability of the CNS to correctly or appropriately process peripheral afferent neuronal information.

After an axon is cut, the part still connected to the nerve cell body seals and forms an end bulb (terminal swelling). Dying back of the axon may occur with an associated disruption of the myelin sheath, or one or more axonal sprouts may emerge from the end bulbs and elongate.

When sprouts reach peripheral target tissue, peripheral receptor activity restarts and growth ends. The regenerating sprouts may elongate from a tangled mass of regenerating sprouts, or buds.

Even if the majority of peripheral nerve function is restored, some sprouts may become trapped somewhere along the nerve and form "neuroma in continuity." If a nerve is only partially transected, axonal regrowth may develop into multiple microneuromas.

Ectopic electrogenesis (pacemakers) may develop in axonal end bulbs and sprouts in a neuroma. These can generate electrical impulses spontaneously, without any initiating stimuli. Impulses may occur secondary to multiple depolarizing stimuli: pressure, temperature changes, ischemia, changes in blood oxygen levels, increased extracellular potassium concentration, and the effects of various peptides and neurotransmitters.

As noted earlier, muscle nociceptive afferents are most typically A-delta and C fibers, which are the fiber types most likely to develop neuromas. The pain, which can also be perceived as deep tissue pain, most probably has contributions from nociceptive afferent fibers from muscle.

Peripheral Neuropathic Pain

Peripheral neuropathic pain (PNP) may be divided into pain secondary to normal activation of the somatosensory pathways and those secondary to neuroma development, which can induce spontaneous ectopic activity at the site of the neuroma, and in the dorsal root ganglion. Neuromas are associated with the induction of clinical pain in the peripheral nerves associated with the stumps of amputated limbs, including phantom limb pain.

Areas of demyelination in otherwise normal peripheral nerves may be associated with the generation of ectopic impulses. Pain from such areas is associated with electrical-like or lancinating pain, which is probably secondary to ephapses, not neuromas.

Peripheral loss of afferent inhibition (demyelination of large peripheral nerves, for example) may contribute to some peripheral neuropathic pain, such as that seen in postherpetic neuralgia.

Neuropathic pain mechanisms must explain episodic, ongoing, and delayed onset pain. Three types of central changes are hypothesized.

1. Changes in afferent impulses, which can induce long-term shifts in central synaptic excitability. This can result in a high enough level of ongoing activity and induce continuous pain.
2. Changes in chemical substances from the periphery produce peripheral sensitization and this produces changes in spinal cord excitability (31). Abnormal hyperexcitability of central nociceptive neurons appears to be highly dependent on the activation of the N-methyl-D-aspartate (NMDA) glutamatergic receptors located on the membrane of spinal cord dorsal horn neurons secondary to massive release of excitatory amino acids (particularly glutamate and aspartate). The use of NMDA receptor antagonists has been shown to induce anti-allodynic effects (32,33).
3. Pathological hyperexcitability may be secondary to changes in central control mechanisms. It is possible that the creation of spinal cord (lamina I), brain stem-spinal cord loops occurs; these loops would be unstable and may explain episodic neuropathic pain.

Other hypotheses exist to explain central modifications that could induce pathological activation of the central nociceptive neurons felt to be responsible for the development of neuropathic pain.

Central disinhibition from loss of modulatory control mechanisms may result in abnormal excitability of central neurons. Decreased levels of inhibitory neurotransmitters [gamma-aminobutyric acid (GABA)] and glycine, both inhibitory neurotransmitters particularly in the spinal cord) with downregulation of GABA receptors are found in the spinal cord dorsal horn after experimental peripheral nerve injury. It is hypothesized that some of the inhibitory interneurons may be destroyed, possibly by excessive stimulation of NMDA receptors, leading to excitotoxic cell death (34).

When peripheral nerve primary afferents are damaged, significant topographic reorganization of the primary afferent terminals in the spinal cord may occur (35). In animal experiments, after peripheral nerve sectioning, some large-diameter primary afferents that typically transmit non-nociceptive mechanoreceptive impulses and which normally terminate in the deep laminae (III and IV) may grow in lamina II, the substantia gelatinosa, which primarily receives input from small-diameter fibers and responds to noxious stimulation (35,36). These non-nociceptive neurons could then become activated by non-noxious stimuli from the larger primary afferents, and respond with nociceptive impulses to non-nociceptive input.

It is notable that the pathogenesis of chronic muscle pain is not very different from that of neuropathic pain. Remembering that we are dealing with the *Neuromuscular System*, both parts of which are intrinsic to each other, gives us reason to hypothesize such interactions—muscle pain and neuropathic, or nerve–related, pain being non-coincidentally conjoined. However, muscle pain from a purely neuropathic lesion is rare.

RADICULOPATHY

Radiculopathic pain is associated with a nerve root lesion. This pain is frequently described as deep and aching, both attributes similar to those described in muscle pain. Radicular pain also includes other attributes: it can be described as sharp, stabbing, and shooting. None of these pain attributes would be attributable to muscle pain. There is also hypoesthesia, or loss of sensation, associated with true radiculopathy.

Electrodiagnotic studies easily identify a radiculopathy. Sensory-evoked potentials (SEPS) are useful in detecting a purely sensory radiculopathy.

Unfortunately, specialists in pain management frequently see patients with the diagnosis of a radiculopathy that is "not surgically amenable to treatment." A thorough history and neurological examination with appropriate attention paid to the musculoskeletal system may frequently find myofascial or myogenic pain, with nociceptive foci in myofascial trigger points. This pseudoradiculopathy is indeed not surgically treatable. An example would be myofascial trigger points found in the piriformis muscle, inducing a "false L_5–S_1 disc syndrome."

Others claim that myofascial trigger points are always found in association with radiculopathy (37).

Complex regional pain syndrome (formerly called reflex sympathetic dystrophy or RSD) will be noted in the chapter on sympathetic aspects of myofascial pain. Research on this entity, and other research (31,38), has shown that physiological neuroplastic changes can occur in the CNS from peripheral nerve lesions and CNS lesions can induce changes in function of the PNS. Again, the close relationship of the CNS, the PNS, the autonomous nervous system (ANS), and the musculoskeletal system would anticipate such findings.

CENTRAL SENSITIZATION

The receptive fields (RF) of specific dorsal horn neurons are anatomically defined by the spatial projection of their dendrites and the topography of the central terminals of primary afferents. When a dorsal horn neuron fires, the stimulus from the periphery must lie within the receptive field of that neuron—the specific area from which a stimulus depolarizes the dorsal horn neuronal membrane at a strength that is above its action potential activation threshold (39). It has been found that after nerve or tissue injury, dorsal horn receptive fields may increase in size, decrease their action potential threshold, and/or increase their responsiveness to nociceptive information in a way that exactly parallels changes in pain sensitivity. These facts are indicative of the fact that the peripheral sensory receptive fields of somatosensory neurons are not fixed, static, or "hard-wired," but are changeable or plastic (40,41).

Repetitive nociceptive input to the spinal cord induces use-dependent or activity-dependent plasticity, in that the spinal cord becomes more and more responsive to subsequent sensory inputs and this leads to hypersensitivity. Modulatory central input (both descending inhibition and excitation) helps determine spinal excitability. Changes in the activity of these descending systems can have significant effects on spinal cord sensory transmission.

Two physiological changes occur, windup and central sensitization.

Windup is a nonlinear increase in the response or output of the dorsal horn neurons, which occurs following repetitive C-fiber stimulation. The response to successive input is continually increased. Windup is accompanied by after-discharges, firing of the cell for many seconds after the end of the train of stimuli. This shows use-dependent functional plasticity that manifests only during pathological states when repeated nociceptive input occurs, indicating that dorsal horn cellular response to nociceptive input is modifiable. A greater increase in the transfer of nociceptive information to the brain occurs following repetitive nociceptive input to dorsal horn cells, which induces a gradual increase in pain sensitivity to the same initiating stimulus (42).

Allodynia, previously noted to be defined as pain induced from normally nonpainful stimuli, and hyperalgesia (amplification of the normal painful response to a noxious stimulus) are features of pain after tissue or nerve injury.

Allodynia could be secondary to any of the following: a decrease in the threshold of A-delta fiber and C-fiber nociceptors in the skin, which would make them fire in response to innocuous low-intensity stimuli (peripheral sensitization), pain resulting from the activation of large low-threshold A-fiber neurons secondary to changes in spinal sensory processing (central sensitization), or a "rewiring" of synaptic connections, where the A-fiber information is being received in the more peripheral laminae (structural plasticity) (42).

Primary hyperalgesia appears to occur after a reduction in the activation thresholds of nociceptors and peripheral sensitization, and is associated with thermal and mechanical hypersensitivity. Secondary hyperalgesia is secondary to central sensitization, with dorsal horn cells being hyperexcitable after nociceptive C-fiber input so that the low-threshold tactile stimulation–activating A-beta fibers are painful and mechanical stimuli, which activate A-delta fibers inducing a much greater pain response (43). The latter changes appear to result from the recruitment of previously weak or subthreshold input to the dorsal horn neurons, secondary to increased excitability of the spinal neuronal membrane (42).

As noted earlier, after tissue injury, central descending modulating systems can induce inhibition or facilitate excitability to the dorsal horn systems. Supposed opioid resistance in neuropathic pain may have several etiologies: a reduction of the inhibitory influence over spinal transmission after nerve injury (44) as a result of decreased opioid receptors on sensory neurons, a decrement in GABA content within the dorsal horn (45), and interneuron transsynaptic cell death following nerve injury (46). The spinal neuronal membrane is thus rendered hyperexcitable secondary to disinhibition, and not increased excitation. Membrane depolarization in the absence of C-fiber input follows, inducing spontaneous discharges, a potential mechanism underlying spontaneous pain seen in neuropathic pain patients (42). Urban and Gebhart (47) have identified descending facilitative systems from areas of the medulla to the superficial dorsal horn. These areas have been implicated in the generation of central sensitization in the dorsal horn after tissue and nerve injury. It appears that changes in supraspinal modulatory influences over spinal transmission have important roles in both the generation and the maintenance of chronic pain states (42).

Mannion and Woolf (42) make the excellent point that in the treatment of chronic pain two things must be accomplished: the identification and treatment of hypersensitivity states and then the primary mechanisms of nociception.

DISTURBANCES IN THE CENTRAL ANTI-NOCICEPTIVE SYSTEMS

Research into the pathophysiology of tension-type headache (see Chapter 12) indicates that chronic painful states are associated with the dysmodulation of central antinociceptive neurotransmitter systems, particularly the serotonergic, noradrenergic, endogenous opiate, and GABAnergic systems (48).

There appears to be a paucity of attention to such central neurotransmitter systems relating to chronic muscle pain. Most probably, such effects will be found to be present, adding another layer of complexity to the treatment of chronic muscle pain states.

REFERENCES

1. Mersky H, Bogduk N. Classification of Chronic Pain: Descriptions of Chronic Pain Syndromes and Definitions of Pain Terms. 2nd ed. Seattle, Wash: IASP Press, 1994.
2. Molander C, Grant G. Spinal cord projections from hindlimb muscle nerves in the rat studied by transganglionic transport of horseradish peroxidase, wheat germ agglutinin conjugated horseradish peroxidase, or horseradish peroxidase with dimethylsulfoxide. J Comp Neurol 1987; 260:246–255.
3. Brimijoin S, Lundberg JM, Brodin E, et. al. Axonal transport of substance P in the vagus and sciatic nerves of the guinea pig. Brain Res 1980; 191:443–457.
4. Lembeck F, Holzer P. Substance P as neurogenic mediator of antidromic vasodilation and neurogenic plasma extravasation. Naunyn-Schmiedeberg's Arch Pharmacol 1979; 310:175–183.
5. Gamse R, Posch M, Saria A, et al. Several mediators appear to interact in neurogenic inflammation. Acta Physiol Hung 1987; 69:343–354.
6. Mense S, Simons DG. Muscle Pain: Understanding its Nature, Diagnosis and Treatment. Baltimore, Md: Lippincott Williams & Wilkins, 2000:30.
7. Ju G, Hokfelt T, Brodin E, et al. Primary sensory neurons of the rat showing calcitonin gene-related peptide immunoreactivity and their relation to substance P, somatostatin-, galanin-, vasoactive intestinal peptide- and cholecystokinin- immunoreactive ganglion cells. Cell Tissue Res 1987; 247:417–431.

8. Hoheisel U, Mense S, Scherotzke R. Calcitonin gene-related peptide-immunoreactivity in functionally identified primary afferent neurones in the rat. Anat Embryol 1994; 189:41–49.
9. Le Greves P, Nyberg F, Terenius L, et al. Calcitonin gene-related peptide is a potent inhibitor of substance P degradation. Eur J Pharmacol 1985; 115:309–311.
10. Duggan AW, Hendry IA, Norton CR, et al. Cutaneous stimuli releasing immunoreactive substance P in the dorsal horn of the car. Brain Res 1988; 451:261–273.
11. Buck SH, Walsh JH, Yamamura HI, et al. Neuropeptides in sensory neurons. Life Sci 1982; 30:1857–1866.
12. Guzman F, Braun C, Lim KS. Visceral pain and the pseudoaffective response to intra-arterial injection of bradykinin and other algesic agents. Arch Int Pharmacodyn 1962; 136:353–384.
13. Franz M, Mense S. Muscle receptors with group IV afferent fibres responding to application of bradykinin. Brain Res 1975; 92:369–383.
14. Fock S, Mense S. Excitatory effects of 5-hydroxytryptamine, histamine and potassium ions on muscular group IV afferent units: a comparison with bradykinin. Brain Res 1976; 105:459–469.
15. Keele CA. Excitants of pain receptors. Acta Neuroveg 1966; 28:392–404.
16. Kaufman MP, Iwamoto GA, Longhurst JC, et al. Effects of capsaicin and bradykinin on afferent fibers with endings in skeletal muscle. Circ Res 1982; 50:133–139.
17. Kumazawa T, Mizumura K. Thin-fibre receptors responding to mechanical, chemical and thermal stimulation in the skeletal muscle of the dog. J Physiol 1977; 273:179–194.
18. Sicuteri F. Vasoneuroactive substances and their implication in vascular pain. In: Friedman AP, ed. Research and Clinical Studies in Headache. Vol.1. New York, NY: Karger, 1967:6–45.
19. Mense S. Sensitization of group IV muscle receptors to bradykinin by 5-hydroxytryptamine and prostaglandin E_2 Brain Res 1981; 225:95–105.
20. Jose PJ, Page DA, Wolstenholme BE, et al. Bradykinin-stimulated prostaglandin E_2 production of endothelial cells and its modulation by anti-inflammatory compounds. Inflammation 1981; 5:363–378.
21. Hoheisel U, Mense S. Leukotriene D4 depresses the mechanosensitivity of group III and IV muscle receptors in the rat. Neuroreport 1994; 5:645–648.
22. Mense S, Hoheisel U. Influence of leukotriene D4 on the discharges of slowly conducting afferent units from normal and inflamed muscle in the rat. Pflugers Arch 1990; 415(suppl 1R):150.
23. Piper PJ. Formation and actions of leukotrienes. Physiol Rev 1984; 64:744–761.
24. Samuelsson B, Dahlen SE, Lindgren JA, et al. Leukotrienes and lipoxins: structures, biosynthesis and biological effects. Science 1987; 237:1171–1176.
25. Samuelsson B. Leukotrienes: mediators of immediate hypersensitivity reactions and inflammation. Science 1983; 220:568–575.
26. Mense S, Simons DG. Muscle Pain: Understanding its Nature, Diagnosis and Treatment. Baltimore, Md: Lippincott Williams & Wilkins, 2000:10–11.
27. Mense S, Simons DG. Muscle Pain: Understanding its Nature, Diagnosis and Treatment. Baltimore, Md: Lippincott Williams & Wilkins, 2000:52.
28. Bahr R, Blumberg H, Janig W. Do dichotomizing afferent fibers exist which supply visceral organs as well as somatic structures? A contribution to the problem of referred pain. Neurosci Lett 1981; 24(1):25–28.
29. Procacci P, Francini F, Zoppi M, Maresca M. Cutaneous pain threshold changes after sympathetic block in reflex dystrophies. Pain 1975; (2):167–175.
30. Reinert A, Mense S. Inflammatory influence on the density of CGRP and SP-immunoreactive nerve endings in rat skeletal muscle. Neuropeptides 1993; 24:204–205.
31. Coderre TJ, Katz J, Vaccarino AL, et al. Contribution of neuroplasticity to pathological pain: review of clinical and experimental evidence. Pain 1993; 52:259–285.
32. Felsby S, Nielsen J, Arendt Nielsen L, et al. NMDA receptor blockade in chronic neuropathic pain: a comparison of ketamine and magnesium chloride. Pain 1996; 64:283–291.
33. Eide PK, Stubhaug A, Oye I, et al. Continuous subcutaneous administration of the N-Methyl-D-aspartic acid (NMDA) receptor antagonist ketamine in the treatment of post-herpetic neuralgia. Pain 1995; 61:221–228.

34. Mao J, Price DD, Zhu J, et al. The inhibition of nitric-oxide activated poly(ADP-ribose) synthetase attenuates transsynaptic alteration of spinal cord dorsal horn neurons and neuropathic pain in the rat. Pain 1997; 72:355–366.

35. Woolf CJ. Molecular signals responsible for the reorganization of the synaptic circuitry of the dorsal horn after peripheral nerve injury: the mechanisms of tactile allodynia. In: Borsook D, ed. Molecular Neurobiology of Pain: Progress in Pain Research and Management. Vol. 9. Seattle, Wash: IASP Press, 1997:171–200.

36. Woolf CJ, Shortland P, Coggeshall RE. Peripheral nerve injury triggers central sprouting of myelinated afferents. Nature 1992; 355:75–78.

37. Gunn CC. Radiculopathic pain: diagnosis and treatment of segmental irritation or sensitization. J Musculoskel Pain 1994; 5(4):119–134.

38. Hoheisel U, Beylich G, Mense S. Effects of an acute muscle nerve section on the excitability of dorsal horn neurons in the rat. Pain 1995; 60:151–158.

39. Willis WD, Coggeshall RE. Sensory Mechanisms of the Spinal Cord. New York, NY: Plenum Press, 1991.

40. Hylden JLK, Nahin RL, Traub RJ, et al. Expansion of receptive fields of spinal lamina I projection neurons in rats with unilateral adjuvant-induced inflammation: the contribution of dorsal horn mechanisms. Pain 1989; 37:239–243.

41. Cook AJ, Woolf CJ, Wall PD, et al. Dynamic receptive field plasticity in rat spinal cord dorsal horn following C primary afferent input. Nature 1987; 325:151–153.

42. Mannion RJ, Woolf CJ. Pain mechanisms and management: A central perspective. Clin J Pain 2000; 16:S144–S156.

43. Koltzenburg M. Painful neuropathies. Curr Opin Neurol 1998; 11:515–521.

44. de Groot JF, Coggeshall RE, Carlton SM. The reorganization of mu opioid receptors in the rat dorsal horn following peripheral axotomy. Neurosci Lett 1997; 233:113–116.

45. Castro-Lopes JM, Tavares I, Coimbra A. GABA decreases in the spinal cord dorsal horn after peripheral neurectomy. Brain Res 1993; 620:287–291.

46. Sugimoto T, Bennett GJ, Kajander KC. Transsynaptic degeneration in the superficial dorsal horn after sciatic nerve injury: effects of a chronic constriction injury, transection and strychnine. Pain 1990; 42:205–213.

47. Urban MO, Gebhart GF. Supraspinal contributions to hyperalgesia. Proc Natl Acad Sci USA 1999; 96:7687–7692.

48. Jay GW. The Headache Handbook: Diagnosis and Treatment. Boca Raton, Fl: CRC Press, 1999:61–62.

4   Myofascial Pain Syndrome

Myofascial pain syndrome (MPS) has long been a clinical subject of interest. Historically, there have been many names for this clinical entity, which has led to a great deal of confusion. These older names included myofibrositis, myofascitis, fibromyositis, myogelosis, and fibrositis, to name a few. Fields (1) noted that many of the most common, persistent, and disabling pain problems are of musculoskeletal origin. He also noted that although MPS was common, many therapists were unaware of its existence. Four years earlier, Travell and Simons (2) had published the criteria for diagnosing MPS.

Unfortunately, the problem of the objectification and awareness of MPS continues to the present day. MPS is diagnostically challenging in that it has multiple guises, and many other clinical entities with supposedly specific diagnoses are actually secondary to MPS.

MPS has been defined by the International Association for the Study of Pain as a regional painful condition associated with the presence of trigger points (TrPs). Myofascial trigger points (MTrPs) are loci of hyperirritability, which when subjected to mechanical pressure, give rise to characteristic patterns of referred pain.

MPS is a very common occurrence in pain clinic populations and is usually diagnostically straightforward. The diagnosis is basically a clinical one, as it is associated with normal radiological studies as well as having no diagnostic laboratory studies.

Yunus noted that one could not meaningfully study the etiology of a condition that is ill defined or nonspecific (4). Over the last decade, a great deal of clinical and scientific data have given greater definition to MPS.

One study of 309 chronic pain patients revealed that MPS with attendant TrPs was found in two-thirds of the patients, and was found to be the most frequent clinical pain syndrome (5).

A more recent study found that there was general agreement across the specialties of pain management providers that MPS was a legitimate diagnosis, with a high level of agreement regarding the signs and symptoms essential to or associated with the diagnosis of MPS (6).

Studies of the prevalence of MPS have some difficulties, when trying to compare them to each other. Specifically, differences in the criteria used to make the diagnosis and the experience and skill of the examiners make this difficult, along with different populations and variations of chronicity.

It has been noted that MPS is seen more frequently in women than men, and it is most often seen in adults between the ages of 31 to 50, although TrPs have also been diagnosed in children and young adults (7,8). Local and referred muscular pain from TrPs has been found to be a major factor in the majority of workers' compensation cases involving pain (9). Women, more frequently than men, appear to develop symptomatic myofascial pain (7).

Recent research indicates that there is only modest genetic influence on the development of chronic musculoskeletal pain (10).

Pain related to chronic MPS can induce disability from not only the attributes of the pain, but also from depression, sleep disturbances, other psychological and behavioral problems, and physical deconditioning secondary to lack of exercise (11).

Fricton et al. (12) studied 164 patients with MPS and found that the mean duration of their pain was 5.8 years for men and 6.9 years for women, with an average of 4.5 clinicians having been seen in the past for their complaints of pain.

This characterization of these patients has not changed in the years since Fricton's study was published.

PHYSIOLOGY

The neuromuscular junction is a synapse that depends on ACh (acetylcholine) as its main neurotransmitter. The nerve terminal receives energy via an action potential from the alpha-motoneuron, which opens the voltage-gated calcium channels. Ionized calcium moves through these channels from the synaptic cleft into the nerve terminal. These channels are found on both sides of the nerve membrane, which releases packets of ACh in response to the ionized calcium. The production of packets of ACh is via a process that uses energy supplied by the mitochondria located in the nerve terminal.

When many packets of ACh are released essentially simultaneously, the amount of ACh overwhelms the cholinesterase (which metabolizes ACh) in the synaptic cleft and the ACh crosses the cleft and reaches the postjunctional membrane of the muscle fiber where the ACh receptors are found. The cholinesterase in the synaptic cleft will metabolize the ACh, which will end its action. This allows the synapse to again respond to another action potential.

When large numbers of vesicles of ACh are released simultaneously in response to an action potential that arrives at the nerve terminal, the postjunctional membrane is depolarized enough for it to reach its threshold for excitation. This will initiate an action potential that will be propagated by the surface membrane, the sarcolemma, throughout the specific muscle fiber.

The motor end plates link the terminal nerve fiber of a motoneuron to a muscle fiber. The endplate zone is the region where motor end plates innervate the fibers of the muscle, also called the motor points.

Myogelosis, an older term, describes small, typically circumscribed areas of firmness and tenderness to palpation found in a muscle or muscles associated with a patient's complaints of pain. This term is essentially synonymous with MTrPs. The focal tenderness, taut bands of muscle, and nodules described in patients with myogelosis are also found to be associated with MTrPs.

A taut band is a grouping of tense muscle fibers that extend from an MTrP to the muscle's attachments. There are three associated features, including the absence of motor unit action potentials, severe, highly localized tenderness in the taut band at the MTrP, and the quick release of the taut band and MTrP-associated tenderness by the inactivation of the TrP. Simons and Travell (2) felt that a local contracture, which was associated with nonelectrical, endogenous shortening of the sarcomere, was secondary to a local energy crisis in the muscle. They postulated that the energy crises would be secondary to the increased metabolic demand of the contractured sarcomeres in the presence of ischemia-induced hypoxia secondary to vigorous sustained contraction. This energy crisis would induce sensitization of contiguous nociceptors (13).

Gerwin reiterates that the entire muscle is not hard or in spasm; the tenderness is present over the hardened taut band (14).

Simons noted shortened sarcomeres in the region of the MTrP with compensatory lengthening of sarcomeres (one of the repeating structural units of striated muscle fibrils) in the same fibers continuing to their attachments. This was associated with an expanded diameter of the shortened sarcomeres in the area of the MTrP with contiguous thinning of the fiber diameters beyond the MTrP, which was related to the increased firmness to palpation of the MTrP itself (13,15).

One of the clinical diagnostic criteria of an MTrP, the taut band, can also be found in patients without TrPs (16). This finding raises the question of whether a symptomatic MTrP represents an additional spread and "propagation" of TrP pathology from several contraction knots to more extensive involvement of more muscle fibers (17). MPS in a single muscle with MTrPs may "metastasize" to involve other muscles, which are both contiguous and in other regions of the body.

Active loci are multiple minute regions that exhibit spontaneous electrical activity (SEA), with endplate noise, in an MTrP that may be associated with spike activity characteristic of single-fiber action potentials on electromyography. It was recognized that some of the end plates in MTrPs were abnormal, as the SEA was abnormal and resulted from an enormously increased release of ACh (13). It was noted by Simons that the active loci occurred predominantly in MTrPs and were the central dysfunction in the MTrP, and were also scattered among normal end plates throughout the MTrP (18). In humans, it was found that active loci are four times more common in TrPs than in the endplate zone outside of a TrP. Also, no active loci were found in the taut band outside of the endplate zone. The SEA type of auditory endplate electrical activity is related to MTrPs (17).

The electromyographic evidence has been variously interpreted, but it is thought by Simons that excessive ACh will induce increased and continuous electrical activity that produces a contraction knot (17) (see following text). This will also create a higher voltage endplate potential, which would be more readily detectable, and much more of the endplate region would be continuously active electrically, and not active intermittently at a few isolated miniscule locations. A contraction knot would increase the target size of the electromyographic (EMG) needle. Normal miniature endplate potentials are more difficult to obtain (17).

An important feature of MTrPs, contraction knots, appeared, on biopsy of dog muscle, to be thick, enlarged, round muscle fibers with extremely contracted sarcomeres, with corresponding swelling of the contiguous muscle fiber. Human biopsy showed on electronmicroscopy an excess of muscle A-band and lack of the I-band, on cross section. It was noted that the complete replacement of the I-band by the A-band only occurs in fully contracted sarcomeres (13).

The local twitch response (LTR) is obtained by mechanical stimulation of an MTrP in a taut band of muscle. It is a transient, fast contraction of the palpable taut band of muscle fibers associated with an MTrP. The LTR may be provoked by mechanical/palpatory impact to the affected muscle, via needle penetration of the TrP and by snapping palpation of the TrP (see following text) (19,20). The LTR is a confirmatory clinical sign. Upon injection into an MTrP, the LTR is seen and this is indicative that the injection should be clinically effective. The LTR is typically extremely painful when elicited, and it is a strong indication of the presence of an MTrP.

The relationship between the elicitation of a painful LTR from successful needling or injection of a TrP suggests that it may originate from stimulation of sensitized nociceptors in the region of the MTrP (21). The alpha-motoneurons associated with end plates with excessive ACh release appear to be responsive to the strong sensory spinal input from these sensitized nociceptors. Snapping palpation may induce an LTR in both the TrPs palpated, as well as in the taut band of another muscle close by (17).

A patient who lost the LTR after a brachial plexus injury, which resulted in total loss of nerve conduction, was found to recover the LTR on EMG associated with the recovery of nerve conduction (22). This is consistent with rabbit literature that shows the LTR to be a direct spinal reflex (20).

Trigger Points

MTrPs are small hyperirritable foci in muscles and fascia, which are most typically found in a taut band of skeletal (striated) muscle. They can also be found in ligaments, tendons, skin, joint capsule, and periostium. They may be localized to a single muscle or found in multiple muscle groups. When pressure is directed onto the active TrP, a local or referred pain pattern is obtained. The referred pain pattern will be consistent for a specific TrP. The "zone of reference" is the region of referred pain in an area distant from the TrP. Patients may also perceive paresthesias or numbness in the zone of reference. Compression of a latent TrP may also induce pain.

The areas of referred pain are not consistent with myotomal, dermatomal, or sclerotomal patterns. Kellgren's work (23) found this consistency after studying the specificity of muscular and ligamentous pain secondary to muscular injections of 0.1 to 0.3 mL of hypertonic saline.

Referred pain does tend to be segmental, in that the referred pain patterns are typically located in sites innervated by nearby or adjacent spinal cord segments (14).

A TrP may be formed, or activated, secondary to mechanical problems from muscle overload, which can be acute, sustained, or repetitive. Nerve compression that can induce obvious neuropathic electromyographic changes is associated with an increased number of active MTrPs. In summary, TrPs may be directly activated by work overload, muscle overwork fatigue, direct trauma, and radiculopathy (24). Indirect TrP activation can occur via other existing TrPs, visceral disease, joint dysfunctions, arthritic joints, and by stress/emotional distress (17).

There are six different classifications of TrPs (17):

Active MTrP is tender and, with direct compression, produces referred pain as well as referred motor phenomena and may induce autonomic phenomena, induces tenderness in the pain reference zone, it will mediate, after appropriate stimulation, an LTR, is associated with a taut band of muscle, and other associated phenomena include muscle shortening, weakness, and decreased range of motion (17).

Latent MTrP is painful only when directly palpated/compressed, but may have all the other clinical characteristics of an active TrP, including decreased range of motion of the muscle, weakness, and muscle shortening. Referred pain is typically not seen (17).

Primary MTrP is centrally located in the muscle, typically activated by an acute or chronic muscle work overload, or by repetitive overuse of the muscle in which it occurs, and not secondary to TrP activity in another muscle (17).

Key MTrP is responsible for activating one or more satellite TrPs in its zone of reference; inactivation will also inactivate associated satellite TrPs (17).

Satellite MTrP is centrally located in the muscle, induced via mechanical or neurogenic stimulation by the activity of a key TrP, inactivated when the key TrP is inactivated, may be found in the key TrP's zone of reference, in an overloaded synergist that is substituting for the muscle in which the key TrP is found, in an antagonist muscle countering the increased tension of the key muscle, or in a muscle linked neurogenically to the key TrP (17).

Attachment TrP is found at the musculotendinous junction and/or where the muscle attaches to the bone; this induces an enthesopathy (see the following text) secondary to unrelieved tension/relative spasm of the taut band produced by a central TrP (17).

Enthesopathy is typically a well-circumscribed area of pain or tenderness found in the specific regions of muscle attachment: musculotendinous junctions or where tendons and ligaments attach to bone. This differs from the more diffuse TrP referred pain that may not be well localized. Enthesopathy may develop into enthesitis, which is typically post-traumatic in nature, found at muscle insertions, and can be associated, with continued muscle stress, with fibrosis and calcification (17).

The central MTrP is found at the center of muscle fibers and is associated with dysfunctional end plates in the motor endplate zone. Contraction knots cause the nodular findings on examination. Both local and referred pain are secondary to sensitized nociceptors via a local energy crisis. Finally, tension from contraction knots causes the taut band beyond the palpable nodule. These TrPs differ greatly in etiology from attachment TrPs, which are found in the attachment zone secondary to taut muscle band tension. An associated inflammatory reaction causes palpable induration, and local and referred pain is secondary to nociceptors sensitized by persistent taut band tension. The taut band at the attachment TrP is secondary to contraction knots in the central TrP.

Active TrPs may spontaneously convert to latent TrPs, and vice versa. Both active and latent TrPs can induce increased muscle tension, shortening of the muscle, and decreased range of motion. These finding are most typically made on examination, as pain is the patient's primary complaint when active TrPs are palpated. Weakness is also seen, as the patient uses other, noninvolved muscles to perform routine tasks—although pain is a frequent complaint, latent TrPs that do not produce spontaneous pain may also cause weakness.

Shah and his group (25,26) have found biochemical changes at the center of the TrP consisting of increased levels of calcitonin gene-related peptide (CGRP), substance P (SP), norepinephrine, interleukin 1 and 6, and tumor necrosis factor-α, all in association with a low pH of 3.0 to 4.0.

Trigger-Point Hypothesis

A TrP consists of many microscopic abnormal regions in extrafusal skeletal muscle fibers. The myofascial pain syndrome with associated MTrPs is a neuromuscular disease.

The integrated pathophysiology of an MTrP would include—as noted by Simon and Travell (17)—the following:

- Excessive production and release of acetylcholine (ACh) at the myo-neural junction (motor nerve terminal) during rest
- Association with sustained depolarization of the postjunctional membrane of the associated muscle fiber, also associated with endplate noise (spontaneous electrical activity, or SEA)
- Continued depolarization inducing, first, a release of calcium ions that are not reabsorbed into the sarcoplasmic reticulum (SR), which then induces more and

more extra-SR calcium associated with continued sarcomere contracture, or shortening

- Continuous contractures inducing an increased need for energy at the site further aggravated by the compression/constriction of small blood vessels by the continuous muscular contracture in the region, which increases an *energy crisis* by prohibiting appropriate oxygen and nutrients to flow from these vessels
- Increased demand for energy in the region (the MTrP) that has an impaired energy supply, which leads to the release of algetic, sensitizing substances that would effect the autonomic, nociceptive, and non-nociceptive sensory nerves in the region, in turn increasing production of ACh from the associated nerve endings
- Local sensitization from the algetic chemicals leading to sensitization of the associated spinal cord dorsal horn region, inducing continuous nociceptive impulses that are sent rostrally
- Spinal cord sensitization that becomes self-sustaining over time, secondary to continuous peripheral nociceptive information from the MTrP
- The continued release of algetic substances, which can contribute to the continued over-release of ACh from the nerve terminal inducing a vicious cycle of energy crisis, release of algetic substances, and release of more ACh

In an extension of this hypothesis by Gerwin et al. (27), it is thought that muscle activity secondary to significant muscle stress, which leads to muscle injury and capillary constriction, is the initiating event. The muscle injury will induce a release of algetic substances, which stimulate muscle nociceptors. Sympathetic nervous system activation occurs in the evolving pathological state. Ischemia occurs from capillary contraction from the muscle contraction and causes hypoperfusion. The regional pH becomes acidic, which will inhibit acetylcholine-esterase (AChE). CGRP, which is released from nociceptors in the injured muscle, will also inhibit AChE, increase Ach release, and upregulate cholinergic receptors. This cascade leads to increased cholinergic activity with increased sarcomere hypercontraction, the formation of taut bands, and increased frequency of miniature endplate potentials.

CLINICAL ASPECTS

The largest single tissue type in the body is skeletal muscle, which accounts for 50% of the body's weight (28). It should come as no surprise that substantial problems can be induced by difficulty in this system.

The term "myofascial pain syndrome" appears to engender some confusion. Simons (29) notes that the term (MPS) has been used specifically with regard to a pain syndrome that is induced by TrPs found in the belly of a muscle, specifically not scar, ligamentous, or periosteal TrPs. The term has also been used generally to indicate many conditions that induce muscle pain without reference to and even in the absence of TrPs, making MPS an ambiguous identifier. He suggests the use of the term "myofascial pain syndrome due to TrPs" to be more specific, and the term "regional muscle pain syndrome" to be used as the more general term. It is thought that this is certainly correct—one of the major difficulties with the entire concept of MPS has been the lack of specifics relating to the diagnosis and the basic terminology of the disorder. It was the Wolfe group (30) who in 1990 developed specific criteria for the diagnosis of fibromyalgia (see Chapter 8). This has yet to be accomplished for MPS with TrPs.

When reference is made to MPS, in this textbook, this is specifically with reference to MPS with TrPs.

Clinically, the patient with MPS may describe muscular pain that is more frequently diffuse, but that can be localized. The attributes for this pain may be deep, dull, aching, and continuous. It is rare to have the more neuropathic attributes such as burning or vascular attributes such as throbbing.

The onset may be post-traumatic, following an acceleration/deceleration injury ("whiplash") or a slip and fall. It may begin insidiously, with the patient having worked at a desk on a computer for many hours or days. Many patients will report that they remember no inciting event. Indeed, as an MPS may be secondary to another medical problem, or even mimic another problem, its diagnosis may commonly be missed secondary to treatment of the purported primary problem (i.e., tooth pain, which is secondary to referred pain from an MTrP).

Case Study 1

The patient was a 46-year-old right-handed Caucasian female who accidentally fell backwards from the ledge of a sunken bathtub and sustained a fracture of the fifth metatarsal of the left foot. The fracture was appropriately set via a closed manipulation of the foot. Healing was very slow. She was placed in a walking boot. When the patient began to do some simple stretching exercises, after she had been told to do them, she developed severe, constant burning pain over the top of the foot, going up to the ankle. She immediately saw her orthopedist, who felt that she might be developing complex regional pain syndrome (CRPS type 1) (also known as reflex sympathetic dystrophy—RSD). She was sent for consultation. Examination and sudomotor (autonomic sweat reflex) testing was normal. She had sustained an acute strain of the flexor digitorum longus, which flexes the distal phalanges of the lateral four toes and assists in plantar flexing the foot. Treatment consisted of nonsteroidal anti-inflammatory medications, icing, and heat. The pain resolved within a week. The patient was seen again five months after the initial fracture with a two-month history of severe pain in the RIGHT low back, buttock, and leg. Examination revealed a new, three-fourth-inch leg length discrepancy, with the right leg shorter than the left. The patient's pelvis was also internally rotated. She had multiple tender TrPs in the piriformis muscle and in the iliotibial band. (Her primary care physician had suggested a heel lift for the right shoe. That seemed to make things worse; so she returned to the clinic.) Treatment consisted of physical therapy, which helped the iliopsoas musculature relax, which returned the leg lengths to normal. TrP injections to the iliotibial band and the piriformis muscle, along with further physical therapy and a consistently performed home exercise program helped to end the pain. Its causation was secondary to muscle spasm and TrP development on the right, secondary to the three to four months during which she wore the walking boot, which caused a significant change in her gait, with the affected muscles responding poorly to the change and muscle overloading inducing the myofascial problems.

Pertinent points include: (*i*) the incorrect assumption of autonomically mediated pain (CRPS/RSD) and (*ii*) the emergence of a painful MPS secondary to another problem. MPS may confound a clinician by mimicking a different clinical entity, in that frequently, diagnosis of one disorder may be, instead, entirely secondary to an MPS.

Aside from pain, other common complaints associated with an MPS may include muscle stiffness, fatigue, tenderness, weakness, sleep disorder, autonomic nervous system symptoms, and even poor balance, dizziness, and ear pain (if the more rostral musculature is affected).

When a patient is seen with a specific complaint, the differential diagnosis must include an MPS if appropriate. Much too frequently, patients are referred to an ear, nose, and throat (ENT) specialist for complaints of ear pain or dizziness for which a full ENT workup can find no etiology. A great deal of time and money is spent before the TrPs in the sternocleidomastoid muscles, which can refer these problems to the ear, are identified. Possibly, more common is the compliant of tooth pain (31), which leads to dental work, including tooth extraction, root canals, and more, with no effect. Referred pain from TrPs in the masseter and temporalis muscles is then identified.

History and Physical Examination

A patient comes into the office with complaints of pain. You take a thorough history and perform a physical examination to obtain a diagnosis. Problems may begin here. First, an MPS must be in the differential diagnosis. Second, to obtain the best history, you have to know the correct questions to ask. To know the correct questions, you have to understand the entire pathophysiology of the problem. For example, if you understand the possible consequences of an alpha wave intrusion into stage 4 sleep, you know to ask about nocturnal awakenings. Finally, and this is getting harder to do all the time, you must spend adequate time to obtain the history and perform the examination. This can average in some clinics at between 30 and 45 minutes, a short period of time to collect the details of a 3- to 10-year (or more) history of pain. Although physicians do not get paid for doing it, a typical full history may take one to two hours or more. There are no real short cuts. Although MPS can mimic multiple medical problems, you must first be certain that those problems are not present before you consider the presence of an MPS.

Several things should be done before and specific questions asked during the pain-related history. Prior to seeing a patient, it is an excellent idea to go through any relevant past medical records. This will give you an idea of the patient's past diagnoses, which tests were done, which medications were tried, and what happened. In spite of having read these documents, it is a given that you must take your own history and do your own evaluation. You should be as thorough as you can when asking about past medical events, past life events, and past diagnoses and treatments.

Some basic questions should examine the history of present illness:

- What are the characteristics, or attributes of the pain?
- When did it start? Was there an initiating event?
- Has the pain been continuous or intermittent?
- Can you point with one finger to the area of pain? Is the pain always in the same place? Does the pain move around? Is the pain in more than one (contiguous) area?

This is usually a good time to have the patients draw their pain on the blank figure of a human form. Have them use different colors to mark severe pain, aching pain, and so on; have them mark areas of paresthesias and/or numbness with a different color. They may number the areas of pain by the sequence in which the pain started and moved to different areas. Repeated pain drawings during treatment are very useful tools to help determine the patient's clinical course.

- Have you ever had this type of pain before?
- What can be done to make the pain better?
- What makes the pain worse?
- Does the pain prevent you from doing anything you typically do?
- What sort of work do you do? Does the pain affect your work? If so, how?
- Do you participate in any athletic activities? What are they? Are you still participating?
- Do you have any problems falling asleep? Do you take any medications to fall asleep? Do you awaken from pain at night? If so, how many times a night?
- What medications are you taking? What medications have you taken in the past? Do you have any side effects from medications? Any allergies to medication?
- Do you feel that you are under any type of stress?
- Is the pain causing any type of problems at your work? At home? With your friends?

These are basic questions. Each positive answer should begin a cascade of associated pertinent questions.

These questions are followed by the rest of the basic history:

- Past medical history: past medical problems, treatments, and hospitalizations, past surgical procedures, trauma, psychological difficulties
- Review of systems (be certain to include questions relating to endocrine symptoms/previously diagnosed disorders, dental problems, etc.)
- Changes in appetite? Changes in libido?
- Current medications
- Allergies

The physical examination would now be done. Before we go over this, specifically regarding the myofascial examination, we need to understand what we are looking for, and how to find it.

Trigger-Point Examination

How does one go about finding a TrP, which is typically 2 to 5 mm in size? There are several techniques that can be utilized to go about this task.

First, some prerequisites: the patient must be warm and comfortable. If the patient is in a cold examination room, the general musculature will become tense, and a TrP examination may be futile. Second, the fingernails on the examiners hands must be short, so as to avoid scraping the patients skin.

Flat palpation is the best way to begin, particularly in large muscles and smaller muscles, which can be palpated from only one side. The fingers are slightly bent, with the fingertips perpendicular to the palm. The patient may be sitting or lying prone. The skin above the region of the suspected TrP is pushed to one side, and the fingertips slowly traverse the area. If the patient is warm, and if the muscle is relaxed, a taut band may be easily palpated, and the TrP likewise easily palpated. If the movement of the fingers is done too quickly (snapping palpation), it is likely to obtain an LTR, which is painful.

Pincer palpation can be used in muscles such as the sternocleidomastoid, which can be grasped between the thumb on one side of the muscle, and the fingers on the other. A taut band can be palpated, as can the TrP, as the muscle is rolled between the fingers. This is helpful for obtaining a more discrete palpatory picture of the taut band and any TrP. As the muscle is released from between the fingers, an LTR may be obtained.

Another important diagnostic exercise is to press directly over an active TrP, which may lead to the development/demonstration of referred pain. The pain should refer to the same place each time a specific TrP is compressed. It is helpful to know the typical TrP referral patterns found for different TrPs. This information is available in the superb "bible" of myofascial pain written by Drs. Travell and Simons (2,17). The current thought regarding the mechanisms of referred pain were discussed in Chapter 3.

Pain related to myofascial TrPs may be aggravated by pressure directly on the TrP, sustained and/or repeated contraction of the involved muscle, passively stretching the muscle, strenuous use of the muscle, particularly when it is in the shortened position, placing the involved muscle in a shortened position for prolonged periods of time, and exposure to cold and drafts. MTrP pain may be decreased by short period of rest, moist heat applied directly to the TrP, slowly passively stretching the involved muscles, short periods of light activity with movement, and by specific myofascial treatment (17).

Painful rolling of the skin is also frequently found.

Depending on the location of active TrPs, patients may develop a number of nonpainful symptoms of MTrPs. These may include pilomotor activity ("goose flesh"), changes in sudomotor activity (sweating), excessive lacrimation, and other autonomic signs and symptoms such as vasoconstriction causing one limb or region to appear "colder" to palpation, as well as dizziness. Dermatographia is the term for using the fingernail or a pencil to write or draw on the skin and then see the areas become red and raised. This is seen most commonly on the skin over musculature affected by active TrPs, particularly over the muscles of the back, shoulders, neck, and torso. Depression and sleep disorders are also commonly seen.

Clinical accuracy in the determination of TrPs is not as easy as it sounds. Hsieh et al. (32) looked at the inter-rater reliability of the palpation of TrPs in the trunk, using as his exam group physiatrists and chiropractors. They were attempting to determine the inter-rater reliability of palpation of three characteristics of TrPs, the taut band, LTR, and referred pain. It was concluded that TrP palpation was not reliable for detecting taut bands and LTRs, and marginally reliable for referred pain, after training both physiatrists and chiropractors.

In another study looking at the reliability of examination of patients with myofascial pain, chronic fibromyalgia, and controls, both dolorimetry (algometry— see following text) and palpation were of sufficient reliability to discriminate control patients from patients with myofascial pain and fibromyalgia, but could not discriminate between patients with myofascial pain and fibromyalgia (33).

Gerwin et al. (34) report two studies in which examiners looked at the distinctive features of MPS, including a TrP in a taut band of muscle, the LTR, patterns of referred pain characteristic of specific TrPs, and the reproduction of the patient's pain during examination. In the first study, the attempt to establish inter-rater reliability failed. The second study by the same examiners included a training period first, and was successful at establishing inter-rater reliability. Interestingly, although present, inter-rater reliability varied among the different features of MPS.

The importance of specific training and experience in the determination of the various aspects of MPS, including taut bands and trigger points, is therefore not to be underestimated.

Pressure algometry (PA) has been used to document the pain threshold and the activity of a TrP along with its response to treatment. An algometer utilizes pressure (in kg/cm²) placed directly over a TrP to determine, aside from the pressure pain threshold, the referred pain threshold and the patient's pain tolerance. It is certainly useful to obtain such information prior to treatment and PA can be utilized to document changes in the pressure pain threshold as the TrP, along with any associated taut bands of muscle, are released (35,36).

The smallest amount of pressure, which induces pain or discomfort, the pressure pain threshold, would appear to represent the degree of sensitization affecting the nerve fibers by sensitizing, or algetic substances.

PA is an excellent method of determining the results of treatment, both short and long term, as it can be expressed in a clear numerical fashion: the amount of pressure expressed by kg/cm² directed over the TrP, or the site of the TrP, needed to evoke pain. This will obviously be lower in patients with active TrPs prior to treatment, and higher (that is, more pressure can be directed over the site without inducing pain) in treated patients.

The main indications for the use of PA is to locate TrPs, then evaluate treatment results, and do so again during later follow-up. The use of PA can also demonstrate progress during treatment and this will help motivate patients to continue with their individualized treatment protocol.

The clinician who uses PA should consider the gender differences of patients, the side-to-side differences, and regional differences. Recognition of low-tolerance pain syndromes is also important.

When using PA, the device should be held vertically over the precise location of the TrP. The speed of pressure increment—1kg/sec—is important, along with the time interval between measurements and the distance between two measured sites (37).

Aside from the patient's complaints of pain, LTRs have also been seen under the tip of the PA device.

The aspects to be considered to make PA reliable include proper equipment and technique, along with sufficient training of the examiner. The patients need to be willing to undergo the measurements, often repeatedly. Finally, particularly if an examiner is looking for any type of statistical information, reliability of PA is improved by repeated measurements (37).

Clinically speaking, this information can be statistically correlated with patients' subjective complaints of pain, making PA a very useful clinical tool.

Other aspects of MPS examination must be kept in mind. Muscles in which TrPs are found also show muscle shortening, decreased range of motion, typically from diminished joint motion, and weakness. These three TrP signs are also found in the presence of latent TrPs, although pain is typically not present unless direct TrP compression is performed.

Therefore, as part of the musculoskeletal examination (MSE), you must look carefully at the following:

- *Muscle strength*: Muscle evaluation must compare both the right and left sides of the body.
- *Muscle spasm*: Spasmed muscles may be rigid, hard, and show diminished flexibility. These problems must be relieved prior to any examination to look for TrPs and/or taut bands.

- *Joint mobility*: Shortened muscles can help in the development of decreased joint mobility and joint contractures. The latter is developed, most often, secondary to decreased usage due to inactivity caused by pain.

The actual physical examination begins when the clinicians greet their patient for the first time. Watching how a patient gets out of a waiting room chair and seeing how the patient extends the arm and hand to shake hands are both important. The author typically invites the patient to walk in front of him as the patient walks to the consultation room. In this way, the patient's posture and gait are being examined before the patient realizes it. During the history, careful observation is made of how the patients are sitting—do they frequently move around in their chair? Do they favor one side when they are seated? Do they grimace while they talk? What other pain behaviors do they exhibit? Do they laugh and joke and show no pain behavior while describing their severe pain, a 10 over 10 on a 0 to 10 scale? Once they get into the examination room and the physical exam is proceeding, does their affect change? Do they begin to demonstrate a great deal of pain behavior? Was their gait normal when they walked into the consultation room, but antalgic when they are examined? Was their handshake firm, but you find grip strength weakness on examination? Some patients feel that they must demonstrate significant pain behaviors to have the physician believe that they have any pain at all. Sometimes this is entirely unconscious on the patient's part. Other times? The physician must judge for himself or herself.

The full physical examination should begin with the general examination, including the head, ears, eyes, nose, and throat (HEENT), cardiovascular system, lungs, abdomen and extremities, thyroid gland, and so on.

This is followed (at least by the author) by the neurological examination. This is important for evaluating strength, sensation, and reflexes, all of which have a bearing on the MSE. The presence or absence of a neuralgia/neuropathy or radiculopathy must be determined. Of course, the cranial nerves and cerebellar functions must also be tested, along with gait and station, heel, toe, and tandem gait, and the Romberg test.

The MSE follows. This is what gives the most pertinent information regarding the presence or absence of an MPS. It is the author's preference to have a mirror in the exam room that the patient can use to see what, if any, asymmetries are found.

The patient must be in a gown. You can then easily observe any physical asymmetries, such as finding one shoulder elevated, or one hip elevated. You can show this to the patients, who need to be educated from the start as to what is going on with them. Without such education, it is difficult for most patients to "just do what the doctor tells them." Patients read a lot, and do a great deal of Internet surfing and read up on what they think or have been told their diagnosis is, and you must be prepared to show your patients exactly what findings cause you to make the diagnosis of an MPS.

Have your patient perform active cervical range of motion (ROM), or lumbosacral ROM in front of the mirror. Many of the patients have no prior idea how decreased their ROM may be.

As your patient, during the history, should have drawn a pain picture, which included the areas of pain, as well as numbness and tingling and/or weakness, you start with a good idea on where to look during the examination. However, you must remember that when dealing with TrPs, the place you are initially looking at may be a zone of reference for the TrP(s) causing their chief complaint.

Pain is, after all, whatever the patient says it is. It is a symptom, not a diagnosis. It is up to the clinician, pain management specialist or not, to determine what the patient is talking about.

Therefore, the MSE must be as thorough as possible, with more care, if necessary, being given to the area of the pain's origin or etiology.

Case Study 2

A 52-year-old right-handed Caucasian female was seen in neurological consultation. She had a nine-month history of pain down the lateral aspect of her left leg associated with low back pain. Her lumbosacral magnetic resonance imaging (MRI) had shown nonspecific degenerative joint disease, with a small anterior herniation of the lumbar segment 5 (L5) disk. The patient had been seen for orthopedic evaluation and, as the pain had persisted beyond six months and was greatly interfering with the patient's life, the physician had recommended surgery. An EMG had been performed, which was negative. The patient's husband had brought her for consultation, as he did not want his wife to have surgery.

History was pertinent for the patient's complaints of low back pain, including left buttock pain, "like I'm sitting on a tennis ball," as well as pain shooting down the lateral aspect of her left leg. The pain in her buttock was the most severe and sitting or standing for more than ten minutes would increase the pain significantly. Neurological examination showed a slight decrement of her left Achilles reflex, as well as minimal sensory changes in the left L5–S1 (sacral segment 1) distributions to pin.

Musculoskeletal evaluation revealed minimal paravertebral muscle spasm in the lumbar region. She had significant pain to palpation of the left sacroiliac joint and to the left piriformis muscle. She had TrPs in the piriformis, as palpation would reproduce her shooting pain, as well as the typical low back, buttock, and leg pain. She had several TrPs in the left iliotibial band.

Diagnostically, she had a piriformis syndrome, also called, in the past, the "false L5–S1 disk syndrome." This explained the sensory changes and the decreased left Achilles reflex.

Treatment consisted of TrP injections into the piriformis musculature with associated physical therapy. After six weeks, she had no complaints of pain and her neurological examination was normal.

She obviously did not need surgery.

Testing for Trigger Points

Two forms of testing for MTrPs have been utilized. The first is diagnostic ultrasound. One study of 11 subjects with clinically identified active MTrPs found no correlation between the clinical identification of the active TrPs and diagnostic ultrasound (38). Gerwin and Duranleau (39) found that active TrPs in the right infraspinatus and right gluteus maximus muscles, which had referred pain on direct palpation and needle insertion into the TrP, elicited a grossly visible LTR of the taut band, which could be visualized, along with contractions of the taut bands, with diagnostic ultrasound.

The second form of testing utilized has been infrared thermography. The results with this clinical tool appear to be more promising. One study indicated that skin hyperthermia as visualized thermographically was found in the zone of reference regions of an active TrP. Latent TrPs produced no such change (40). These findings were different from those in another study, which found that activating an MTrP by direct pressure produced cooling of the skin in the zone of reference and beyond (41). A third study showed similar findings. The authors of this study (42) used a cold immersion test of patients' hands and found that the hand/arm with active TrPs took a significantly longer amount of time to recover to their preimmersion temperatures. Cold immersion looks at changes in the autonomic nervous systems vascular control abilities.

Clinical work found hyperthermia over an active TrP, and hypothermia in the regions of referred pain. The hyperthermia was gone 24 hours after the TrP was injected and the patient received follow-up physical therapy.

Surface EMG (sEMG), which came into clinical use in the 1920s, does not test for TrPs. It is a diagnostic tool, not a test, which can be utilized via a number of different applications to obtain physiological data from the surface of the skin, which reflects the underlying electromyographic as well as electrophysiologic potentials. Needle EMG studies look at one motor unit within a muscle. This does not give any indication of the general muscle function. The sEMG looks at gross motor rather than fine motor activity. It can do static assessments, which look at patterns of antalgia, or dynamic, movement-oriented evaluations that look at general or regional firing patterns of the neuromuscular system. Muscle asymmetries, muscle fatigue, irritability, and even the effects of associated emotional responses can be evaluated with this technique. sEMG is a clinically appropriate tool to help evaluate the "intangibles" of patient complaints, which do not show up on computed axial tomography (CAT) scan or magnetic resonance imaging (MRI). It is frequently used with biofeedback to teach patients muscle retraining. However, this 50+-year-old therapy is now looked at, by some insurance companies, as experimental.

A major practical problem is obtaining authorization from insurance companies to use these tools and tests for enhancing clinical determination of the presence and the post-treatment differentiation of the patients' clinical condition.

Sleep Disorders and Pain

The relationship between sleep disturbance and pain is complex (43). Studies of sleep disturbance in patients seen in pain clinics indicate that chronic myofascial pain patients report significant problems with sleep disturbance.

One study (44) of patients with myofascial pain who were seen in a multidisciplinary pain center found that 65% indicated that they were "poor sleepers," who had longer periods of sleep latency, or initial insomnia, more frequent nocturnal awakenings, longer duration of these nocturnal awakenings, and fewer total hours of sleep. They also described increased pain intensities as compared to the "good sleepers" in the study.

Another study (45) showed similar results, with patients in an inpatient pain program. The sleep disturbances of these myofascial pain patients showed delayed sleep onset, decreased "quality" of sleep and fewer hours slept. In this study, sleep disturbance was found to correlate with increased measures of depression and anxiety.

In an older study (46), which used polysomnography (an electroencephalographic sleep study) to evaluate chronic pain patients, patients with insomnia and psychiatric disorders, or just those with insomnia, the chronic pain patients had sleep difficulties similar to those noted in the above two studies. Eight chronic pain patients showed an alpha wave intrusion in non-REM (nonrapid eye movement) sleep. The authors suggested that pain tolerance in chronic pain patients decreases, secondary to lack of sleep.

Briefly, to review, sleep is divided into five stages: 1, 2, 3, 4, and REM. Alpha- and beta-wave activity is associated with wakefulness. Stages 1 through 4 are non-REM stages of sleep. Stages 3 and 4 are commonly called slow wave, or delta, sleep.

An alpha-wave intrusion into delta sleep has been hypothesized as the mechanism of sleep disturbance in chronic myofascial pain patients (47).

Chronic pain patients have also been found to have other, comorbid, primary sleep disorders, including sleep apnea, restless legs syndrome, and periodic limb movements, also called nocturnal myoclonus, during sleep (46,48–51).

Depression is frequently associated with chronic pain (52,53) Depressed patients also have frequent nocturnal awakenings, longer sleep latencies, and REM disturbances (54).

Other studies have found a relationship between muscle pain, sleep disturbance, and depression (55).

The majority of the research looking at pain and the alpha–delta sleep abnormality has been done in fibromyalgia patients. This is covered in Chapter 8.

Serotonin is important to a number of processes. Decreased levels of serotonin can induce increased pain perception, depression, sleep disorder, and abnormal hypothalamic hormone secretion. The serotonergic system originates in the brain stem and specifically the nucleus raphe magnus, and projects to the cortex in the broadest possible way, with multiple projections.

Serotonin helps promote REM sleep. When it is depleted with p-chlorophenylalanine (PCPA), research has shown symptoms of pain, nonrestorative sleep, and somatic and neurovegetative signs of depression (56) (changes in appetite, sleep, and libido).

Serotonin appears to be involved in both sleep induction and wakefulness via activity at different receptors in different brain regions as well as interactions with other neurotransmitters (57).

As both the endogenous opiates and serotonin work in concert, along with other neurotransmitters, to help achieve antinociception, it is not surprising that the endogenous opiate system also has a role in sleep. The nucleus of the solitary tract, located in the posterior part of the reticular formation, appears to enhance delta sleep when injected with opioid. It contains the highest concentrations of opioid receptors in the medulla (58).

ACh also affects both pain and sleep. Cholinergic neurons help modulate REM sleep (59).

Psychological Aspects

A number of "vicious cycles" exist in the pathophysiology of the TrP and in the relationship between muscle pain and spasm and psychological or affective difficulties.

Psychological factors have been found to have a role in the abnormal recruitment of paraspinal muscles in patients with chronic low back pain (60). "Psychogenic" trapezius muscle tension found on surface EMG to have low variability and low amplitude may be secondary to prolonged activity in specific motor units, rather than frequent shifts of activity between different units in a larger, existent pool of motor units. If the same motor units are constantly firing, overload may follow with a resultant metabolic/energy crisis (61).

Patients with a chronic MPS, when compared to patients with fibromyalgia are found to have similar psychological measures, although the fibromyalgia patients' were more severe and disabling. The fact that trauma was a common initiating factor of MPS seemed to be related to its chronicity (62). A similar study (63) found that some features, including fatigue, poor sleep, and headaches are found much less frequently in patients with an MPS.

Mersky (64) notes that chronic muscular pain is not a life stress syndrome in and of itself, but it must be looked at in terms of being an organic disorder made worse by psychological factors, and not the other way around.

When MPS was compared to a significantly more severe chronic pain problem, CRPS type 1 or RSD, MPS patients had higher scores on the Minnesota Multiaxial Personality Inventory, including hypochondriasis, depression, hysteria, while being lower than CRPS patients on the hypomania scale (65).

When patients are living with chronic myofascial face pain, the pain contributes to the development of depression, from mild up to a major depressive disorder (66). The development of depression in other forms of chronic MPS appears to be less psychologically devastating.

The facts seem to address the development of depression and anxiety as a function of MPS. MPS is not, by definition, a psychogenic disorder. More information regarding the psychology of pain is discussed in Chapter 15.

Differential Diagnosis of Myofascial Trigger Points and Other Disorders
Facial Pain
The first essential step here, as easy as it may sound, is to determine if you are dealing with a headache or facial pain or both. Although the temporalis, upper trapezius, and the sternal division of the sternocleidomastoid muscles can cause tension-type headache, they can also cause atypical facial pain with neuralgic aspects. Temporomandibular joint dysfunction (TMJ) may be overdiagnosed, with patients receiving splints and surgery(s) among other treatments for what is essentially a masseter muscle problem. This has also been called myofascial pain dysfunction syndrome (MPDS) when it applies to the face. It is obviously important to know the regions of referred pain from head and neck muscle TrPs.

TrPs in the temporalis muscles (and the masseter) may refer pain to the teeth, leading the patient on a futile dental odyssey, complete with root canals, extracted teeth, and expensive caps. Then, when the dental work has been done, and no one knows what is causing the continuing pain, the patient is sent to a tertiary care pain specialist.

TrPs may be associated with radicular pain.

Case Study 3
The patient, a 39-year-old right-handed female, was seen two-and-a-half years after she developed headache and facial pain. The facial pain had been initially diagnosed as trigeminal neuralgia, and a Janetta procedure was performed (a neurosurgical procedure where titanium was placed between the trigeminal ganglion ipsilateral to the pain and an artery that may have been lying on the ganglia, inducing the trigeminal neuralgia). This did not help the facial pain, or the headache. A second surgery was performed a week later to repair a CSF (cerebral spinal fluid) leak. Several months later, a Gamma Knife procedure was performed [using radiation to stop, in this case, the semilunar (trigeminal) ganglion from functioning]. This induced facial dysesthesias or painful numbness in all three divisions of the ipsilateral (same side) trigeminal nerve. Months later, the patient was seen at one of

the country's better known medical centers. There, another surgery was performed to stop another CSF leak. The patient was diagnosed with hemicrania continua, a relatively rare form of headache that is exquisitely sensitive to indomethacin. However, the indomethacin did not help at all; so almost a dozen more medications were tried, none of which was helpful.

When initially seen, the patient had three main complaints: a constant generalized headache, on the right side more than the left side of her head, severe "jabbing" pain located over her right eyelash that was the same pain previously diagnosed as trigeminal neuralgia, and significant discomfort of the right side of her face, secondary to the trigeminal nerve dysfunction post-Gamma Knife procedure, which made it very uncomfortable for her to put makeup on that side of her face and take a shower, as the water striking her face was dysesthetically painful.

Examination revealed a woman in obvious pain. She had a cervical MPS, with TrPs on the ipsilateral (same side as her pain) more so than the contralateral (other) side, in the trapezius, deltoids, and cervical paravertebral muscles, which actively referred pain to the head. This would certainly explain her "daily general headache." She had hyperesthesias to pin in parts of the right side of her face, explainable by the postoperative Gamma Knife trigeminal nerve dysfunction. Most importantly, she had a positive Tinel's sign over the right supraorbital nerve, which means that when fingers or a reflex hammer lightly percussed the area, it reproduced the "jabbing" pain that had been her initial complaint.

Treatment, over the course of several weeks, consisted of physical therapy to break down the significant muscle spasm in the cervical region; she was placed on tegretol, which, over time, markedly ameliorated the facial dysesthesias and a specific right supraorbital nerve block was performed, which stopped her "jabbing" pain completely, for a six-day period. That specific pain returned, but was not considered as severe as it was prior to the nerve block. A TrP deep in the right cervical paravertebral muscles was injected, and the "jabbing" pain again went away. The next day, in physical therapy, manual pressure to the region of the TrP again stimulated the pain.

A second supraorbital nerve block will be performed if the severe "jabbing" pain returns, and if necessary, a radio frequency ablation of the nerve may be considered. However, primarily, conservative treatment, including physical therapy, Tegretol, Elavil, and a home exercise program were successfully utilized.

The myofascial aspects of tension-type headache are discussed in Chapter 12.

Dizziness and ear pain, which had been given a significant ENT workup, without any diagnosis or help for the patients, can be secondary to TrPs in the clavicular division of the sternocleidomastoid muscle and the scalenus muscles.

Herniated disks in the cervical region may be assumed to cause arm pain that is secondary to TrPs in the supraspinatus and infraspinatus muscles. Cervical arthritis may also be part of the differential diagnosis.

TrPs in the upper rectus abdominis musculature and the thoracic paravertebral muscles can cause midback pain, frequently mimicking disk disease or herniation. Low back pain may be secondary to the lower aspects of the rectus abdominis muscles and the thoracolumbar paraspinal muscles. The piriformis muscle may also induce sciatic pain that may be assumed to be secondary to a herniated lumbar disk. Pain down the lateral aspect of the lower extremities may be diagnosed as a herniated disc; however, the presence of TrPs in the gluteus medius, tensor fascia, and even the gastrocnemius muscles must be evaluated.

The clinician should look for TrPs after an appropriate examination has been performed and spinal MRIs and/or EMG/nerve conduction velocity (NCVs), if clinically indicated, have been done. Although TrPs are common, you must rule out other clinical causes of a problem first. A caveat is that many times patients with a herniated disc(s) will also have an MPS with TrPs referring pain. The problem that may cause the most severe pathological difficulties should be dealt with first. This does not mean that all patients with a herniated disk need to have surgery first. In fact, it may be clinically more appropriate to treat these patients conservatively with physical therapy and TrP injections first. Clinically, it has been found that these patients may not need surgery over 80% of the time. The neurological indications that would mandate surgery include muscle weakness and atrophy, reflex changes, and chronic, intractable pain. If you can ameliorate the pain, and there are no other neurological abnormalities (even in the presence of a diminution of a reflex, not an absence), you can prevent the need for surgery for quite a while, if not obviate the need for it.

Endocrine Disorders Associated with Myofascial Pain

It is not uncommon to find dozens of patients who present with muscle pain, spasm, and TrPs that are secondary to a primary endocrine disorder. The two most common are hypothyroidism and menopause. It is a good practice to perform a confirmatory lab test, and if your suspicions are correct, the patient may need to see an endocrinologist.

Some of the most common endocrine problems associated with myofascial pain include the following:

Hypothyroidism is secondary to a lack of thyroid hormone production [levothyroxine (T_4) and liothyronine (T_3)] secondary to a problem with the hypothalamic–pituitary–thyroid (HPT) axis. Clinically, the patients are frequently overweight. Their eyelids may be puffy, their voice hoarse. The thyroid gland may be enlarged. Their muscles are stiff, tender, and, on occasion, weak. They may display muscle hypertrophy. TrPs are common. Their primary complaint may be diffuse muscle tenderness. The Achilles reflex may show delayed relaxation. Laboratory testing typically shows low serum thyroxine (T_4), free thyroxine index, and a high thyroid-stimulating hormone (TSH) level.

The most common complaints found in hyperthyroidism include muscle weakness and pain, TrPs, heat intolerance, increased sweating, thinning hair, increased appetite, emotional/mental difficulties, and sexual dysfunction. The physical findings may reveal a goiter, proptosis, loss of convergence, lid lag, increased deep tendon reflexes, tachycardia, cardiac arrhythmias, and a fine, fast tremor of the hands/fingers. Laboratory findings include high levels of T_3 (triiodothyronine), T_4, and free thyroxine index. The TSH is typically low.

Menopause, secondary to estrogenic insufficiency may be difficult for the patient and associated with myofascial pain and TrPs, sweats, and "hot flashes." On occasion, muscle pain, and/or joint pain may be the primary complaints. Associated symptoms may include anxiety, weakness, depression, emotional difficulties, and loss of libido. These symptoms typically all improve with exogenous estrogen replacement.

"Male menopause," secondary to significant decreases in serum testosterone, may be associated with myofascial pain and TrPs, along with weakness and depression. Exogenous testosterone may relieve these symptoms.

Muscle weakness, wasting, spasm, and pain are frequently associated with Cushing's disease [secondary to an adrenocorticotropic hormone (ACTH)-secreting tumor of the pituitary, with associated adrenal hyperplasia] and Cushing's syndrome (secondary to a primary adrenal tumor or ectopic production of ACTH). Other signs and symptoms include female facial hirsutism, round, red facies, purple abdominal striae, thin skin with easy bruising, thinning scalp hair, and osteoporosis. Hypertension and mild diabetes mellitus along with affective changes and spinal fractures (secondary to osteoporosis) may also be seen. Laboratory testing shows elevation of a 24-hour urinary free cortisol level and a high morning plasma cortisol. Treatment includes surgical removal of the tumor and chemotherapy.

Primary adrenal insufficiency, or Addison's disease, may present with muscle pain, spasm or, on occasion, knee contractures. It can be associated with increased skin pigmentation on examination, low blood pressure, orthostatic hypotension, weakness, and cachexia. Laboratory testing can demonstrate abnormalities of the electrolytes and an increased serum ACTH.

Pituitary–adrenal insufficiency typically is found to be caused by adrenal atrophy secondary to tumor, hemorrhage, or even infarction of the pituitary. The presenting symptoms not infrequently include myofascial pain and TrPs. The examination should show poor muscle development, weakness, testicular atrophy, loss of libido, and an eunuchoid appearance.

Hypoparathyroidism, secondary to surgical damage or removal (or by spontaneous causation), may be associated with acute muscle spasms and even tetany secondary to decreased serum calcium. Hyperparathyroidism is associated with an increased level of serum calcium, secondary to increased serum parathyroid hormone. Muscle weakness, or myopathy that may be secondary to elevated calcium.

Perpetuating Factors

Once an MPS with TrPs has manifested, there are a number of things that may perpetuate the syndrome. It is important to identify these mechanical and/or systemic problems and deal with them appropriately.

Mechanical factors may include tight collars, tight brassiere straps, carrying heavy purses or bags over the shoulders, compressing the hamstring muscle by the hard edges of chairs, and ergonomic problems associated with work, such as having a computer monitor that is too high or a keyboard that is not properly placed or too difficult for a patient to utilize comfortably. These issues are relatively simple to correct. Ergonomic issues may be dealt with via an occupational therapist.

Postural abnormalities must be identified and corrected.

Other common problems include inherent structural inadequacies, such as the short leg syndrome (one leg shorter than another) and a small hemipelvis (secondary to an asymmetry in the height of the two halves of the pelvis).

Case Study 4

A 13-year-old right-handed female was seen for the chief complaint of numbness in her legs when she danced in practice or competition. The girl practiced hard, on a daily basis. Her mother noted that she could tell when her daughter's legs became numb, as she would have trouble dancing and even have to stop. Examination revealed that the patient's head was thrust forward, her shoulders were high and forward, her right shoulder higher than the left, with significant spasm in the trapezius and deltoid muscles as well as the cervical paravertebral muscles. Her hips were uneven, with the top of the left iliac crest higher than the right. Her left leg was shorter than the right. There was iliopsoas and piriformis spasm and pain to palpation, with active TrPs. When these problems were explained to the patient and her mother, both expressed amazement. Upon inquiry regarding trauma, there was none. Finally, when the initial consultation and examination were finished and the mother and daughter got up to leave, the patient put on a backpack that was obviously heavy. About 40 pounds! To keep herself balanced, she had to lean forward with the backpack perched high on her shoulders. The answer was then obvious. Discussion revealed that any alternative method of carrying her books, such as a wheeled piece of luggage, or something similar, would create animosity from her schoolmates. Treatment consisted of physical therapy and a recommendation to consider an alternative method of carrying her books.

Systemic perpetuating factors include endocrine or metabolic factors (discussed earlier), folic acid deficiency, and low iron levels. Muscle can also be stressed and show impaired healing secondary to toxic, inflammatory, and nutritional difficulties.

Chronic muscle pain associated with exercise intolerance may not be secondary to MPS (or even fibromyalgia syndrome). The problem's differential diagnosis may include Lyme disease, deficiencies of vitamin D, or even a mutation in the cytochrome b gene of mitochondrial DNA (mtDNA) (14,67).

Psychological stressors are of equal importance in terms of perpetuating a myofascial problem. Although the other perpetuating factors noted in this section may be found on examination or via laboratory testing, psychological problems may not "come out" easily, as a patient may have no understanding of the ability of such problems to be part of a psychophysiological muscle pain problem. This is one important reason for the utilization of an interdisciplinary treatment team needed to deal with chronic myofascial and other forms of chronic pain.

The presence of unidentified psychological/psychophysiological factors will undermine appropriate treatment, and if unidentified, they will continue the patients' cycles of continued pain in spite of appropriate diagnosis and treatment. The "entire patient" must be treated, physically, mentally, and emotionally.

A CONFLUENCE OF THE PATHOPHYSIOLOGICAL AND THE CLINICAL

It appears that tenderness and referred pain related to chronic musculoskeletal pain may well result from peripheral and central sensitization, which can then be instrumental in transitioning acute to chronic pain.

The fact that chronic musculoskeletal pain is associated with central sensitization has been noted in several recent studies including chronic whiplash related pain (68,69), and other forms of chronic myofascial pain (70–72).

It has also been noted that patients with referred hyperalgesia had experienced pain for at least six years, although patients in pain for six months had not developed hyperalgesia (3). Teleologically, it would take time for constant nociceptive input to induce central sensitization. Widespread musculoskeletal pain commonly begins with localized pain described as deep, also indicating that the development of central sensitization occurs over time (74).

Other studies appear to have found a relationship between the development of central sensitization and the number of clinically palpable TrPs in myofascial pain (75,76). It is also noted that in the presence of central sensitization, low-intensity input could induce pain when a possible latent TrP is activated; this may also indicate at least one causal relationship between a localized painful condition and its spread or development of generalized pain (74).

SUMMARY

MPS with TrPs may fool the clinician—typically, it has already fooled the 5.6 physicians patients see before going to a tertiary pain management center. A great deal of time, money, failed hopes, medication reactions, unnecessary surgeries, and pain have been wasted by the time a patient has had all of the "bad diagnoses" such as herniated disks ruled out. Hopefully, they will find a physician who knows that because all of the other, obvious diagnoses have been ruled out, and the patient still has pain, something else must be going on. And then the musculoskeletal system is examined.

The differential diagnosis of pain should always include MPS. Although it is not a diagnosis of exclusion, as it may be found in the presence of other pathological conditions, it should not be dismissed out of hand.

MPS with TrPs is an important problem to look for: it is actually something we can help with, as there are many things we can do to decrease a patient's pain if it is secondary to this pathophysiological entity.

REFERENCES

1. Fields H. Pain. New York, NY: McGraw-Hill, 1987:209–229.
2. Travell J, Simons D. Myofascial Pain and Dysfunction: The Trigger Point Manual. Baltimore, Md: Williams and Wilkins, 1983.
3. Mersky H, Bogduk N, eds. Classification of Chronic Pain: Descriptions of Chronic Pain Syndromes and Definition of Pain Terms. 2nd ed. Seattle, Wa: IASP Press, 1994:47.
4. Yunus MB. Understanding myofascial pain syndromes: a reply. J Musculoskel Pain 1994; 2(1):147–149.
5. Lidbeck J, Hautkamp GIM, Ceder RA, Naslund ULO. Classification of chronic pain at a multidisciplinary pain rehabilitation clinic. Pain Res Manag 1998; 3(1):13–22.
6. Harden RN, Bruehl SP, Gass S, Niemiec C, Barbick B. Signs and symptoms of the myofascial pain syndrome: a national survey of pain management providers. Clin J Pain 2000; 16(1):64–72.
7. Kraft GH, Johnson EW, LaBan MM. The fibrositis syndrome. Arch Phys Med Rehabil 1968; 49:155–162.
8. Sola AE, Rodenberger MS, Gettys BB. Incidence of hypersensitive areas in posterior shoulder muscles: a survey of two hundred young adults. Am J Phys Med 1955; 34:585–590.
9. Fricton JR, Awad EA, eds. Advances in Pain Research and Therapy. Vol. 17. New York: Raven Press, 1990.
10. Kato K, Sullivan PF, Evengard B, Pedersen NL. Importance of genetic influences on chronic widespread pain. Arthritis Rheum 2006; 54(5):1682–1686.
11. Moldofsky H, Scarisbrick P, England R, et al. Musculoskeletal symptoms and non-REM sleep disturbance in patients with "fibrositis syndrome" and healthy subjects. Psychosom Med 1975; 37:341–351.
12. Fricton JR, Kroening R, Haley D, et al. Myofascial pain syndrome of the head and neck: a review of clinical characteristics of 164 patients. Oral Surg 1985; 60:615–623.
13. Simons DG. Myofascial trigger points: the critical experiment. J Musculoskel Pain 1997; 5(4):113–118.
14. Gerwin RD. A review of myofascial pain and fibromyalgia—factors that promote their persistence. Acupunct Med 2005; 23(3):121-134.
15. Simons DG. Myofascial pain syndrome due to trigger points. In: Goodgold J, ed. Rehabilitation Medicine. St. Louis, Mo: C.V. Mosby Co., 1988:686–723.

16. Wolfe F, Simons DG, Fricton J, et al. The fibromyalgia and myofascial pain syndromes: A preliminary study of tender points and trigger points in persons with fibromyalgia, myofascial pain syndrome and no disease. J Rheumatol 1992; 19:944–951.

17. Simons DG, Travell JG, Simons LS. Travell and Simons' Myofascial Pain and Dysfunction: The Trigger Point Manual. Volume 1. Upper Half of Body. 2nd ed. Baltimore, Md: Williams & Wilkins, 1999.

18. Simons DG, Hong C-Z, Simons LS. Nature of myofascial trigger points, active loci. J Musculoskel Pain 1995; 3(suppl 1):62.

19. Simons DG, Dexter JR. Comparison of local twitch responses elicited by palpation and needling of myofascial trigger points. J Musculoskel Pain 1995; 3(1):49–61.

20. Hong CZ, Torigoe Y. Electrophysiological characteristics of localized twitch responses in responsive taut bands of rabbit skeletal muscle. J Musculoskel Pain 1994; 2(2):17–43.

21. Hong CZ. Lidocaine injection versus dry needling to myofascial trigger points: the importance of the local twitch response. Am J Phys Med Rehabil 1994; 73:256–263.

22. Hong CZ. Persistence of local twitch response with loss of conduction to and from the spinal cord. Arch Phys Med Rehabil 1994; 75:12–16.

23. Kellgren JH. A preliminary account of referred pains arising from muscle. Br Med J 1938; 2:325–327.

24. Travell JG. Myofascial trigger points: clinical view. In: Bonica JJ, Albe-Fessard D, eds. Advances in Pain Research and Therapy. Vol. 1. New York, NY: Raven Press, 1976: 919–926.

25. Shah JP, Phillips TM, Danoff JV, Gerber LH. An in vivo microanalytical techniques for measuring the local biochemical milieu of human skeletal muscle. J Appl Physiol 2005; 99(5):1977–1984.

26. Shah JP, Phillips TM, Danoff JV, Gerber LH. A novel microanalytical technique for assaying soft tissue demonstrates significant quantitative biochemical differences in 3 clinically distinct groups: normal, latent and active. Arch Phys Med Rehabil 2003; 84:A4.

27. Gerwin RD, Dommerhold J, Shah, JP. An expansion of Simons' integrated hypothesis of trigger point formation. Curr Pain Headache Rep 2004; 8(6):468–475.

28. Clemente CD. Gray's anatomy of the human body. 30th ed. Philadelphia, Pa: Lea and Febiger, 1985:429.

29. Simons DG. Myofascial pain syndrome: One term but two concepts; a new understanding. J Musculoskel Pain 1995; 3(1):7–13.

30. Wolfe F, Smythe HA, Yunus MB, et al. The American College of Rheumatology 1990 criteria for the classification of fibromyalgia. Arthritis Rheum 1990; 33:160–172.

31. Kim ST. Myofascial pain and toothaches. Aust Endod J 2005; 31(3):106–110.

32. Hsieh CY, Hong CZ, Adams AH, et al. Interexaminer reliability of the palpation of trigger points in the trunk and lower limb muscles. Arch Phys Med Rehabil 2000; 81(3): 258–264.

33. Tunks E, McCain GA, Hart LE, et al. The reliability of examination for tenderness in patients with myofascial pain, chronic fibromyalgia and controls. J Rheumatol 1995; 22(5):944–952.

34. Gerwin RD, Shannon S, Hong CZ, et al. Interrater reliability in myofascial trigger point examination. Pain 1997; 69(1–2):65–73.

35. Hong CZ. Algometry in evaluation of trigger points and referred pain. J Musculoskel Pain 1998; 6(1):47–59.

36. Fischer AA. Algometry in diagnosis of musculoskeletal pain and evaluation of treatment outcome: an update. J Musculoskel Pain 1998; 6(1):5–32.

37. Pontinen PJ. Reliability, validity, reproducibility of algometry in diagnosis of active and latent tender spots and trigger points. J Musculoskel Pain 1998; 6(1):61–71.

38. Lewis J, Tehan P. A blinded pilot study investigating the use of diagnostic ultrasound for detecting active myofascial trigger points. Pain 1999; 79(1):39–44.

39. Gerwin RD, Duranleau D. Ultrasound identification of the myofascial trigger point. Muscle Nerve 1997; 20:767.

40. Diakow PR. Differentiation of active and latent trigger points by thermography. J Manip Physiol Ther 1992; 15:439–441.

41. Kruse RA Jr, Christiansen JA. Thermographic imaging of myofascial trigger points: a follow-up study. Arch Phys Med Rehabil 1992; 73:819–823.

42. Neoh CA, Jawan B, Lee JH. Thermography in the diagnosis of trigger points-induced forearm pain. Chinese J Pain 1993, 3:51–57.
43. Skevington SM. Activities as indices of illness behaviour in chronic pain. Pain 1983; 15:295–307.
44. Morin CM, Gibson D, Wade J. Self-reported sleep and mood disturbance in chronic pain patients. Clin J Pain 1998; 14:311-314.
45. Haythornthwaite JA, Hegel MT, Kerns RD. Development of a sleep diary for chronic pain patients. J Pain Symptom Manage 1991; 6:65–72.
46. Wittig RM, Zorick FJ, Blumer D, et al. Disturbed sleep in patients complaining of chronic pain. J Nerv Ment Dis 1982; 170:429–431.
47. Yunus MB, Masi AT, Aldag JC. A controlled study of primary fibromyalgia syndrome: clinical features and associations with other functional syndromes. J Rheumatol 1989; 16(suppl 19):62–71.
48. Mahowald MW, Mahowald ML, Bundlie SR, Ytterberg SR. Sleep fragmentation in rheumatoid arthritis. Arthritis Rheum 1989; 32:974–982.
49. Sahota PK, Dexter DM. Sleep and headache syndromes: a clinical review. Headache 1990; 30:80–84.
50. Atkinson JH, Ancoli-Israel S, Slater MA, et al. Subjective sleep disturbance in chronic low back pain. Clin J Pain 1988; 4:225–232.
51. Moldofsky H, Tullis C, Lue FA. Sleep related myoclonus in rheumatic pain modulation disorder (fibrositis syndrome). J Rheumatol 1986; 13:614–617.
52. Fishbain DA, Cutler R, Rosomoff HL, Rosomoff RS. Chronic pain-associated depression: antecedent or consequence of chronic pain: a review. Clin J Pain 1997; 13:116–137.
53. Turk DC, Okifuji A, Scharff L. Chronic pain and depression: role of perceived impact and perceived control in different age cohorts. Pain 1995; 61:93–101.
54. Gillin JC, Duncan W, Pettigrew KD, et al. Successful separation of depressed, normal, and insomniac subjects by EEG sleep data. Arch Gen Psychiatry 1979; 36:85–90.
55. Ursin R, Endresen EM, Vaeroy H, Hjelmen AM. Relations among muscle pain, sleep variables and depression. J Musculoskel Pain 1999; 7(3):59–72.
56. Menefee LA, Cohen MJM, Anderson WR, et al. Sleep disturbance and nonmalignant chronic pain: a comprehensive review of the literature. Pain Med 2000; 1(2):156–172.
57. Portas C, Bjorvatn G, Ursin R. Serotonin and the sleep/wake cycle: special emphasis on microdialysis studies. Prog Neurobiol 2000; 60:13–35.
58. Reinoso-Barbero RM, Andres IP. Effects of opioid microinjections in the nucleus of the solitary tract on the sleep-wakefulness cycle states in cats. Anesthesiology 1995; 82: 144–152.
59. Perry E, Walker M, Grace J, Perry R. Acetylcholine in mind: a neurotransmitter correlate of consciousness? Trends Neurosci 1999; 22:273–280.
60. Watson PJ, Booker CK, Main CJ. Evidence for the role of psychological factors in abnormal paraspinal activity in patients with chronic low back pain. J Musculoskel Pain 1997; 5(4):41–56.
61. Waersted M, Eken T, Westgaard RH. Psychogenic motor unit activity: a possible muscle injury mechanism studied in a healthy subject. J Musculoskel Pain 1993; 1(3/4): 185–190.
62. Roth RS, Bachman JE. Pain experience, psychological functioning and self-reporting disability in chronic myofascial pain and fibromyalgia. Clin J Pain 1993; 9:189–195.
63. Inanici R, Yunus MB, Aldag JC. Clinical features and psychological factors in regional soft tissue pain: comparison with fibromyalgia syndrome. J Musculoskel Pain 1999, 7(1/2):293–301.
64. Merskey H: Chronic muscular pain—A life stress syndrome? J Musculoskel Pain 1993; 1(3/4):61–69.
65. Nelson DV, Novy DM. Psychological characteristics of reflex sympathetic dystrophy versus myofascial pain syndromes. Reg Anesth 1996; 21(3):202–208.
66. Dohrenwend BP, Raphael KG, Marbach JJ, Gallagher RM. Why is depression comorbid with chronic myofascial face pain? A family study test of alternative hypotheses. Pain 1999; 83(2):183–192.
67. Andreu AL, Hanna MG, Reichmann H, et al. Exercise intolerance due to mutations in the cytochrome b gene of mitochondrial DNA. N Eng J Med 1999; 341(14):1037–1044.

68. Curatolo M, Petersen-Felix S, Arendt-Nielsen L, et al. Central hypersensitivity in chronic pain after whiplash injury. Clin J Pain 2001; 17:306–315.
69. Johansen MK, Graven-Nielsen T, Olesen AS, Arendt-Nielsen L. Generalized muscular hyperalgesia in chronic whiplash syndrome. Pain 1999; 83:229–234.
70. Graven-Nielsen T, Arendt-Nielsen L, Svensson P, Jensen TS. Stimulus-response functions in areas with experimentally induced referred muscle pain: a psychophysical study. Brain Res 1997; 744:121–128.
71. Leffler AS, Kosek E, Lerndal T, et al. Somatosensory perception and function of diffuse noxious inhibitory controls (DNIC) in patients suffering from rheumatoid arthritis. Eur J Pain 2002; 6:161–176.
72. Svensson P, List T, Hector G. Analysis of stimulus-evoked pain in patients with myofascial temporomandibular pain disorders. Pain 2001; 92:399–409.
73. Leffler AS, Kosek E, Hansson P. The influence of pain intensity on somatosensory perception in patients suffering from subacute/chronic lateral epicondylalgia. Eur J Pain 2000; 4:57–71.
74. Arendt-Nielsen L, Graven-Nielsen T. Central sensitization in fibromyalgia and other musculoskeletal disorders. Curr Pain Headache Reports 2003; 7:355–361.
75. Carli G, SUman AL, Biasi G, Marcolongo R. Reactivity to superficial and deep stimuli in patients with chronic musculoskeletal pain. Pain 2002; 100:259–269.
76. Bajaj P, Bajaj P, Graven-Nielsen T, Arendt-Nielsen L. Trigger points in patients with lower limb osteoarthritis. J Musculoskel Pain 2001; 9:17–33.

5

Sympathetic Aspects of Soft-Tissue Pain

MYOFASCIAL PAIN SYNDROME

Myofascial pain syndrome (MPS) is an important source of musculoskeletal pain. It is also one of the most common sources of chronic pain. Clinically, MPS involves a localized or regional pain complaint that is associated with tender trigger points with referred pain upon palpation, which are located in taut banks of skeletal muscle.

The localized, hypersensitive regions of muscle associated with trigger points are secondary, at least in part, to sensitization of the afferent peripheral nerve endings in the muscle by prostoglandins, bradykinin, histamine, substance P, and other nociceptive or algetic neurochemicals. Histologically and conceptually, there is evidence of an "energy crisis" found, which is identified by a decrease in high-energy phosphates and an associated increase in low-energy phosphates, as well as local hypoxia, secondary to local vascular and microvascular disturbances. The local, peripheral sensitization also is associated with a central, spinal cord sensitization in regions of the dorsal horn.

Trigger points induce several difficulties in the muscles in which they are found. These include increased stiffness, fatiguability, weakness, and restricted range of motion. These muscles may be shortened and exhibit increased pain when stretched. Patients typically protect these muscles by adopting poor posture with sustained reflex muscle contraction. These self-inflicted muscular restrictions may both perpetuate existing trigger points and induce development of more trigger points in the same or in other contiguous musculature.

Palpation of trigger points will cause referred pain in reproducible patterns that are specific for a particular trigger point. Autonomic dysfunction, including ipsilateral injection and lacrimation, may be induced by palpation of trigger points in the sternal division of the sternocleidomastoid muscle.

As noted earlier, referred pain from trigger points may be mediated by any of four experimentally postulated mechanisms: (i) convergence–projection, in which pain may be initiated by muscle nociceptors but then referred to another area served by other somatic receptors, which converge on the same region of the spinothalamic tract, (ii) convergence–facilitation, in which impulses from one somatic zone are facilitated or amplified in the spinal cord by other activity originating in nociceptors from a trigger point in another area of the body, and (iii) peripheral branching of primary afferent nociceptors, in which the brain may misinterpret activity from nociceptors in one part of the body as originating from nerves coming from another part of the body.

The fourth, more relevant hypothesis is that of the sympathetic modulation of peripheral nociceptors including increased sympathetic modulation of peripheral nociceptors inducing increased sympathetic activity that causes an increase in substances, which sensitize primary afferent nerve receptors in the area of referred pain and the site of initial peripheral sensitization. There are clinical correlations of this hypothesis, making it more clinically factual, which will be discussed in the following text.

SYMPATHETICALLY MAINTAINED PAIN

Sympathetically maintained pain, as described by Roberts (1), may begin after even minor soft-tissue or peripheral nerve trauma. The initial nociceptive impulses are transmitted via the unmyelinated C fibers to the Rexed layers in the dorsal horns, where they stimulate fibers of the wide-dynamic-range neurons and induce hypersensitivity in that region. The wide-dynamic-range neurons also become sensitized, or more responsive to all subsequent afferent stimuli.

Over time, the wide-dynamic-range neurons will continue to give a vigorous response to mechanical input from A-fiber mechanoreceptors. This may cause hypersensitivity to touch or movement (allodynia). The wide-dynamic-range neurons are also directly connected to the lateral horn cells, which enervate sympathetic structures in the periphery. Studies documenting these concepts appear to explain the sometimes extreme sensitivity found in involved tissues, including nodularity (trigger points) found in painful myofascial areas, as well as vasomotor changes (2–5).

The hypersensitivity reaction may also be induced in the area of trauma if nerves are injured. Compensatory pain and vasomotor symptoms of complex regional pain syndrome (CRPS, previously called reflex sympathetic dystrophy, or RSD) are dependent on local levels of norepinephrine (NEP), which fluctuate, in part, by stress-induced increased sympathetic release of NEP (6). It has also been noted that the same increased response of the sympathetic nervous system occurs in the presence of uncontrolled stress, along with increased plasma adrenocorticotropic hormone (7).

SYMPATHETICALLY MAINTAINED PAIN AND MYOFASCIAL PAIN SYNDROME

From the two entities, sympathetically maintained pain and MPS, it is clinically possible, if not probable, that of the multitude of patients with soft-tissue injuries leading to MPS those who do not recover within a short period of time (one to three months) of appropriate physical therapy may have developed secondary sympathetically maintained pain.

Research data indicate that some receptors in skin and skeletal muscle can be influenced by sympathetic activity. It appears that the sympathetic influence on muscle receptors is functional in pathological states, but *not* under normal physiological conditions (8).

It has also been established that, with prolonged afferent input, central mechanisms may lead to skeletal muscle motor reactions, autonomic reactions, and distorted sensory phenomena including paresthesias and neurogenic pain (8).

Motoneurons, after changes in stimulation, may induce abnormal activity in thin myelinated and unmyelinated afferents from skeletal muscle and tendons, secondary to uncoordinated and tonic contraction (9).

Sympathetically maintained pain in many patients is not associated with tissue dysfunction (2,10). It has been suggested that signs of sympathetic dystrophy seen in sympathetically maintained pain result from disuse atrophy and extreme muscular guarding behaviors, not sympathetic hyperfunction (11). Over time, the painful areas of sympathetically maintained pain do not expand (12).

Patients with MPS also develop and maintain abnormal, guarded postures to prevent muscle stretch-induced pain. They also experience, the expansion of the area of pain, secondary to this guarding, and the development of adjacent muscle spasm, pain, and trigger points, which are associated with sympathetically maintained pain.

Other aspects of MPS may be explained by sympathetically maintained pain, including painful skin rolling, hypersensitivity of the skin and muscles to touch and pressure, vasomotor changes including pallor, hyperemia, subjective coldness, and hyperhidrosis, and the marked central and neuropharmacological reactions to emotional stress.

Patients with MPS also exhibit significant sleep abnormalities, typically an alpha intrusion into stage 4 sleep, also seen in asymptomatic patients with significant emotional stress and depression. Serotonin and NEP are implicated in sleep pathophysiology and in depression.

The emotional or stress-related aspects noted earlier as possibly etiological in the establishment of sympathetically maintained pain and/or CRPS are also frequently noted in patients with MPS. As many of these patients experience trauma such as a motor vehicle accident, anxiety, fear, and stress, and the possible development of the post-traumatic stress disorder, emotional difficulties are prevalent. These admittedly situational stressors related to the trauma may be amplified by the loss of material goods, continued pain, loss of work, and, therefore, income as well as litigation, making them apparent "setups" for the development of sympathetically maintained pain.

Clinically speaking, how can the diagnoses of these two entities be differentiated? First, on examination, the clinician may find painful skin rolling, dermatographia, and hyperhidrosis, particularly on sudomotor or sweat testing, and, on the face, scleral injection, lacrimation, ipsilateral rhinorrhea, even a partial Horner's syndrome, with ptosis and meiosis, but not anhidrosis. Further examination of the skin may reveal flushing over the painful areas, with associated warmth and extreme sensitivity to palpation.

Also, treatment shows the various diagnoses. In cases of obvious myofascial pain with trigger points, a sympathetic block will decrease the pain, but not the elements of the MPS, which can then be treated appropriately with an excellent outcome.

CASE STUDY

MS was a 38-year-old right-handed male sent to the clinic with the diagnosis of right upper extremity CRPS/RSD. He had been injured in a work-related accident eight months earlier, essentially striking his arm and shoulder against some wood. When initially seen, the claim of CRPS was immediately suspect, as the patient wore his watch on the affected arm. He wore a long-sleeved shirt without difficulty. On examination, he had significant hypersensitivity, but not true allodynia. Sudomotor testing was positive for increased sympathetic activity in the right arm and hand. He had significant trigger point findings in the ipsilateral trapezius, deltoid, and pectoralis muscles. His right upper extremity did not show any dystrophic changes, including loss of hair, thinning of the skin, or changes in his fingernails.

When physical therapy was attempted, for the second time, the first being four months earlier, the therapist was not able to touch the patient's skin or do any muscle work secondary to strenuous complaints of pain. Neuropharmacological treatment did not help this problem.

The patient received an ipsilateral stellate ganglion block. The painful areas became numb enough to enable the physical therapist to begin performing appropriate MPS treatment. The block was repeated once more, in ten days, when the patient again became insistent about severe pain. Simple physical therapy was continued, the patient was weaned off of his narcotics and left on the tricyclic antidepressants, and the patient's pain was gone within a month.

Of note was the fact that the patient had previously received a series of three stellate ganglion blocks, which had the same effect then, as when he was in the clinic, thus accounting for his diagnosis of CRPS/RSD. In reality, the sympathetically maintained pain was being treated by the blocks, but the MPS was not treated until he reached the clinic. When the MPS had been appropriately treated, the sympathetically maintained pain had resolved. Also, of note, was the fact that the patient had no true signs of CRPS/RSD on initial examination. He did, however, show signs of increased sudomotor or sweat activity, a measure of increased sympathetic nervous system involvement.

Clinically, there are many similarities in the diagnosis and the treatment of the MPS and sympathetically maintained pain. An interdisciplinary treatment approach is most effective in patients who have a history of chronic myofascial pain, especially if aspects of sympathetically maintained pain are also found. Physical therapy to break down the myofascial aspects of the pain is necessary, along with exercises to stretch, strengthen, and recondition the musculature and maintain normal joint and muscle mobility. The use of stress-loading activities may also be necessary, particularly if there is significant sympathetically maintained pain. Psychotherapy may be needed, along with stress management, including biofeedback-enhanced neuromuscular re-education and muscle relaxation. Neuropharmacological treatment is obviously also of extreme importance. The use of methodologies to deal with sympathetically maintained pain specifically may be needed to enable MPS to receive the needed therapy.

It appears that sympathetically maintained pain may be secondary to many of the pathophysiological abnormalities of MPS. This must be part of the differential diagnosis when dealing with patients with chronic MPS with significant hyperalgesia.

Ge et al. (13) also note evidence of sympathetic aspects of mechanical sensitization and local and referred muscle pain.

In reality, it is felt that we are just now realizing the importance of sympathetic aspects of myofascial pain and sympathetic aspects of other chronic pain syndromes.

REFERENCES

1. Roberts WJ. A hypothesis on the physiological basis for causalgia and related pains. Pain 1986; 24:297–311.
2. Tabmoush AL. Causalgia: redefinition as a clinical pain syndrome. Pain 1981; 10:187–197.
3. Bonica JJ. Causalgia and other reflex sympathetic dystrophies. In: Bonica JJ, Liebeskind JC, Albe-Fessard DG, eds. Proceedings of the Second World Congress on Pain, Advances in Pain Research and Therapy. Vol. 3. New York, NY: Raven Press, 1970:141–166.

4. Van Houdenhove B, Basquez G, Onghena P, et al. Etiopathogenesis of reflex sympathetic dystrophy: a review and biopsychological hypothesis. Clin J Pain 1992; 8:300–306.
5. Bruel S, Carlson CR. Predisposing psychological factors in the development of reflex sympathetic dystrophy. Clin J Pain 1992; 8:287–299.
6. Ecker A. Norepinephrine in reflex sympathetic dystrophy: a hypothesis. Clin J Pain 1989; 5:313–315.
7. Breier A, Albus M, Pickar D, et al. Controllable and uncontrollable stress in humans. Alterations in mood and neuroendocrine and psychophysiological function. Am J Psychiatry 1987; 144:1419–1425.
8. Janig W. The sympathetic nervous system in pain: physiology and pathophysiology. In: Stanton-Hicks M, ed. Pain and the Sympathetic Nervous System. Boston, Ma: Kluwer Academic Publishers, 1990:17–90.
9. Mense S. Slowly conducting afferent fibers from deep tissues: neurobiological properties and central nervous system actions. Vol. 6. Progress in Sensory Physiology. New York, NY: Springer Verlag, 1986:139–219.
10. Nathan PW. On the pathogenesis of causalgia in peripheral nerve injuries. Brain 1947; 70:145–170.
11. Ochoa JC, Torebjork E, Marchettini P, et al. Mechanisms of neuropathic pain. In: Fields HC, Dubner R, Cervero F, eds. Vol. 9. Proceedings of the Fourth World Congress on Pain. Advances in Pain Research and Therapy. New York, NY: Raven Press, 1985:431–450.
12. Loh L, Nathan PW. Painful peripheral states and sympathetic blocks. J Neurol Neurosurg Psychiat 1978; 41:664–671.
13. Ge HY, Fernandez-de-Las-Penas C, Arendt-Nielsen L. Sympathetic facilitation of hyperalgesia evoked from myofascial tender and trigger points in patients with unilateral shoulder pain. Clin Neurophysiol 2006; 117(7):1545–1550.

6

Medical Management of Myofascial Pain Syndrome

GENERAL

Myofascial pain syndrome (MPS), a common musculoskeletal pain syndrome, can be acute or chronic, local, regional, or generalized. Commonly, it is a primary disorder including local or regional pain syndromes; it may be clinically a secondary problem occurring as a consequence of another medical problem. It is treatable. It responds to manual techniques, while other factors—postural, ergonomic, and structural—must be dealt with appropriately (1).

A national survey of pain management providers found general agreement across specialists that MPS is a legitimate diagnosis that is distinct from the fibromyalgia syndrome (FMS). There was a high level of agreement regarding signs and symptoms essential to or associated with the diagnosis of MPS (2).

Another study looked at patient satisfaction. MPS patients have less accurate knowledge regarding their pain symptoms and express lack of satisfaction with physicians' efforts to treat their pain. The importance of patient education as a significant component of intervention in their chronic pain treatment is immense (3).

This chapter discusses the various conservative treatment options/modalities that can be used in the treatment of MPS. Aspects of the individual conservative treatments available will be covered, but it is not the intent of this work to act as a physical therapy (PT) or psychological textbook.

As will be noted in the following text, the most time- and cost-effective treatment paradigms are interdisciplinary in nature. These are discussed in detail in Chapter 17.

CONSERVATIVE CARE

Only after the clinical diagnosis of MPS has been made, and the physician has ruled out any endocrinopathies or other primary problems, can the patient begin therapy.

Patients who are injured (in a motor vehicle accident, slip and fall, or other injury) should be evaluated earlier rather than later. Initial examination must rule out spinal cord/nerve root problems, with an MRI (magnetic resonance imaging) performed if needed. In the presence of a nerve or nerve root injury, it will take at least three weeks before the electromyogram (EMG)/nerve conduction study (NCV) is positive from the acute injury. Examination should be neurologically and orthopedically within normal limits.

Palpable muscle spasm with associated tenderness is typically found. MPS with myofascial trigger points (MTrPs) does not usually immediately follow acute soft-tissue pain frequently, given the acute diagnosis of cervical, thoracic, or lumbosacral strain/sprain.

However, not infrequently MTrPs and taut bands may be found in the patient with acute soft-tissue pain, but they may frequently have been pre-existing (or of insidious onset) and may act as a physiological "set up" for the acute to chronic soft-tissue pain disorder, extending the injury and making it more severe.

The most conservative treatment approach is the initial use of medication. Acute muscle relaxants will not affect a pre-existing MPS; nor will a nonsteroidal anti-inflammatory medication (NSAID). However, in the presence of an acute soft-tissue injury, these medications may be helpful. A simple muscle relaxant (see following text) such as methocarbamol, metaxalone, or chlorzoxazone may be prescribed with the patients' understanding that they must be taken as directed to obtain a therapeutic plasma level.

NSAIDs such as ketoprofen or ibuprofen should be used to help patients maintain their ability to function, as bed rest is not a beneficial treatment.

It may take at least 48 hours after a traumatic injury for the patients' resulting soft-tissue pain to maximize. This should be explained to them.

In cases of severe soft-tissue trauma, physical therapy (PT) may be necessary within a week of injury, when the initial tenderness has possibly remitted to some degree. The purpose of PT is to decrease edema, spasm, and pain, and improve muscle pain/spasm and joint range of motion.

Patients with MTrPs may need trigger-point injections (TrPIs) (see Chapter 7).

The majority of patients can be placed on appropriate medications, taught the appropriate muscle stretching exercises, and within several weeks regain their preinjury status.

The most important reason to make the correct diagnosis and perform appropriate treatment as early as possible is to prevent the development of chronicity. Ten percent to 15% of these patients may utilize/need 80% or more of the health care dollars needed to treat these than chronic MPS patients.

After the onset of MPS, pre and/or postsoft tissue injury, the development of chronicity may stem from: (*i*) poor/inaccurate diagnosis, (*ii*) too much time passing prior to beginning care, (*iii*) poorly done PT, (*iv*) inappropriately recommended bed rest for days to weeks, (*v*) ignorance of the medical diagnosis of MPS, and (*vi*) iatrogenic overutilization of narcotic analgesics. After initial, acute trauma, narcotics may be used if needed to enable maintenance of function, for a 7- to 10-day period.

When patients with chronic MPS are seen, prior to initiating treatment, they should be evaluated for depression, anxiety disorder, iatrogenic medication overutilization, and their psychosocial milieu must be detailed to enable the development of a full, appropriate individualized, interdisciplinary pain management program (see Chapter 17).

To hope to successfully provide therapy for chronic MPS patients, all of the identified clinical–organic, psychological, and psychosocial aspects of their pain problem must be treated simultaneously, most appropriately in a full program provided under one roof.

The various aspects of treatment of MPS follow.

MEDICATIONS

The simple analgesics are easily chosen by the patient, if not the physician. They are inexpensive and easy to obtain. They include aspirin and acetaminophen. Aspirin appears to work by inhibiting the synthesis of prostaglandin by blocking the action of cyclo-oxygenase (COX), an enzyme that enables the conversion of arachidonic acid to prostaglandin to occur. Prostaglandins are synthesized from cellular membrane phospholipids after activation or injury, and sensitize pain receptors.

Aspirin, the prototypical NSAID, has anti-inflammatory and antipyretic properties, along with its pain-relieving properties. The recommended adult dose for
treatment is 650 mg every six hours. Taking the aspirin with milk or food may
decrease gastric irritation. Aspirin can also double bleeding time for four to seven
days after taking 0.65 g. Peak blood levels are found after 45 minutes. The plasma
half-life is two to three hours.

Acetaminophen usage is common. It provides about the same amount of
analgesia as aspirin, but does not have the gastrointestinal (GI) side effects. That
acetaminophen may work by inhibition of prostaglandin synthesis in the central
nervous system (CNS) has been suggested. It has much weaker anti-inflammatory
activity than aspirin. Peak plasma levels occur between 30 and 60 minutes. Its
plasma half-life is two to four hours. New information has indicated that patients
taking 4 g of acetaminophen a day for 14 days or more may induce elevations in
serum alanine aminotransferase (ALT), a hepatic enzyme (4).

Ibuprofen, an NSAID, is also available over the counter in doses of 200 mg per
tablet. It can cause significant GI distress. It has a half-life of two to four hours, with
peak plasma levels attained in one to two hours. The adult dosage is 200 to 400 mg
every four to six hours, with a maximum of 1200 mg per day.

These medications are frequently sold in combination with other drugs such
as caffeine, which exert no specific analgesic effects, but may potentiate the analgesic effects of aspirin and acetaminophen. There are aspirin–caffeine combination
drugs (Anacin®) and aspirin, acetaminophen, and caffeine combinations (Excedrin
Extra-Strength®, Excedrin Migraine®, and Vanquish®). The recommended dosage is
two tablets every six hours as needed.

The biggest problem is that taking aspirin, acetaminophen, or combination
tablets daily or even every other day for a week or more (possibly less) can induce
the problem of analgesic-rebound headache in those patients with tension-type headache (which is discussed in Chapter 12).

As with birth control pills, when the clinician asks a patient what medications
they are taking, they may "forget" that the birth control pill, or aspirin, or acetaminophen (which are nonprescription) are medications, and forget to tell you, or even
be too embarrassed to tell you because they are taking a large number of pills each
day; so the clinician must be certain to ask specifically.

There are a number of NSAIDs that are prescribed. Because of the variability in
their efficacy, pharmacokinetics, and side effects, patients may need to be tried on
more than one, sequentially, not in combination, to determine the best one for them.

The NSAIDs work, as noted before, by interfering with the action of COX
(both I and II) in the synthesis of prostaglandins. GI side effects are common, in up
to 15% to 20% of patients, and may include epigastric pain, nausea, heartburn, and
abdominal discomfort. A history of GI bleeding or ulcerations should indicate that
great caution must be used, if these medications are used at all.

The most frequently prescribed NSAIDs include:

Naproxen sodium (Anaprox®), which reaches peak plasma levels in one to
two hours, and has a mean half-life of 13 hours. It can be taken at 275 or 550 mg
every six to eight hours, with a top dosage of 1375 mg per day.

Ibuprofen (Motrin®) is prescribed in dosages of 600 and 800 mg per tablet.
The suggested dosage for mild to moderate pain is 400 mg every four to six hours
as needed.

Ketoprofen (Orudis®) is a COX inhibitor, but also stabilizes lysosomal membranes and possibly antagonizes the actions of bradykinin. Its peak plasma level is

reached in one to two hours and has a two-hour plasma half-life. It is now over the counter (12.5-mg tablets), but is best used as 50 to 75 mg capsules. The recommended daily dosage is 150 to 300 mg a day in three or four divided doses. GI side effects are generally mild. Care should be taken when given to a patient with impaired renal function.

Keterolac tromethamine (Toradol®) can be given orally or parentally for moderate to severe acute pain. Peak plasma levels occur after intramuscular (IM) injection in about 50 minutes. Its analgesic effect is considered to be roughly equivalent to a 10-mg dose of IM morphine. The typical injectable dose is 60 mg. Because of its potentially significant hepatic/renal side effects, the FDA has stated that Toradol should be given orally, after an IM injection of 60 mg, at 10 mg, every eight hours, for a maximum of five days.

The COX 2 inhibitors (celecoxib, rofecoxib, and valdecoxib) are NSAIDs that also have analgesic properties without, for most patients, the typical GI problems associated with NSAIDs. They appear to work by inhibiting prostaglandin synthesis, via inhibition of COX 2, which corresponds to its improved GI side effect profile, although not affecting the COX 1 isozyme, responsible for its anti-inflammatory functions. Because of issues of cardiovascular problems, both rofecoxib and valdecoxib have been taken off of the market. Celecoxib may be taken twice a day, 100 to 200 mg bid, whereas rofecoxib is taken once a day, at dosages ranging from 12.5 to 50 mg and valdecoxib once a day, at 10 or 20 mg.

Muscle relaxants are given for acute soft-tissue spasm/pain by some clinicians. They are probably best utilized during the first one to three weeks post injury. They may be useful in patients with significant muscle spasm and pain. They are used appropriately after the development of muscle spasm after an injury such as a slip and fall, motor vehicle accident, work and athletic injuries, or over stretching.

These medications work via the development of a therapeutic plasma level. Their exact mechanism of action is unknown, but they do not directly affect striated muscle, the myoneural junction, or motor nerves. They produce relaxation by depressing the central pathways, possibly through their effects on higher CNS centers, which modifies the central perception of pain without effecting the peripheral pain reflexes or motor activity.

Carisoprodol (Soma®) is a CNS depressant that metabolizes into a barbiturate, which makes it both addictive and particularly inappropriate to use for patients with pain from muscle spasm in addition to minor traumatic brain injury. It acts as a sedative and it is thought to depress polysynaptic transmission in interneuronal pools at the supraspinal level in the brain stem reticular formation. It is short lived, with peak plasma levels in one to two hours and a four- to six-hour half-life. Dosage is 350 mg every six to eight hours. It should not be mixed with other CNS depressants. It is also marketed in two other combined forms, (with aspirin as Soma Compound) and with codeine, for additional analgesic effects.

Chlorzoxazone (Parafon Forte DSC®) is a centrally acting muscle relaxant with fewer sedative properties. It is reported to inhibit the reflex arcs involved in producing and maintaining muscle spasm at the level of the spinal cord and subcortical areas of the brain. It reaches it peak plasma level in three to four hours, and duration of action is three to four hours. It is well tolerated, and side effects are uncommon. Dosage is 500 mg three times a day.

Metaxalone (Skelaxin®) is a centrally acting skeletal muscle relaxant that is chemically related to mephenaxalone, a mild tranquilizer. It is thought to induce muscle relaxation via CNS depression. Onset of action is about one hour, with peak blood levels in two hours, and duration of action is four to six hours. The recommended dose is 2400 to 3200 mg a day in divided doses (tablets are 400 mg each). It should be used carefully in patients with impaired liver function and should not be used at all in patients with significant renal or liver disease and a history of drug-induced anemias. Side effects include nausea, vomiting, GI upset, drowsiness, dizziness, headache, nervousness, and irritability as well as rash or pruritis. Jaundice and hemolytic anemia are rare.

Methocarbamol (Robaxin®) is a centrally acting skeletal muscle relaxant. It may inhibit nerve transmission in the internuncial neurons of the spinal cord. It has a 30- to 45-minute onset of action. Peak levels are found in about two hours, and its duration of action is four to six hours. It comes as 500- and 750-mg tablets. Tablets containing methocarbamol and aspirin (Robaxisal) are also available. The recommended dose of Robaxin is 750 mg three times a day. As with all of these medications, it should be taken for 7 to 10 days. It is well tolerated, with initial side effects that resolve over time, including lightheadedness, dizziness, vertigo, headache, rash, GI upset, nasal congestion, fever, blurred vision, urticaria, and mild muscular incoordination. In situations of severe, seemingly intractable muscle spasm, Robaxin may be given intravenously in doses of about a gram every 8 to 12 hours.

Orphenedrine citrate (Norflex®, Norgesic®) is a centrally acting skeletal muscle relaxant with anticholinergic properties thought to work by blocking neuronal circuits, the hyperactivity of which may be implicated in hypertonia and spasm. It is available in injectable and oral formulations. The IM dose of Norflex is 2 mg, whereas the intravenous dosage is 60 mg in aqueous solution. The oral formulation (Norflex) is given in 100-mg tablets—one tablet every 12 hours. Norgesic is a combination form, including caffeine and aspirin and should be given one or two tablets every six to eight hours. Norgesic Forte, a stronger combination, is given one half to one tablet every six to eight hours. Because of its anticholinergic effects, it should be contraindicated in patients with glaucoma, prostatic enlargement, or bladder outlet obstruction. Its major side effects are also secondary to its anticholinergic properties and include tachycardia, palpitations, urinary retention, nausea, vomiting, dizziness, constipation, and drowsiness. It may also cause confusion, excitation, hallucinations, and syncope.

Many of these medications are given in combination with other drugs, including barbiturates (butalbatal and meprobamate) and narcotics (codeine, oxycodone, propoxyphene, etc.). This is probably not a good idea, as the barbiturates and narcotics can easily help develop patient dependence.

A useful combination may include methocarbamol 750 mg three times a day for ten days in patients with significant spasm, accompanied by ketoprofen, 75 mg, every six to eight hours as needed, with food as needed. For the acute post-traumatic soft-tissue injury, one tablet of each taken together every six to eight hours for two to three doses works very well.

Again, narcotic medications should not be used for the patient with acute soft-tissue injury as a first-line medication, as the risk of tolerance/dependence is too great.

The tricyclic antidepressants (TCAs), are a very useful treatment choice for chronic MPS.

The TCA medication of choice is amitriptyline, a sedating TCA. Like all of the tricyclics, it works in the synapse to decrease reuptake of serotonin and, depending on the individual medication, norepinephrine. Amitriptyline, unlike the other TCAs, also works to repair the damage in stage 4 sleep architecture. It is the most sedating tricyclic. The typical dosage is between 10 and 50 mg at night. The author has found it rare for more than 20 or 30 mg to be necessary.

Doxepin is also a frequently used tricyclic. Anticholinergic side effects such as sedation are reduced (but not by much) when compared to amitriptyline. It does *not* work on the sleep architecture. It is used at the same dosage levels of amitriptyline.

Notice that the tricyclics are not used in their antidepressant dosages, anywhere from 100 to 350 mg a day. Even though the doses are low, their effectiveness in the treatment of chronic post-traumatic tension-type headache is there.

The SSRIs include Prozac®, Paxil®, and Zoloft®, among others. These medications are not typically sedating (although for some patients they may be) and with the exclusion of those patients, they are energizing. They should be given in the morning. Prozac and Paxil should start at 10 to 20 mg a day and they can be increased to 60 to 80 mg. Zoloft should be given at 25 to 50 mg in the morning, up to 150 mg in divided doses. The doses should be divided, giving one when the patient gets up in the morning (around 7:00 am) and one at noon. Patients should understand that taking these medications later than noon can, in many cases, cause problems with sleep.

The clinician can also safely combine 10 to 40 mg of Prozac or Paxil, or 50 mg of Zoloft given in the morning with a small dose of amitriptyline or doxepin (10 to 30 mg) at night. Inappropriate dosages of these two forms of medications can, rarely, induce the serotonin syndrome.

There are other excellent antidepressants such as Wellbutrin, Serzone, and Effexor. These should be considered as needed.

Do not combine these medications with the monamine oxidase (MAO) inhibitors.

Another excellent medication is Clonazepam®, a fifth-generation form of benzodiazepine. It is GABAnergic in effect. It works at the level of the internuncial neurons of the spinal cord to enhance muscle relaxation. It helps centrally with anxiolysis. It has a side effect of sedation. In doses of 4 to 12 mg a day, it works as an anticonvulsant. At smaller doses, 0.5 to 1 mg—up to 3 mg—given at night, it is very useful in the treatment of patients with chronic tension-type headache. The sedation lasts for a shorter time than the sedation from tricyclics, and this itself is useful.

If the acute use of skeletal muscle relaxant medications is not enough to end the problem, Tizanidine is a good choice of medication after the first three weeks or so has gone by and the patient is still exhibiting painful neuromuscular spasm. Tizanidine is an alpha$_2$ noradrenergic agonist (5,6). It has supraspinal effects by inhibiting the facilitation of spinal reflex transmission by the descending noradrenergic pathways, as it decreases firing of the noradrenergic locus ceruleus (7). It acts presynaptically in the spinal cord inducing a polysynaptic reduction in released excitatory transmitters (8). It also decreases hyperexcitability of the muscle without acting on the neuromuscular junctions or muscle fibers (9). Short acting, its maximum plasma concentrations are reached within one to two hours (9). It has a large first pass metabolism, with a half-life of 2.1 to 4.2 hours (10). Dosages should be slowly increased, starting at 1 to 2 mg at night and slowly increasing to 20 to 24 mg. Maximum dosage is 36 mg in divided dosages, typically found in patients who need an antimyotonic. Interestingly, this medication appears to decrease muscle pain while providing its antimyotonic effects.

A meta-analysis found that antidepressant medications (ADMs) are more effective when compared to placebo in decreasing pain severity, but not functional status, in patients with chronic low back pain (11).

Tricyclic antidepressant medications (TCAs), such as amitriptyline, desipramine, and imipramine, for example, block the induction of long-term potentiation by inhibiting actions on N-methyl-D-aspartate (NMDA) receptors (12).

A randomized controlled trial (RCT) indicated that amitriptyline reduces the transmission of painful stimuli from myofascial tissue rather than reducing overall pain sensitivity. It was felt that this effect was secondary to a segmental reduction of central sensitization in combination with peripheral antinociceptive actions (13). Topical (percutaneously applied) anesthetics may also be utilized (14).

Complementary medical therapies have been used for the treatment of MPS. Studies supporting this are poor—they have only anecdotal effectiveness for the most part (acupuncture, biofeedback, ultrasound, lasers, massage)—but most are not rigorously investigated, secondary to the poor research quality (lack of appropriate controls, sample sizes, and blending measures) (15).

TRIGGER-POINT INJECTION THERAPY

Chapter 7 describes the physiology and treatment aspects of the needling and infiltration (N & I) of MTrPs.

A systematic review in the Cochrane Database indicates that there is little convincing clinical evidence regarding the effects of interventional therapy (facet joint and epidural, short- and long-term efficacy) for low back pain (16) (see Chapter 16).

In a multicenter RCT, patients injected with sterile water reported a more painful treatment response than those injected with saline. Neither injectable showed a better clinical outcome in patients with chronic MPS (17).

Of interest is McNulty's study (18) showing increased needle EMG activity during stress, although two adjacent muscles remained electrically silent. These results suggest, at least, a mechanism by which emotional factors influence muscle pain, showing significant implications for the psychophysiology of pain with MTrPs.

An RCT indicated that needle EMG at trigger points (TrPs) on myofascial bands tended to improve symptoms. Needling these points elicits motor end plate activity and local twitch responses and induces far more relief than that seen when needling random points in the muscle (19).

A systematic review from the Cochrane Database found that the efficacy of needling therapies (direct and indirect dry and wet needling) in the treatment of pain from MTrPs is neither supported nor refuted by research (23 trials, N=955 patients) (20). Inspite of objective clinical practice, this review showed no differences between TrPIs with various injectates or between wet or dry needling. In spite of this, the authors of this review recommend that the method employed be the safest and most comfortable for a patient. Unfortunately, this form of equivocation appears to make so-called evidence-based medicine (EBM) systematic reviews less than, clinically, a "gold standard."

A systematic review (NIN Consensus Development Panel on Acupuncture) found acupuncture, or deep, dry needling, useful in the treatment of myofascial pain (and fibromyalgia) (21). A different RCT found that Japanese acupuncture associated with heat will yield a modest pain reduction in patients with myofascial neck pain. Previous patients' experience with acupuncture and their confidence in it helped to predict beneficial clinical outcomes (22).

PHYSICAL THERAPY
Vapocoolants/Spray and Stretch
Ethyl chloride was the first vapocoolant thought to be a good conservative treatment for musculoskeletal pain with or without associated joint sprains (23). Travel and Rinzler (24) noted how best to utilize the vapocoolant to deactivate MTrPs. Problems existed with ethyl chloride: it could act as a general anesthetic, it was flammable, its vapor was toxic, and at 4% to 15% of vapor mixed with air, it was potentially explosive.

Travel (25) helped develop flouri-methane, a much safer alternative that, while possibly not as cold as ethyl chloride, was not flammable or explosive.

Spray and stretch, although a good adjunctive post-MTrP injection treatment, is also an alternative noninvasive approach to the treatment of MTrPs (23,26,27).

The purpose of the vapocoolant (or plain ice) is to provide an area of hypoesthesias around a TrP and associated shortened muscle, which would allow muscle stretching with less pain. Routinely, spray and stretch is performed until muscle length has been normalized.

Electrical Stimulation
Electrical Stimulation (E-Stim) is frequently used to relieve muscle spasm and pain of MTrPs both pre- and post-TPI. Transcutaneous electrical nerve stimulation (TENS) is felt, at low frequencies (60–90 Hz), to work via the gate control theory in the spinal cord. At the very low levels (1–4Hz) galvanic or tetanizing current can work well to induce muscle relaxation. At both of these levels, endogenous opiates are stimulated. High-frequency TENS (up to 1000–2000 Hz) appears to have a more serotonergic system effect. Ultra-high frequency (15,000 Hz) TENS, which in the past was known as "cortical electrical stimulation" (CES), has been found to change the neurochemical milieu of the brain (27).

Phonophoresis and Iontophoresis
Electricity and ultrasound are used to move medication through the skin (28).

Stretching
Both active and passive stretching should begin early and proceed throughout treatment as a major part of all patients' home exercise program (29).

Soft-Tissue Treatment
There are varying forms of soft-tissue treatment (SST), including contraction and relaxation techniques, (30,31) muscle energy techniques, TrP pressure release, deep stroking massage, and myofascial release (31). Modalities, including therapeutic ultrasound, moist heat, high-voltage galvanic stimulation, and interferential current are also important, at least initially, in treatment (31).

One of the most frustrating problems seen is the administration of poor PT, which is one of the most common reasons for a patient referral to a tertiary care pain management center. Specifically, trying to strengthen spasmed, tight, contracted muscle will only potentiate the problem, and thus guarantee the development of a chronic nonmalignant pain syndrome based on a chronic MPS.

Relaxation
There are various forms of relaxation training including muscular tense–relax, (32,33) autogenic training and biofeedback-enhanced neuromuscular re-education and muscle relaxation, (34,35) and hypnosis and self-hypnosis.

Strengthening
As muscle relaxation occurs, strengthening is increased incrementally. Like stretching, strengthening should be part of every patient's home exercise program.

EVIDENCE-BASED MEDICINE REVIEWS

One RCT (36) indicated that ultrasound (US) gave no pain relief, but massage and exercise decreased the number and pain intensity of MTrPs.

A meta-analysis of the use of US therapy in musculoskeletal disorders (37) (from the Cochrane Database) indicated that the results comparing US with sham-US were not significant, and the comparison of US with non-US treatment or no treatment were not undertaken. Although finding an unimportant effect of U.S. treatment, it was noted that there were "problems in doing a meta-analysis of many different musculoskeletal diseases, where ultrasound may have a different impact. However, although the pathogenesis varied, the cause of pain is to some extent always inflammation" (37). Finally, "no attempt was made to distinguish between acute and chronic disorders."

Several other systematic reviews from the Cochrane Database were noted, both of which looked at TENS.

One review tried to evaluate the effectiveness of TENS in chronic pain. Nineteen RCT (randomized controlled trials) from 107 were evaluated. The "results of this review are inconclusive; the published trials do not provide information on the stimulation parameters which are not likely to provide optimum pain relief, nor do they answer questions about long term effectiveness (38)." Larger randomized studies were suggested.

Finally, another Cochrane Database systematic review looked at the efficacy of TENS in the treatment of chronic low back pain. Five trials were included ($N = 170$ patients receiving sham-TENS and $N = 251$ patients receiving active TENS). It was concluded that the results of the meta-analysis found no evidence to support the use of TENS in the treatment of chronic low back pain. It also notes that the meta-analysis "lacked data on how TENS effectiveness is affected by four important factors: type of application, site of application, treatment duration of TENS, optimal frequencies and intensities" (39).

The appropriateness of EBM guidelines based on poor experimental literature is questionable.

PSYCHOLOGICAL TREATMENT

There is absolutely no "one-size-fits-all" psychological approach to the chronic pain patient. Although many clinicians feel that a behavioral management program is appropriate, utilizing the Fordyce (40) paradigm of behavior "modification" by not rewarding pain behaviors, most now favor cognitive behavioral therapy (CBT).

CBT involves restructuring of a patient's maladaptive beliefs regarding his/ her ability to cope with the pain or control it and the reduction of pain behaviors; building healthy behavioral patterns and relaxation training are also parts of this treatment strategy (41,42).

These various aspects of the treatment of MPS should be applied to patients on an individualized, patient-specific basis, whether the patient has acute soft-tissue pain/MPS or a chronic MPS.

REFERENCES

1. Gerwin RD. Classification, epidemiology, and natural history of myofascial pain syndrome. Curr Pain Headache Rep 2001; 5(5):412–420.
2. Harden RN, Bruehl SP, Gass S, Niemiec C, Barbick B. Signs and symptoms of the myofascial pain syndrome: a national survey of pain management providers. Clin J Pain 2000; 16(1):64–72.
3. Roth RS, Horowitz KI, Bachman JE. Chronic myofascial pain: knowledge of diagnosis and satisfaction with treatment. Arch Phys Med Rehabil 1998; 79(8):966–970.
4. Watkins PB, Kaplowitz N, Slattery JT, et al. Aminotransferase elevations in healthy adults receiving 4 grams of acetaminophen daily: a randomized controlled trial. JAMA 2006; 296(1):87–93.
5. Sayers AC, Burki HR, Eichenberger E. The pharmacology of 5-chloro-4-(2-imidazolin-2gamma-1-amino)-2,1,3-benzothiadiazole (DS 103 282), a novel myotonic agent. Arzneimittelforschung 1980; 30:793–803.
6. Coward DM, Davies J, Herrling P, Rudeberg C. Pharmacological Properties of Tizanidine (DS 103-282). New York, NY: Springer-Verlag NY Inc., 1984:61–71.
7. Palmeri A, Wiesendanger M. Concomitant depression of locus coeruleus neurons and of flexor reflexes by an alpha$_2$-adrenergic agonist in rats: a possible mechanism for an alpha$_2$-mediated muscle relaxation. Neuroscience 1990; 34:177–187.
8. Davies J, Johnson SE, Lovering R. Inhibition by DS 103-282 of D-(^{3}H)aspartate release from spinal cord slices. Br J Pharmacol 1983; 78:2P.
9. Wagstaff AJ, Bryson H. Tizanidine: a review of its pharmacology, clinical efficacy and tolerability in the management of spasticity associated with cerebral and spinal disorders. Drugs 1997; 53:435–452.
10. Koch P, Hirst DR, von Wartburg BR. Biological fate of sirdalud in animals and man. Xenobiotica 1989; 19:1255–1265.
11. Salerno SM, Browning R, Jackson JL. The effect of antidepressant treatment on chronic back pain: a meta-analysis. Arch Intern Med 2002; 162(1):19–24.
12. Watanable Y, Saito H, Abe K. Tricyclic antidepressants block NMDA receptor-mediated synaptic responses and induction of long-term potentiation in rat hippocampal slices. Neuropharmacology 1993; 32:479–486.
13. Bendtsen L, Jensen R. Amitriptyline reduces myofascial tenderness in patients with chronic tension-type headache. Cephalalgia 2000; 20(6):603–610.
14. Argoff CE. A review of the use of topical analgesics for myofascial pain. Curr Pain Headache Rep 2002; 6(5):375–378.
15. Harris RE, Clauw DJ. The use of complementary medical therapies in the management of myofascial pain disorders. Curr Pain Headache Rep 2002; 6(5):370–374.
16. Nelemans PJ, Bie RA de, Vet HCW de, Sturmans F. Injection therapy for subacute and chronic benign low back pain (Cochrane Review). In: The Cochrane Library, Issue 4, Oxford: Update Software, 2002.
17. Wreje U, Brorsson B. A multicenter controlled trial of injections of sterile water and saline for chronic myofascial pain syndromes. Pain 1995; 61(3):441–444.
18. NcNulty WH, Gevirtz RN, Hubbard DR, Berkoff GM. Needle electromyographic evaluation of trigger point response to a psychological stressor. Psychophysiology 1944; 31(3):313–316.
19. Chu J. Does EMG (dry needling) reduce myofascial pain symptoms due to cervical nerve root irritation? Electromyogr Clin Neurophysiol 1997; 37(5):259–272.

20. Cummings TM, White AR. Needling therapies in the management of myofascial trigger point pain: a systematic review. Arch Phys Med Rehabil 2001; 82(7):986–992; (The Cochrane Database System Rev, 2002, 4:04414).
21. NIN Consensus Development Panel on Acupuncture. JAMA 1998; 280:1518.
22. Birch S, Jamison RN. Controlled trial of Japanese acupuncture for chronic myofascial neck pain: assessment of specific and nonspecific effects of treatment. Clin J Pain 1998; 14(3):248–255.
23. Kraus H. The use of surface anesthesia in the treatment of painful motion. JAMA 1941; 116:2582–2583.
24. Travel J, Rinzler SH. The myofascial genesis of pain. Postgrad Med 1952; 11:425–434.
25. Travel J. Office Hours: Day and Night. New York, NY: World Publishing Company, 1968.
26. Hong CZ. Considerations and recommendations regarding myofascial trigger point injection. J Musculoskel Pain 1994; 2(1):29–58.
27. Cassuto J, Liss S, Bennett A. The use of modulated energy carried on a high frequency wave for the relief of intractable pain. Int J Clin Pharmacol Res 1993; 13(4):239–241.
28. Kahn J. Principles and Practice of Electrotherapy. 2nd ed. New York: Churchill Livingstone, 1991.
29. Borg-Stein J. Treatment of fibromyalgia, myofascial pain and related disorders. Phys Med Rehab Clin N Am 2006; 17(2):491–510.
30. Voss DE, Ionta MK, Myers BJ. Proprioceptive Neuromuscular Facilitation. 3rd ed. Philadelphia, Pa: Harper and Row, 1985.
31. Simons DG, Travell JG, Simons LS: Myofascial Pain and Dysfunction: The Trigger Point Manual. Volume 1. Upper Half of Body. 2nd ed. Baltimore, Md: Williams & Wilkins, 1999:94–177.
32. French AP, Tupin JP. Therapeutic application of a simple relaxation method. Am J Psychother 1974; 28:282–287.
33. Bernstein DA, Borkovee TD. Progressive Relaxation Training. Champaign, Ill: Research Press, 1973.
34. Grzesiak RC. Biofeedback in the treatment of chronic pain. Curr Concepts Pain 1984; 2:3–8.
35. Nouwen A, Solinger JW. The effectiveness of EMG biofeedback training in low back pain. Biofeedback Self Regul 1979; 4:8–12.
36. Gam AN, Warming S, Larsen LH, et al. Treatment of myofascial trigger-points with ultra-sound combined with massage and exercise—a randomized controlled trial. Pain 1998; 77(1):73–79.
37. Gam AN, Johannsen F. Ultrasound therapy in musculoskeletal disorders: a meta-analysis. Pain 1995; 63(1):85–91 (The Cochrane Database Syst Rev 4:05520, 2002).
38. Carroll D, Moore RA, McQuay HJ, et al. Transcutaneous electrical nerve stimulation (TENS) for chronic pain (Cochrane Review). In: The Cochrane Library, Issue 4, Oxford: Update Software, 2002.
39. Milne S, Welch V, Brosseau L, et al. Transcutaneous electrical nerve stimulation (TENS) for chronic low back pain (Cochrane Review). In: The Cochrane Library, Issue 4, Oxford: Update Software, 2002.
40. Fordyce WE, Fowler RS, deLateur BJ. Application of behavior modification technique to problems of chronic pain. Behav Res Ther 1968; 6:105–107.
41. Turk DC, Meichenbaum D, Genest M. Pain and Behavioral Medicine: A Cognitive-Behavioral Perspective. New York, NY: Guilford, 1983.
42. Ciccone DS, Grzesiak RC. Chronic musculoskeletal pain: A cognitive approach to psycho-physiologic assessment and intervention. In: Eisenberg MG, Grzesiak RC, eds. Advances in Clinical Rehabilitation, Vol. 3. New York, NY: Springer, 1990:197–215.

7   Trigger-Point Injections

In the previous chapter, various conservative treatment modalities for myofascial pain syndrome (MPS) were discussed. In many patients, particularly those who have developed a chronic non-cancer pain syndrome secondary to a chronic MPS, a more invasive treatment technique may be needed. If conservative treatments such as spray-and-stretch and various physical therapy techniques do not deactivate existent myofascial trigger points (MTrPs), deep, invasive techniques become necessary.

Trigger-point injection (TrPI) therapy is possibly the most frequently performed interventional technique. Prior to performing this procedure, clinical imperatives include: (*i*) the ability to examine the patient and find taut bands and MTrPs in the primary affected muscles, but also identify secondary MTrPs in the primary muscle's synergistic/antagonistic muscles as well as satellite MTrPs in the primary and secondary MTrPs' zones of referred pain, (*ii*) a thorough understanding of the local and regional anatomy of the areas to be injected, (*iii*) the ability to anticipate, recognize, and treat any complications that may arise, and (*iv*) the knowledge of maximal dosages for injected local anesthetics to avoid systemic toxicity.

When treating patients with chronic MPS, it is appropriate to treat conservatively first and then utilize a multitreatment protocol. If, after one to two weeks, corresponding to three to six physical therapy sessions in patients with continued problems with MTrP-induced muscle weakness, shortening, increased fatigability, and pain, MTrP injections (MTPIs) may be felt to be appropriate.

TECHNIQUE

Once the mechanics of the procedure, along with possible side effects (hematoma, infection, and pneumothorax, among others), are explained to the patient, a consent is signed. As the patient's need for TPIs is anticipated, they should be taken off of aspirin and aspirin-containing compounds for a week prior to the injections to help eliminate any related propensity to bleed or show prolonged clotting times.

Aside from the patient's clinic nurse, the physical therapist is frequently in attendance when TrPIs are performed. This is important as it gives the clinician in charge of the patient's physical rehabilitation input into which MTrPs should be injected at a particular time. Whenever possible, patients who receive TrPIs should be seen in physical therapy within two to four hours after injection. The presence of the physical therapist also allows them and the physician to talk about how and when to advance a patient's individualized physical therapy program, including home exercises.

The patient is placed in a gown to allow easy access to the region to be injected. The primary, secondary and satellite TrPIs are identified and marked with an indelible marker (not used on the face or neck). The patient is placed in a seated position (if they have had prior injections), or a lateral or prone position, to minimize vasovagal episodes and the marked MTrPs are cleaned with betadine and then alcohol.

A 3-cc syringe with a 25 or 27 gauge, 1.5-inch needle is used. The needle used to draw up the injectate, typically lidocaine 0.5% to 1.0% without epinephrine, is exchanged with the needle to be used for injecting the patient.

The clinician is gloved and uses two fingers from the nondominant hand to stabilize the MTrP. The small-gauge needle is moved through the skin and into the MTrP. For optimal outcome, a local twitch response (LTR) should be obtained. After aspiration, a small amount of local anesthetic (0.1–0.3 cc) is injected. The author has found that the most positive clinical outcome occurs when the MTrP is needled and injectate infiltrated (N&I) at least three times, with, frequently, the production of an LTR each time. The needle is not removed each time. The tip of the needle is withdrawn, no higher than the region of subcutaneous tissue, moved 1 to 2 mm to either side before it re-enters the MTrP, aspiration occurs, and a small amount of injectate is again infiltrated.

When the needle is removed from the skin, cotton gauze is used to apply pressure over the injection site to minimize hematoma and help with local anesthetic spread.

The next MTrPs are injected in similar fashion.

The author typically limits injections to six MTrPs during a session; injections may be performed weekly with a series of three, with follow-up physical therapy until all active MTrPs are deactivated. It is the author's practice to use no more than 4 to 6 cc of lidocaine without epinephrine during each session to prevent toxic reactions.

The patient is observed for several minutes after pressure is removed from the last injected TrP and then, typically, he/she is seen in physical therapy.

CHOICE OF INJECTATE

The author prefers to use lidocaine 0.5% to 1.0%, without epinephrine, as it is an amide with correspondingly rare anaphylactic reactions; it has a rapid onset of action and it is more potent than procaine hydrochloride 0.5%. The latter is frequently used; it is an ester and more likely to produce an anaphylactic reaction than lidocaine or bupivacaine 0.125% to 0.25%, also an amide with longer lasting effectiveness compared to lidocaine. Long-acting local anesthetics may be more likely to induce muscle necrosis. Epinephrine induces local vasoconstriction and may contribute to local ischemia. It is not recommended in any local anesthetic injectate for MTrPs.

The use of corticosteroids when injecting MTrPs is not recommended as there is typically no associated inflammatory process associated with MTrPs and repeated corticosteroid injection may damage soft tissue; overuse can be associated with muscle atrophy and dimpling of the associated soft-tissue region. For similar reasons, injections of nonsteroidal anti-inflammatory drugs (NSAIDs) are not recommended (1,2).

Saline has also been used alone and, compared to local anesthetic, with varying results (3,4).

MECHANISM OF PAIN RELIEF POST MYOFASCIAL TRIGGER-POINT INJECTION

A number of different mechanisms have been postulated, which may contribute to the deactivation of a MTrP by injection. These include:

- local anesthetic-induced interruption of feedback mechanisms (5),

- fluid injectates that dilute endogenous algetic substances (5),
- nerve fiber depolarization, secondary to the release of intracellular potassium secondary to mechanical disruption of muscle fibers (5),
- mechanical disruption of the TIP, secondary to disrupting muscle elements or nerve endings (5),
- increased fluid pressure from within the TIP that enables disruption, made easier with added external pressure, and
- mechanical disruption of involved end plates signified by single or multiple LTRs.

CONTRAINDICATIONS TO TRIGGER-POINT INJECTIONS

TPIs should not be performed on patients with systemic or local infection, a bleeding disorder or patients on an anticoagulant regime, or those who are pregnant.

REASONS FOR TRIGGER-POINT INJECTION FAILURE

There are a number of reasons one may encounter persistence of MTrP activity post injection. Lack of recognition and treatment of hypothyroidism, folic acid deficiency, or low levels of iron in patients with MPS may cause continued difficulty. Similarly, structural disorders such as a leg length discrepancy or pelvic asymmetry may be reason enough for perpetuation of MPS.

Other reasons for postinjection perpetuation of MPS include (6):

- inability of patients who receive TrPIs to participate in proper postinjection care,
- patients with significant muscle spasms not ameliorated by physical therapy with or without medications prior to TrPIs,
- patients with low pain thresholds who develop a marked anxiety reaction to TrPIs,
- patients who are emotionally unstable,
- limiting injections to only primary TrPs or just to secondary/satellite TrPs,
- incorrect diagnoses, that is, significant radiculopathy without associated TrPs,
- injecting more than one TrP area at a time causing increased muscle spasm,
- patients in litigation,
- patients who are unemployed secondary to pain, long duration of pain, constant pain, poor analgesic effectiveness, changes in social activity, and poor coping skills (7), and
- concurrent use of calcium channel blockers (8).

POST-INJECTION PHYSICAL THERAPY PROGRAM

Clinically, it is a mistake to use TrPIs as a form of monotherapy for patients with MPS. It is the ability to provide proper follow-up care post-TPIs that helps to ensure therapeutic success (5, 9–11).

Significant differences can be found in treatment outcome in many patients who obtain follow-up care with physical therapy post injection as compared to those who are unable to receive appropriate follow-up care [secondary to poor insurance, poorly educated case manager/adjustor, HMO/PPO (health maintenance organization/preferred provider organization) rules].

A post-MTrP injection physical therapy program is very important. It should include at a minimum: vapocoolant spray and gentle limbering exercises (spray and stretch), active and passive stretching techniques, and a home exercise program (HEP). Electrical stimulation may be used (11–14).

TPIs are given weekly, as needed, with physical therapy follow-up the day of injection and, optimally, on a three times-a-week basis. Most patients need a series of TPIs weekly for three weeks to thoroughly deal with all forms of active TIPs in one region. As noted earlier, the author limits TPIs to six during a session.

PATIENT INSTRUCTIONS POST TRIGGER-POINT INJECTIONS

As with all interdisciplinary pain management programs, patients must be educated and act as a part of their treatment team. Patients should know that after TPIs (6):

- pain relief may be temporary,
- the patients may feel sore for 24 to 48 hours,
- they must look for redness, pain, warmth, and swelling—signs of infection at the site of injection,
- after TIPs, other nearby MTrPs may become symptomatic—these secondary TIPs may also need to be injected,
- it is best to have all treatment under one roof (in a multidisciplinary pain management center) rather than have patients travel long distances for treatment with physical therapy, as this can increase muscle spasm and hinder therapeutic effectiveness, and
- the patients should practice their HEP two to three times a day.

DRY NEEDLING

Acupuncture, the insertion of needles into MTrPs for pain relief, is an "old" treatment utilized for centuries (15,16).

In 1979, Lewit noted the "needle effect in the relief of myofascial pain" (17), noting that 86.8% of 241 patients had pain relief from the needling of MTrPs.

Intramuscular stimulation, also known as deep dry needling (DDN) relates dry needle insertion to pain relief (18). Gunn (19) notes that a solid 30-gauge acupuncture needle with a pointed tip is less traumatic to use than the beveled edge of a hollow needle.

The main problem with this technique is that it may be more painful than MTrP injection with anesthetic. Another difficulty is that DDN may damage nerves, blood vessels, and other soft-tissue structures. Bleeding secondary to DDN contributes to the high percentage of patients with significant post-treatment pain and soreness (19).

Superficial Dry Needling

Superficial dry needling (SDN) involves inserting the needle into the subcutaneous tissue immediately over the MTrP. After insertion, the needle remains for five to ten minutes or more, as needed, in situ. The efficacy of SDN has been noted in patients with MPS in the lumbar region (20).

SDN, being relatively painless, does appear to have better clinical utilization criteria when compared to DDN.

EVIDENCE-BASED MEDICAL LITERATURE

There is a substantial paucity of RCTs that would contribute to the evidence-based medical studies involving the best overall techniques to deactivate MTrPs.

One reason for this is the previously acknowledged difficultly noted in making the clinical diagnosis of MPS. If finding MTrPs is difficult for both trained and untrained clinicians, how much more difficult would deactivating MTrPs be?

A second reason is the difficulty in determining accurate (nonsubjective) pain levels in patients after MTrP deactivation. How can the information be objectively collected?

Finally, just how does one go about developing blinded, controlled, randomized trials dealing with invasive methods of deactivating MTrPs?

Evidence-based medicine, again, may not be the primary evidence to be assessed here—clinical efficacy is.

BOTULINUM TOXIN

The use of botulinum toxin (BTX) has increased markedly over the last decade. It has been used for headache (21) of various types, blepharospasm, dystonia, soft-tissue pain, for cosmetic reasons, and multiple other reasons.

There are seven subtypes of BTX, only two of which are currently in use. The oldest form is BTX Type A, known as in the United States and Dysport in Europe, and the most recent FDA-approved form, BTX Type B—Myobloc®, or, manufactured by Solstice Neurosciences. It must be noted that using either form of BTX for treatment of MPS is considered "off label" and would not be a first line form of treatment. It should be used in patients in whom conservative care, including physical therapy and local anesthetic TPIs have failed, leaving the patients with continued muscular pain and spasm.

The BTX molecule is relatively large, with a heavy chain bound to a light chain by a disulfide bond. Via endocytosis, the molecule is taken into the presynaptic cell in the myoneural junction, where both forms induce a blockade of acetylcholine release at the motor end plates, essentially terminating their ability to express acetylcholine for at least three months (average), therefore decreasing muscle spasms. This helps prove that the MTrP is associated with the neuromuscular junction (22,23).

BTX Type A ships in a lyophilized form, which must be reconstituted with preservative free normal saline. It has a relatively short active life after reconstitution. Many physicians use all of a vial once reconstitution has occurred. BTX Type B comes in a multiuse vial and can be stored for nine months on the shelf and 30 months or more if refrigerated.

There is a paucity of double-blind, randomized controlled trials with BTX and MPS. Older existent trials may be subject to interpretation.

When used to inject MTrPs, the technique is identical to local anesthetic MTrP injection. However, BTX Type A and B have very different dosage schemata. The toxic dose of BTX Type B is higher than that of BTX Type A.

Treatment with either form of BTX should not be performed more frequently than every three to four months if necessary. It is possible for patients to develop antibodies to a particular form of BTX, making it necessary to use the other type before possibly returning to the initial subtype used.

The most common side effects of BTX include pain at the injection site, and a short-lasting flu-like syndrome. Patients taking aminoglycoside antibiotics should not use BTX. BTX Type A is also contraindicated in patients with human albumin allergies. Both subtypes must be avoided in patients with disorders of neuromuscular transmission such as myasthenia gravis or the Lambert Eaton syndrome.

The results from the use of BTX vary. For example, one group using Dysport® found significant improvement in pain levels four to six weeks post treatment for upper back MPS (24). Another recent study using Dysport® found no difference between the effect of small doses of BTX Type A when compared to physiological saline in the treatment of MPS (25).

REFERENCES

1. Drewes AM, Andreasen A, Poulsen LH. Injection therapy for treatment of chronic myofascial pain: a double-blind study comparing corticosteroid versus diclofenac injections. J Musculoskel Pain 1993; 1(3/4):289–294.
2. Bourne IHJ. Treatment of chronic back pain comparing corticosteroid-lignocaine injections with lignocaine alone. Practitioner 1984; 222:333–338.
3. Hameroff SR, Crago BR, Blitt CD, et al. Comparison of bupivacaine, etidocaine and saline for trigger point therapy. Anesth Analg 1981; 60:752–755.
4. Sola AE, Williams RL. Myofascial pain syndromes. Neurology 1956; 6:91–95.
5. Simons DG, Travell JG, Simons LS. Myofascial Pain and Dysfunction: the Trigger Point Manual. Volume 1. Upper half of body. 2nd ed. Baltimore, Md: Williams & Wilkins, 1999.
6. Rachlin ES, Rachlin IS. Myofascial Pain and Fibromyalgia: Trigger Point Management. St. Louis, Mo: Mosby, 2002:231–258.
7. Hopwood MB, Abram SE. Factors associated with failure of trigger point injections. Clin J Pain 1994; 10(3):227–234.
8. Shenoi R, Willibald N. Trigger points related to calcium channel blockers. Muscle Nerve 1996; 256.
9. Fricton JR. Etiology and management of masticatory myofascial pain. J Musculoskel Pain 1999; 7(1/2):143–160.
10. Fischer AA. Treatment of myofascial pain. J Musculoskel Pain 1999; 7(1/2):131–142.
11. Marini I, Fairplay T, Vecchiet F, Checci L. The treatment of trigger points in the cervical and facial area. J Musculoskel Pain 1999; 7(1/2):239–245.
12. Cheng PT, Hsuen TC, Hong CZ. The immediate effectiveness of electrical muscle stimulation and electrical nerve stimulation on myofascial trigger points. Am J Phys Med Rehabil 1997; 76(2):162.
13. Imamura ST, Fischer AA, Imamura M, et al. Pain management using myofascial approach when other treatments failed. Phys Med Rehab Clin N Am 1997; 8:179–196.
14. Hong CZ. Considerations and recommendations regarding myofascial trigger point injection. J Musculoskel Pain 1994; 2(1):29–58.
15. Kho HG, Robertson EN. The mechanisms of acupuncture analgesia: review and update. Am J Acupuncture 1997; 25(4):261–281.
16. Wong JY, Rapson LM. Acupuncture in the management of pain of musculoskeletal and neurologic origin. Phys Med Rehabil Clin N Am 1999; 10(3):531–545.
17. Lewit K. The needle effect in the relief of myofascial pain. Pain 1979; 6:83–90.
18. Gunn CC. Treating Myofascial Pain: Intramuscular Stimulation (IMS) for Myofascial Pain Syndromes of Neuropathic Origin. Seattle, Wash: Health Science Center for Educational Resources, University of Washington, 1989.
19. Gunn CC. Acupuncture and the peripheral nervous system. In: Filshie J, White A, eds. Medical Acupuncture. A Western Scientific Approach. Edinburgh, UK: Churchill Livingstone, 1998:137–150.
20. Macdonald AJR, Macrae KD, Master BR, Rubin AP. Superficial acupuncture in the relief of chronic low-back pain. Ann R Coll Surg Engl 1983; 65:44–46.
21. Jay GW, Jay SJ. Botulinum Toxin Type-B (Myobloc™) in the Treatment of Episodic and Chronic Tension-Type Headache and Migraine. In Press.

22. Simons DG. Clinical and etiological update of myofascial pain from trigger points. J Musculoske Pain 1966; 4(1/2): 81–85.
23. Yue SK. Initial experience in the use of Botulinum toxin A for the treatment of myofascial related muscle dysfunctions. J Musculoskel Pain 1995; 3(suppl 1):22.
24. Gobel H, Heinze A, Reichel G, et al. Efficacy and safety of a single botulinum type A toxin complex treatment [Dysport (R)] for the relief of upper back myofascial pain syndrome: Results from a randomized double-blind placebo-controlled multicentre study. Pain 2006; 125(1–2):82–88.
25. Ojala T, Arokoski JP, Partanen J. The effect of small doses of botulinum toxin a on neck-shoulder myofascial pain syndrome: a double-blind, randomized, and controlled crossover trial. Clin J Pain 2006; 22(1):90–96.

8 Fibromyalgia: Clinical Aspects and Pathophysiology

For several centuries, medicine has dealt with the problem of widespread musculo-skeletal and soft-tissue pain problems without having any definitive idea of specific diagnosis (1,2). Gowers first used the term "fibrositis" in 1904 to describe what he felt was muscle pain secondary to inflammation (3). Traut (4) used the term fibrositis to describe generalized musculoskeletal aching, poor sleep, fatigue, and multiple tender points (TPs). The first controlled study of the clinical characteristics of the fibromyalgia syndrome (FMS) was published by Yunus et al. (5). In this study, multiple symptoms including pain, poor sleep, fatigue, paresthesia, irritable bowel syndrome (IBS), and headaches were, with multiple TPs, more common in fibromyalgia patients than in age, sex, and race-matched normal controls. This study brought FMS to clinical consciousness. The multicenter criteria study performed by the American College of Rheumatology (ACR) helped establish the validity of FMS (6).

FMS, most simply, is characterized by chronic widespread musculoskeletal pain, stiffness, and tenderness to palpation at specific TPs (5–8). Fibromyalgia has been classified as primary and concomitatant (9).

Primary fibromyalgia indicates that there is no underlying or concomitant medical condition that might have contributed to a patient's pain. FMS is considered concomitant if another condition such as osteoarthritis (OA), rheumatoid arthritis (RA), systemic lupus erythematosus (SLE), or hypothyroidism is present, and, in turn, contributes to a patient's pain or fatigue. There are no specific differences existent between primary and concomitant FMS. When the concomitant condition is treated appropriately, there is no significant change in a patient's clinical picture of FMS. It is felt that the term secondary fibromyalgia should not be used instead of concomitant, as there is no change in a patient's FMS after the successful treatment of the underlying condition (10).

The diagnosis of FMS has been warily accepted, especially as there is no "gold standard" test that can confirm it. This, in association with the ever-growing numbers of patients given this diagnosis who appear unable to work and frequently request disability have made the diagnosis, to some, suspect (11). Others believe that FMS is a functional, or psychological problem, while still others do not believe FMS exists (12,13).

Chronic widespread pain, a general diagnosis indicative of chronic generalized musculoskeletal pain (in the majority of cases) with no underlying diagnosis, with or without TPs, is an enormous problem. While between 14% and 26% of the American adult population suffers from chronic pain or arthritis, about 11% complain of chronic widespread pain (14–16). Generalized musculoskeletal pain itself encompasses between 10.6% and 17% of the adult population (17).

There appears to be a spectrum of patients with chronic widespread pain, including those patients with and without TPs. It has been felt that it was not useful to use TPs to differentiate between chronic widespread pain and FMS (18). Other authors note that patients with chronic widespread pain and high numbers of TPs were different from patients with chronic widespread pain alone. They felt that the patients with chronic widespread pain and high numbers of TPs had a higher female prevalence, more fatigue, worse function, and distress (19–21). They questioned whether these patients (FMS) were the extreme part of a spectrum of chronic widespread pain, or whether there was a real dichotomy between FMS and chronic widespread pain (22).

Russell (23) felt it would be useful to consider FMS separate from chronic widespread pain. He used the analogy of FMS and chronic widespread pain being similar to other continuous variables such as hypertension, in that although blood pressure is the continuous variable, when it reaches medically significant regions of current or potential morbidity, it becomes a distinct entity. Another similar continuous variable would be blood glucose levels, with significant pathological entities at either end of that spectrum.

White and Harth (19–22) felt that the patients classified as having FMS were clearly worse in many ways than patients who had chronic widespread pain but not FMS, and, therefore, they considered FMS as a separate syndrome from chronic widespread pain.

While FMS patients seen at a tertiary care interdisciplinary pain center are mostly between 20 and 40 years of age, other authors have described FMS as occurring most commonly in women between 40 and 60 years of age (5,6,8) Roizenblatt et al. (24) and Yunus (25) have both described juvenile forms of FMS; FMS has also been noted to occur in the elderly (26).

Wolfe et al. (27) noted that the prevalence of FMS in Wichita, Kansas, was found to be 2% in the community. The prevalence of FMS in women in the New York/New Jersey metropolitan area was 3.7%, with a higher rate among racial minorities (28). White et al. (29) found the prevalence of FMS in London, Ontario, Canada to be 3.3%. In the Wichita study, the prevalence among women was 3.4% versus 0.5% in men. The London Ontario study also found a larger female prevalence, 4.9% compared to 1.6% in men.

A more recent Canadian study using the Canadian Community Health Survey, Cycle 1.1 (2000) found the Canadian prevalence rate to be 1.1% with a 6:1 female: male ratio (30).

Weir et al. (31) found that patients with FMS (females more likely than males) were 2.14 to 7.05 times more likely to have at least one comorbid condition including: depression, anxiety, headache, IBS, chronic fatigue syndrome (CFS), SLE, and RA. In another study, a high incidence of FMS was found in female, but not male, migraine patients (32).

CLINICAL ASPECTS

FMS is a common condition, which has been associated with significant disability (33). Patients with FMS complain of widespread pain, frequently stating that they "hurt all over." Most of these patients also complain of stiffness (about 85%) (5), pain in the cervical region, the low back, the major joints, pain in their hands and feet, and chest wall.

Their pain and stiffness can be typically aggravated by overuse or underuse/inactivity-induced deconditioning, weather (cold or humid), trauma, poor sleep, stress, and loud and/or continuous noise (5,6).

A subset of FMS patients complain of peripheral arthralgias, with some pain found on palpation, but no objective swelling, as one would expect with an inflammatory arthritis (34).

Other common symptoms of FMS patients include severe fatigue, sleep difficulties, morning fatigue, or nonrestorative sleep, paresthesia, psychological distress, cognitive difficulties ("fibromyalgia fog"), and a swollen feeling in their distal extremities.

Fatigue is found to be moderate or severe in 75% to 90% of patients (5,6). This may be secondary to poor sleep, excessive physical activity, deconditioning, or psychological factors (5,35).

Nonrestorative sleep is also common. Approximately 75% of FMS patients have sleep problems (7,8). Morning fatigue is noted in 75% to 90% of patients (5,6). Poor sleep is frequently a combination of initial insomnia, multiple nocturnal awakenings, light sleep or restless legs syndrome, and periodic limb movement abnormalities (10). Poor sleep correlated with fatigue and psychological distress, as well as increased pain (5,6,10,35).

Moldofsky (36) noted diurnal variations in the pain of FMS patients. Their "worst" times were in the early morning, late afternoon, and evenings. They felt best between 10 am and 2 pm. Seasonal effects were also noted, with FMS patients feeling better in spring and summer, but experiencing more pain and diminished energy and poor mood in November and March.

Psychological distress has also been correlated with increased severity of pain (21).

Other associated features include headache, IBS, restless legs syndrome, "female urethral syndrome" or interstitial cystitis, a thyroid disorder (typically hypothyroidism), and primary dysmenorrhea (6).

FMS has been reported to be associated with RA, OA, SLE, and Sjogren's syndrome. It is important to note that these inflammatory conditions are not thought to cause FMS, as appropriate treatment of these concomitant conditions does not decrease or ameliorate a patient's symptoms of FMS.

Although there may be a higher occurrence of FMS with these disorders, the actual mechanistic relationship between them is unknown. It may be possible that in subgroups of FMS patients with these disorders, the concomitant problems themselves, such as arthritis or other forms of peripheral inflammation, may be the initial source of continuous peripheral nociception to the CNS which may lead to central sensitization (CS) with its associated neuroplastic changes yielding amplified pain and FMS.

The ACR's classification criteria for FMS was published in 1990 (6). It was not initially meant as diagnostic criteria, but has been used for this purpose. The FMS criteria included widespread pain for three months or more and the presence of 11 TPs among 18 specific TP sites (Table 1). Pain was to be found in all four body quadrants, including the limbs and the axial skeleton.

On clinical evaluation it appears that the number of TPs [(which differ greatly from myofascial trigger points (MTrPs), in that TPs do not refer pain)] although clinically a reflection of the FMS criteria, may not have a direct correspondence with a patient's level of disability. As a clinical measure, TPs appear to be a gross measure of a patient's discomfort and possibly a general or generic measure of the depths of a patient's FMS-associated function, in the same way a sedimentation rate is a general test that may indicate that there is something going on clinically,

TABLE 1 Tender Point Regions Used in the Diagnosis of
Fibromyalgia Syndrome

Suboccipital muscle
Anterior cervical region at C6
Upper trapezius
Supraspinatus muscle
Parasternal at the 2nd intercostals space
Lateral epicondyle
Upper outer quadrant of the gluteal muscles
Greater trochanter
Medial fat pad of the knee (or vastus medialis muscle)

Note: Each noted point is evaluated bilaterally.

but it is not diagnostic. This is not meant to indicate that TPs are not extremely important in the diagnosis of FMS—they are. However, even during treatment, which ameliorates a patient's symptoms, the clinical TP count may not change.

To attempt to make the reliability of the TP count a more valid measure of a patient's overall pain and ability to function, more specific criteria have been found that attempt to more appropriately validate the severity of TP tenderness.

The tender point index (TPI) (37,38) (also called the total myalgic score) is clinically simple to do. A possible problem is that it may incorporate some elements of a patient's subjective complaints. To obtain the TPI, the examiner sequentially presses the thumb or finger against the 18 TPs noted in the ACR criteria. The intensity should be equivalent to 4 kgs/cm^2, or enough pressure to cause the examiner's fingernail to blanch. With each site that is examined, a tenderness severity scale is applied: nontender=0, tender without physical response=1, tender plus wince or withdrawal=2, exaggerated withdrawal=3, too painful to touch=4. The myalgic score may also be done on a 0 to 3 basis. The sum of all the TP tenderness scores is the TPI. This measure may be repeated sequentially during treatment. The TPI has good inter-rater reliability with the average pain threshold, or APT.

The APT (39) is obtained by the use of an algometer, or dolorimeter. As per the usual use of this tool, the probe is placed perpendicularly over the TP and pressure is increased gradually by 1 kg/s. When the patient states that they feel pain, rather than pressure, the reading on the algometer is taken as the pressure pain threshold for that site. The average of the pressure pain thresholds obtained at all 18 TP sites is the APT. If the APT is less than 4 kg in a patient with a history of chronic widespread pain, or FMS, it is consistent with the finding of 11 of 18 palpably active TPs corresponding to the examination criteria for FMS.

Other typical clinical findings on examination include joint tenderness, but no swelling (unless there is coexistent OA or RA), decreased range of motion of the neck and other joints secondary to pain, and even in the face of complaints of paresthesia, a normal neurological examination is found.

Abnormal skin tenderness, possibly reflective of global hyperalgesia may be noted; another indication of a central pain disorder. The examiner may also find tenderness over the tibia (shin) and other bony regions.

Although FMS has been used as a "wastebasket" diagnosis, it should be diagnosed by its own clinical characteristics, and not as a diagnosis of exclusion. Concomitant disorders (OA, RA, SLE, hypothyroidism) should not influence the diagnosis, as patients with FMS frequently have such concomitant or concurrent diagnoses.

Certain diseases can mimic FMS, but none have a sufficient number of TPs to satisfy the ACR criteria. These disorders may include arthritis, polymyalgia rheumatica, hypothyroidism, ankylosing spondylitis, disc herniation, and cardiothoracic pain. (See following text.)

Yunus (40) notes a significant gender difference in patients with FMS, finding that only 10% of FMS patients are men. Women had more fatigue, nonrestorative sleep, a greater number of symptoms overall, and a greater number of TPs.

In another study comparing 536 new patients with FMS, where 469 were women and 67 were men, it was found that the latter group had statistically less frequent feelings of "hurt all over," fatigue, nonrestorative sleep, and IBS. Fewer TPs were found in the men than in women. It was felt that the number of TPs was the most powerful discriminator between men and women with FMS (35).

Another study performed in Israel found men had greater pain, fatigue, and functional disability, as well as a poorer quality of life, making the point that sociocultural factors were implicated in gender differences (41).

Issues of anxiety and depression were not significantly different between men and women in several studies (42,43).

Yunus notes that gender differences in FMS are due to a composite of biological, psychological, and sociocultural factors, with the relative contribution of each factor varying from patient to patient (40). Celentano et al. (44) note that women are more likely to consult a health care provider, therefore utilizing more medical resources and, finally, are more likely to report disability.

Finally, Yunus (40) notes hormonal differences that may affect gender differences in pain perception: estrogen modulates noradrenergic sensitivity to arterioles, cognitive function and mood, as well as serotonin (5-HT) tonus and vascular tone. Further, he notes that the rate of 5-HT synthesis is 52% higher in men than women and that androgen seems to be protective in FMS.

PATHOPHYSIOLOGY

FMS has also been called myalgic encephalomyelitis (45). It appears to have "graduated" from a disease with a simple etiology to engender a new paradigm of pathoetiology based on scientific data.

While FMS is recognized as a chronic pain disorder with the common multiple dimensions of all chronic pain problems (biological-psychological-sociological), it is also associated with CS, neuroendocrine, and autonomic nervous system (ANS) dysfunction. It appears that the main problem is central in origin.

It is the trigger or pathoetiology to the disorder that seems to be unknown.

Patients with FMS have psychophysiological evidence of hyperalgesia to mechanical, thermal, and electrical stimulation. This leads to the assumption of both peripheral and central nociceptive abnormalities. Peripheral nociceptive systems in the skin and musculature change significantly, with sensitization of vanilloid receptors, acid-sensing ion channel receptors, and purino-receptors. Tissue modulators of inflammation and nerve growth factors (NGFs) can excite these receptors, leading to significant changes in pain sensitivity (46,47) In FMS patients, however, there is no consistent evidence of inflammatory soft-tissue abnormalities, leading the search for the pathoetiology to the CNS (47,48).

Both abnormal temporal summation of second pain, or windup (WU), and CS have been described in FMS. Both of these entities rely on CNS mechanisms. They occur after prolonged C-fiber nociceptive input and depend on the activation of specific nociceptive neurons and wide-dynamic-range (WDR) neurons in the dorsal horn of the spinal cord. Other abnormal pain mechanisms are associated, including dysfunction of the diffuse noxious inhibitory controls. These pain inhibitory mechanisms rely on both spinal cord and supraspinal mechanisms, which both facilitate and inhibit pain (48).

Brain-imaging techniques that can detect neuronal activation after nociceptive stimulation also give evidence for abnormal central pain mechanisms in FMS. Brain images corroborated augmented pain experienced by FMS patients during experimental pain stimuli. Thalamic activity, for example, which contributes to pain processing, is found to be decreased in FMS patients (48). It has also been demonstrated that dysfunction of central pain mechanisms is not only secondary to neuronal activation, but also, possibly, neuroglial cell activation, which appears to have an important role in the induction and maintenance of chronic pain (48).

The perceived pain in FMS patients appears to be related to bio–psycho–social factors, along with changes in the ANS and hypothalamic–pituitary–adrenal (HPA) axis. FMS patients have demonstrated reduced reactivity in the central sympathetic systems, which can be equated to changes or perturbations in the sympathetic–parasympathetic balance (49).

The evidence for central pain processing abnormalities in FMS patients is increasing, with research demonstrating in these patients: hyperalgesia, allodynia, abnormal temporal summation of second pain, neuroendocrine abnormalities, ANS abnormalities, and activation of pain-related cerebral regions. Some authors have noted the characteristics of FMS, which are similar to a neuropathic pain syndrome including many of these characteristics such as hyperalgesia and the association of FMS with ineffective responses to many analgesics (50).

Psychophysiology

Quantitative sensory testing has shown that cold and heat pain, but not perception thresholds, differed significantly between a group of FMS patients and a normal, healthy control (NHC) group. Based on thermal pain thresholds, two subgroups could be identified, with a clinical difference in pain intensities, number of TPs, and sleep qualities noted. Cold pain threshold was especially linked to these clinical aspects (51). Looking at the pain threshold, they found that the threshold to perception of warm and cold stimuli was the same in both groups. However, the threshold to pain—both heat and cold-induced—was much lower in FMS patients than in controls. Looking at the FMS patients, they found that there was one subgroup that demonstrated a lowered pain threshold to both heat and cold pain, and another subgroup that had a lowered pain threshold to cold alone. The researchers noted that the FMS subgroup with lowered pain thresholds to both heat and cold also had a trend toward more disturbed sleep and a greater number or TPs. They raised an important question—could the FMS group with only a decreased cold pain threshold be an "intermediate" group between normal subjects and the more significantly affected FMS patients?

Using laser-evoked potentials (LEP), heat pain thresholds were measured and suprathreshold magnitude estimates of heat pain stimulation were obtained, along with the extent local tissue responses were induced by previous stimulation. Ultralate LEPs indicated the presence of peripheral C-fiber sensitization, mostly at TPs. This was felt to be combined with generalized CS of pain pathways in the FMS patients (52).

TABLE 2 Psychophysiological Abnormalities in
Fibromyalgia (Summary)

Hyperalgesia to mechanical, thermal, and electrical stimulation
Central sensitization
↓ Sympathetic nervous system response to pain
Generalized diffuse pain to minimal mechanical pressure
↓ Perception of heat and cold pain but not perception thresholds

Montoya et al. (53) looked at event-related potentials (ERPs) elicited via either tactile or auditory-paired stimuli via electroencephalogram (EEG) and found abnormal information processing in FMS patients, possibly characterized by a lack of inhibitory control to repetitive nonpainful somatosensory information.

Another study looked at randomized thermal and tactile stimulation in both FMS patients and NHCs. It was found that the perceptual thresholds for cold pain, heat pain, cold pain tolerance, and heat pain tolerance were significantly lower in the FMS patients than in the NHCs. The combination of cold hyperesthesia, cold dysesthesia, and multimodal hyperalgesia suggested a selective dysfunction at a particular level of CNS integration of nociception—the insular cortex. It was noted that the aberrations revealed by supraliminal sensory evaluation may be generic for FMS patients. Finally, the aberrations found in all of the FMS patients for perceived quality and intensity of cold sensory changes may be a diagnostic criterion for FMS patients (54).

See Table 2 for a summary of the psychophysiological abnormalities.

Pain Processing

In Chapter 1, we covered the basic neuroanatomy and physiology of pain. The concept of peripheral sensitization (the reduction in the threshold of nociceptive afferent receptors induced by a local change in the sensitivity of sensory fibers initiated by tissue inflammation or damage resulting from the local production of algetic substances) was also discussed in Chapter 3.

Primary hyperalgesia, or an increased region of pain sensitivity including an area of tissue damage, is typically associated with a second zone or area of increased pain sensitivity, which is the surrounding area of uninjured tissue (zone of secondary hyperalgesia) and which is particularly sensitive to mechanical stimuli. The region of primary hyperalgesia, or sensitivity, is associated with changes of the properties of the area's primary nociceptive afferents. Secondary hyperalgesia is associated with functional, neuroplastic changes in the CNS, starting with the dorsal horn region of the spinal cord.

Although there are some minimal changes in the peripheral regions in FMS patients (see following text), there are no specific inflammatory or other soft-tissue changes found in the FMS patient group (55). There is essentially little, if any, evidence of primary hyperalgesia in the FMS. Some findings are suggestive of peripheral sensitization, including increased amounts of substance P (SP) found in the nerve fibers of FMS muscle tissue. This excitatory neurotransmitter is typically not detectable in peripheral nerves, and could possibly indicate an involvement of the peripheral afferents in the production of the pain seen in the FMS patients (56).

Central Sensitization

CS involves several neurophysiological aspects, including enhanced spinal cord dorsal horn neuronal excitability, which is associated with increased spontaneous neuronal activity, enlarged receptive fields, and an augmentation of stimuli transmitted by both large and small-diameter primary afferent fibers. Activation of muscle nociceptors, more so than skin nociceptors, is much more likely to induce CS (57).

We have previously discussed in detail (Chapter 1) the regions or laminae of the spinal cord dorsal horn, which are involved in pain processing and the rostral transmission of nociceptive information. We also described the modulation of nociceptive information via different neurotransmitter systems. To briefly recap, excitatory neurons in the spinal cord are associated with various excitatory/algetic neurotransmitters including glutamate, SP, aspartate, vasoactive intestinal peptide (VIP), neurotensin, calcitonin gene-related peptide (CGRP), and cholesystokinin (CCK), among others. This excitatory system is "down modulated" by inhibitory dorsal horn interneurons that produce gamma-amino butyric acid (GABA), which acts to inhibit nociceptive neurons.

CS may also be secondary to the activation of glial cells by neurotransmitters, cytokines, or chemokines, and this may also contribute to the neurophysiological enhancement of CNS mechanisms, which lead to CS (57).

Another important process begins with peripheral nociceptive stimulation—the release of SP at the synapse in pre- and postsynaptic dorsal horn neurons, particularly in laminae II. The release of SP enables the removal of the magnesium block of the N-methyl-D-aspartate (NMDA) receptors, which allows excitatory amino acids such as glutamate and aspartate to activate the postsynaptic NMDA receptors. This process permits changes in cell membrane permeability, leading to the influx of calcium and further excitement of secondary neurons. An increased expression of NMDA receptors found in the skin of FMS patients was thought to be indicative of a possibly more generalized increase in other peripheral nerves (58). The activation of NMDA receptors currently appears to be very important for the induction and maintenance of CS (59).

Opioid receptors are closely related to the NMDA receptors. Both have been detected on primary afferent neurons (60). Opioids can modulate NMDA receptor activity both directly and indirectly, the former aspect leading to the search for usable NMDA receptor antagonists, which can decrease opioid tolerance and possibly increase opioid potency.

The activation of NMDA receptors is linked to nitric oxide (NO) production (61). NO is a gaseous molecule that can diffuse into and activate adjacent neurons and glia (62). Its release in lamina I and II of the spinal cord dorsal horn, secondary to nociceptive activity, can, it has been postulated, induce the release of SP and CGRP from C-fibers, one mechanism of CS, which would then be followed by further dorsal horn neuronal changes leading to hyperexcitability, hyperalgesia, and allodynia (63).

Referring back to the initial chapter of this text, repetitive stimulation of C-fibers will increase the discharges from second-order neurons in the spinal cord. This will induce pain amplification related to the temporal summation of second pain, or WU. WU is a progressively increased response of the secondary dorsal horn neurons, which follows repeated and brief stimulation of the peripheral C fibers: with each proceeding stimulus, the activated neuronal response increases and becomes stronger than after the prior stimulus. The NMDA receptors mediate WU, which is also inhibited by NMDA receptor antagonists. The concept of temporal summation in humans is similar to WU, as demonstrated in animals (64). WU has also been demonstrated in humans, with the further finding that WU results from a central, not a peripheral pathophysiological mechanism, as input from C-fibers declines or stays the same with peripheral stimulus repetition (65,66).

Clinically, first pain is typically described as sharp or lancinating, whereas second pain, most commonly seen in association with chronic pain, is described as dull, aching, or burning.

CS may be relevant to FMS pain because it is frequently associated with extensive secondary hyperalgesia and allodynia. Psychophysiological studies, as noted earlier, show evidence that input to central nociceptive pathways are abnormally processed in FMS (51–54).

Ketamine, an NMDA receptor antagonist, has been shown in placebo-controlled studies to reduce both temporal summation and muscle pain, indicating the importance of NMDA receptors in the pathophysiology of FMS (67,68).

Finally, Yunus questions the possibility of an "intrinsic" CS in susceptible FMS patients, a *central sensitivity* rather than central sensitization, which would occur, possibly, without a peripheral nociceptive stimulus. He notes that this might occur secondary to defective inhibitory systems or a hyperstimulated facilitatory pathway and/or generalized hyperexcitment of peripheral nociceptors (69).

Other Pathophysiological Aspects of FMS
Muscle Studies
Two groups have recently looked at the blood flow in muscle. Using contrast enhanced ultrasound imaging of muscular blood flow during and after exercise, Elvin et al. (70) found that FMS patients had a lesser muscle vascularity level following dynamic exercise and during static exercise when compared to controls. They suggest that muscle ischemia can contribute to pain in FMS by helping to maintain CNS changes such as CS.

Ischemia is associated with muscle fatigue. Kasikcioglu et al. (71) described production abnormalities of NO, which might lead to symptoms of fatigue as a long-term effect. They describe a cycle initiated by decreased production of NO in the endothelium. This decreased level of NO may induce microcirculation abnormalities in muscular regions, with muscular fatigue and exercise intolerance progressively developing in FMS.

A controlled electron microscopic study of muscle performed by Yunus failed to show any histologic abnormality that would be specific for FMS (72). Other studies that showed some changes in red fibers showed nothing pertinent to FMS (73,74) Still other studies, some showing decrements in muscle ATP and muscle oxygenation, as well as abnormal findings in the skeletal muscle of FMS patients found by nuclear magnetic resonance spectroscopy, were found to be essentially normal when general muscle deconditioning, frequently seen in FMS, was taken into consideration (75–77) The lack of peripheral muscle abnormalities was one of the reasons that attention was focused on the CNS as the source of the pain associated with FMS.

Autonomic Nervous System Dysfunction
Similar to the ANS changes found in chronic tension-type headache (see Chapter 12), FMS is also associated with changes in ANS function.

Using power spectral analysis of heart rate fluctuation, which provides a measure of ANS function in terms of quantitative beat-to-beat control of cardiovascular functioning, a study looked at sympathetic–parasympathetic balance in a group of FMS patients and a second group of NHCs. Their heart rate variability was assessed using a high-resolution electrocardiogram (EKG) although the patients were both supine and standing. Results showed significant differences between the two groups, particularly in the low-frequency band of power analysis following movement to an upright position, suggesting an abnormal sympathetic function with an impairment of the expected sympathetic vascular input after an orthostatic stress—standing up; while lying flat, the sympathetic component was significantly increased (78).

Typically, the diurnal pattern of heart rate is obtained by dividing the slow (sympathetically mediated) spectral band by the faster (parasympathetically mediated) spectral band. The ratio, normally, decreases significantly at night and rises again in the morning. In FMS patients, there appeared to be a nocturnal predominance of low-frequency component of the spectral band as compared to the controls (78).

In another study, FMS patients and controls had 24-hour ambulatory EKG recordings done to look at heart rate variability. The FMS patient group was found to have decreased heart rate variability and had lost their circadian variation of sympathetic/vagal balance. They also demonstrated an increased nocturnal predominance of the low-frequency component in the spectral analysis, which suggested an exaggerated sympathetic modulation of the sinus node (79).

Heart rate variability as a manifestation of ANS dysfunctional regulation in FMS was also documented by Clauw (80) and felt to be important by Ozgocmen et al. (81).

Tilt table testing studies have shown clinically significant decrements in the blood pressure of some patients with FMS (82).

In a randomized pilot study, norepinephrine-evoked pain was found in FMS patients, which would support the hypothesis that FMS may be a form of sympathetically maintained pain syndrome (83).

There appears to be common clinical manifestations, course of disease, and demographic characteristics of complex regional pain syndrome (CRPS), a primary sympathetic nervous system disorder, repetitive strain injury, and FMS (84).

Intramuscular hypoperfusion was noted in both regional myofascial pain and, to a lesser degree, in fibromyalgia; one theory for this being agonist-induced B-adrenergic receptor desensitization, another possible ANS dysfunction noted (85).

It has also been noted that the increased nocturnal sympathetic activity found in FMS patients may be a contributor to sleep arousal and therefore enhance poor sleep and morning fatigue, two common FMS complaints (86).

Hypocapnia has been noted in patients with FMS in 9% to 27% of patients (vs. 0–2% of controls) on tilt table testing. Hyperventilation appeared to be the major abnormal response to postural challenges via tilt table, in sustained hypocapnia. It is thought that hypocapnia is common in FMS, and capnography should be part of the FMS evaluation (87).

See Table 3 for a summary of the ANS abnormalities.

TABLE 3 Autonomic Nervous System Abnormalities in Fibromyalgia (Summary)

Abnormal sympathetic function after stress in heart rate fluctuations
↓ Heart rate variability and loss of circadian variation of sympathetic/vagal balance
↑ Noradrenergically evoked pain
↑ Nocturnal sympathetic activity

Neurotransmitter Dysfunction

5-HT, as indicated earlier, is an important part of the antinociceptive neurotransmitter systems. It is also involved in sleep and depression. It regulates circadian fluctuations of the HPA axis (88), and it appears to play a role in stimulating the release of corticotrophin-releasing factor/hormone (CRH) from the hypothalamus (89).

Its role in antinociception is of importance, as in FMS it appears that there is abnormal metabolism of 5-HT and tryptophan, its precursor. Decreased serum levels of 5-HT and decreased cerebrospinal fluid (CSF) 5-hydroxyindoleacetic acid (5-HIAA) have been found, both suggesting 5-HT deficiency (90–95). One study indicates that decreased serum 5-HT in FMS may be secondary to low levels of 5-HT in peripheral platelets (96).

The transport ratio of plasma tryptophan, an indicator of brain entry of tryptophan, has been found to be decreased (93). Twenty-four-hour 5-HIAA excretion in FMS patients is also significantly lower than that of controls (97).

While CSF 5-HT levels have not yet been reported, its precursor, 5-hydroxytryptiophan and its metabolite 5-HIAA are decreased in CSF (95,98).

Low CSF levels of the metabolite of norepinephrine, 3-methoxy-4-hydroxyphenethylene glycol (MHPG) and of dopamine and homovanillic acid (HVA) have also been found (95).

Endogenous opioids are also obvious parts of the human antinociceptive system. Beta-endorphin levels were reported to be normal in serum and CSF (99,100). A more recent study looked at peripheral blood mononuclear cell levels of beta-endorphin, which is known to be involved in the regulation of immune system function, and found that beta-endorphin concentrations were significantly lower in patients with FMS or CFS than in NHCs or depressed patients. The levels were found to be higher in the depressed patients than in the controls (101). It has been noted, because of the paucity of finding opioid changes in the serum that opioid peptides were unlikely to be involved directly with pain modulation in FMS. It was also shown that after an intravenous infusion of morphine in a double-blind, placebo-controlled study, neither pain intensity nor number of TPs in FMS patients improved (102).

Dynorphin, an opioid peptide typically found in the spinal cord (SC), is antinociceptive in low dosages (103). Increasing concentrations of dynorphin-induces protracted hyperalgesia, an effect attributed to interactions with NMDA receptors (104–106). Dynorphin is found to be increased in the CSF of FMS patients (107).

SP is an important nociceptive/excitatory neurotransmitter. It decreases the threshold of synaptic excitability, as noted in Chapter 1, and helps engender sensitization of second-order spinal cord neurons. Also, as noted earlier, activation of NMDA receptors causes increased release of SP into the spinal cord dorsal horn. This activation of NMDA receptors in the spinal cord induces release of SP and neuroplastic structural changes in the dendrites of neurons with SP receptors (108). Increased production of SP within the spinal cord in seen in the CSF of patients with pain (109). SP synthesis is upregulated in chronic, inflammatory pain conditions (110). It has been associated with the development of chronic pain and hyperalgesia, but its role in acute pain mediation appears to be small.

A significant increase in CSF SP has been found, and replicated in other studies (111–114). Russell et al. repeated the collections of CSF from 28 medication-free FMS patients an average of 12 months after they were initially evaluated. These researchers found an increase in both symptoms and CSF SP, which appeared to be correlated (115).

Finally, evidence suggested that SP levels in FMS sera were inversely correlated with levels of serum tryptophan and 5-HIAA (116).

NGF is a neurotrophin that is responsible for upregulating SP synthesis during chronic pain (117). Intravenous NGF given to humans induces muscle pain in a dose-dependent manner, affecting women more so than men (118). The mean concentration of CSF NGF is found to be elevated in patients with primary fibromyalgia, but not concomitant FMS (119).

Aside from elevated CSF SP, as noted earlier, CSF CGRP is also elevated in FMS patients (120).

Neuropeptide Y (NPY), which inhibits SP release in the spinal cord is diminished in FMS (121). Diminished NPY may help explain why there is a lack of sympathetic response to stress, such as exercise (122) and orthostatic challenge (78) in FMS.

The establishment of a number of nociceptive neurochemicals in the CSF can, perhaps, have an effect on the abnormal pain sensitivity found in FMS (123).

Yunus et al. (124) looked at a combination of several amino acids and urinary dopamine and felt that this "evaluative grouping" would better classify FMS than alone, with a sensitivity of 86% and specificity of 77% as compared to NHCs.

There are other aspects of the possible pathophysiology of FMS that may contribute to its nociceptive pathophysiology. The effects of NO were discussed earlier, including its ability to increase hyperalgesia and allodynia (57). Pall hypothesized that increased levels of NO and its oxidant product peroxynitrite in FMS, CFS, multiple chemical sensitivities, and post-traumatic stress disorder (PTSD) were significantly linked to all of the processes in a mechanistic manner (125).

Spinal cord glial cells (microglia, astrocytes, and oligodendrocytes) may contribute to abnormal pain sensitivity in FMS via release of neuroactive substances including prostaglandins, excitatory amino acids (EAAs), NGF, and NO (126). Glia are known to play key roles in neuromodulation and neuroimmunicity of the CNS (127,128). In FMS patients, it appears that there are reduced levels of CSF glial cell line-derived neurotrophic factor (GDNF), and in chronic migraineurs (129).

In FMS patients, increases over time in serum levels and/or peripheral blood mononuclear cell-stimulated activity of soluble factors, whose release was stimulated by SP, have been found. Interleukin-8 (IL-8) and IL-6 were increased in FMS patients, the latter after two years or more of FMS. IL-8 promotes sympathetic pain and IL-6 induces hyperalgesia, fatigue, and depression. They may play a role in the modulation of pain related to FMS (130).

Brain-derived neurotrophic factor (BDNF) is an endogenous protein involved in synaptic plasticity of the CNS and peripheral nervous system (PNS) as well as with the structural and functional plasticity of nociceptive pathways in the CNS and within the dorsal root ganglia and the spinal cord. Laske et al. (131) have found that mean serum levels of BDNF are significantly increased in FMS patients versus healthy controls and may increase susceptibility to pain in FMS patients.

Finally, Gi proteins are known to be involved in the modulation of pain perception (132,133). Patients with FMS were found to have hypofunction of the Gi protein systems, but this was not found in patients with neuropathic pain, RA, or OA. FMS patients also showed a higher basal level of cAMP (adenosine monophosphate) than controls (134). Gi protein hypofunction may be looked at as a possible marker of FMS. Another study found Gi protein hypofunction in both migraine and cluster headache patients (135).

See Table 4 for a summary of the neurotransmitter abnormalities.

Abnormal metabolism of serotonin
  ↓ Serum levels
  ↓ CSF levels of 5-hydroxyindoleacetic acid
  ↓ Platelet serotonin
↓ Serum beta-endorphin concentration
↑ CSF dynorphin
↑ CSF substance P
↑ CSF nerve growth factor in patients with primary fibromyalgia
↑ CSF calcitonin gene-related peptide
↓ Neuropeptide Y
↑ Interleukin 6 and 8
↑ Serum brain-derived neurotrophic factor
GI protein hypofunction

Abbreviation: CSF, cerebrospinal fluid.

Neuroendocrine Dysfunction

The mild to moderate decrements in function, or a decreased ability to react to activity in a number of the hypothalamic–pituitary–peripheral gland axes, along with alterations in ANS function in FMS appear to be a dysfunction of their ability to respond to stimuli, rather than a primary defect at the glandular level. Moreover, in a clinical sense, multiple, mild impaired responses to stimuli may induce more significant physiological and clinical difficulties than if there was a problem with a single system.

The pituitary hormone adrenocorticotropic hormone (ACTH), which is secreted in a pulsatile fashion, is stimulated by both arginine vasopressin and CRH. ACTH stimulates the adrenal glands to release cortisol, which is involved in a negative feedback loop to inhibit ACTH.

Research with FMS patients has shown that there are changes in the HPA axis. There is a decreased 24-hour urinary-free cortisol level in FMS patients (136–139). There is also a loss of diurnal cortisol fluctuation and increased evening cortisol levels noted in FMS patients (138,140).

In spite of similar cortisol levels between FMS patients and controls, there is an exaggerated ACTH response to CRH in FMS patients (139,141,142). A relative hypocortisolemia is found in relation to increased ACTH secondary, most probably, to central mechanisms (137,139,142). This response is consistent with chronically low hypothalamic CRH levels.

Also noted is a delayed release of ACTH after stimulation with IL-6. IL-6 stimulates the HPA axis by increasing its activity via stimulation of hypothalamic CRH. The delayed release is possibly secondary to a dysfunction of the hypothalamic neurons (143). It appears possible that this impairment of the hypothalamic–CRH–pituitary ACTH axis may induce a decreased cortisol response to stress.

Growth hormone (GH) is decreased in FMS patients (139,144,145). Insulin-like growth factor-1 (IGF-1) is stimulated by GH and is a primary mediator of GH action. It has been noted that symptoms common to GH deficiency are similar to some FMS symptoms: fatigue, muscle weakness, decreased cognition, and poor exercise tolerance (146). IGF-1 levels in FMS have been found to be decreased (141,147). It is not known if decreased GH levels in FMS are symptomatic of a CNS or hypothalamic induced dysfunction or if this is secondary to sleep disorder (148) [as GH is secreted during stage 3 and stage 4 sleep, which has been found to be disrupted in FMS (149)], physical deconditioning (150), low estrogen production (151), or obesity (152), all factors associated with decreased GH levels (146), Bennett et al. (153) performed a double-blind, controlled study in which FMS patients received subcutaneously injected GH. The patients who received the GH demonstrated an improvement in function, feelings of well–being, and decreased number/pain of TPs.

FMS patients generally have normal levels of thyroid-stimulating hormone (TSH) (154). Other studies have demonstrated a blunted TSH response to thyrotropin-releasing hormone (TRH) in FMS patients (141,154). Decreased free triiodothyronine has also been found (141).

Nocturnal melatonin secretion appears to be normal in FMS. Various studies have found discrepant levels—high, low, and normal, but have a number of methodological differences (155–157).

See Table 5 for summary of neuroendocrine abnormalities.

Sleep Disorders

Nonrestorative sleep is one of the most common complaints in patients with FMS. Moldofsky et al. (149) were the first to describe the sleep abnormality most commonly associated with FMS—the intrusion of fast alpha waves into slow wave (non–rapid-eye-movement) sleep, specifically into sleep stages 3 and 4, the alpha–delta sleep abnormality.

Other EEG abnormalities have also been noted—increased alpha waves in stage 1, decreased delta waves in sleep stages 3 and 4 (most indicative of nonrestorative sleep), and increased nocturnal awakenings and arousals (158–160).

The alpha–delta sleep abnormality is not found in all patients with FMS. It is not specific to FMS, as it has also been found in patients with RA and other painful chronic clinical problems (161,162).

Multiple forms of noxious stimuli applied during slow wave sleep (SWS) will induce decreased delta waves and an increase in alpha and beta wave frequencies (163). In normal subjects, auditory stimuli that disrupts SWS causes nonrefreshing sleep, fatigue, tenderness, and diffuse musculoskeletal pain. Alpha–delta sleep, along with periodic limb movement disorder, restless legs syndrome, and sleep-related breathing disorder occur in some patients with FMS, OA, and RA. There appears to be a reciprocal relationship between sleep quality and pain (163).

Functional Cerebral Abnormalities

At this time, it is possible to measure resting brain activity or the brain's response to experimental stimuli via single photon emission computed tomography (SPECT),

---

TABLE 5   Neuroendocrine Abnormalities in Fibromyalgia (Summary)

Hypothalamic-pituitary-adrenal axis changes
↓ 24-hour urinary free cortisol
↓ Diurnal cortisol fluctuation and decreased evening cortisol levels
↑ ACTH response to corticotropin releasing hormone
↓ Cortisol relative to increased ACTH
↓ Release of ACTH after stimulation of interleukin-6
↓ Growth hormone
↓ T hyroid-stimulating hormone to thyrotropin-releasing hormone
↓ Free triiodothyronine

Abbreviation: ACTH, adrenocorticotropic hormone.

positron emission tomography (PET), and functional magnetic resonance imaging (fMRI). Both PET and SPECT, after stimuli to the brain, measure changes in regional cerebral blood flow (rCBF). PET scans also show levels of neurotransmitter functioning. fMRI, after cerebral activation, shows images of pain-related changes in neuronal activity by registering signal changes of blood deoxyhemoglobin concentration and blood volume (164).

A SPECT study of FMS patients and NHCs during a resting state was performed (165). It showed that when compared to NHCs, FMS patients demonstrated significantly lower levels of rCBF (a marker for synaptic activity) in the thalamus and caudate nucleus, both of which are associated with pain modulation (166,167). Other studies have also demonstrated thalamic hypoperfusion in FMS patients and "nonpatients," community residents with FMS who had not sought medical treatment, who showed decreased caudate rCBF (167).

Normal, healthy individuals respond to painful, phasic pressure stimulation with increased rCBF in the contralateral thalamus, anterior cingulated cortex, the insula, and the primary and secondary somatosensory (SII) cortices (168). With increased stimulus intensity, bilateral activation occurs in the thalamus, anterior cingulated cortices, SII, insula, and the putamen and cerebellum (169).

One study (170) found that FMS patients demonstrated a different pattern of cerebral activation than did healthy controls to phasic, unilateral painful stimulation calibrated to the subjects' pain threshold. With right-sided stimulation, control subjects demonstrated significantly increased rCBF in the left somatosensory cortex, thalamus, and anterior cingulated cortex; FMS patients demonstrated bilateral activation of these structures. The FMS patients rated the intensity of the stimulation as twice as great as the control group, in spite of the FMS patients receiving significantly lower levels of stimulation than the controls. Patients with major depression, but not pain, demonstrated responses in rCBF to pressure stimulation that were similar to controls.

In another study (171), rCBF in FMS patients in the hemithalamic region was lower than that of NHCs.

The decreased response to pain by the thalamus and caudate in FMS patients appears to demonstrate tonically reduced activity in these regions in FMS (171).

Gracely et al. (172) utilized fMRI to evaluate the pattern of cerebral activation corresponding to painful pressure. This controlled study used 16 FMS patients and 16 matched controls, all right hand dominant. Pressure was applied to the left thumbnail beds in two conditions: "stimulus pressure control," where the FMS patients and controls received similar levels of pressure, and "subjective pain control," where the stimulus intensity was increased to deliver a subjective level of pain similar to that of patients. In the first condition, NHCs had 19 regions of increased rCBF compared to 12 regions in patients. Increased fMRI signal was found in seven similar regions in both groups. When the "subjective pain control" condition was met, with the same amount of pressure given to controls that caused pain in the FMS patients, the controls demonstrated only two regions of increased signal, neither of which coincided with an activated region in the FMS patients. Statistically, the FMS patient group had 13 regions of increased activation, as compared to one region of greater activation in this experimental condition in the control group.

These data appear to indicate that FMS is characterized by cortical or subcortical augmentation of pain processing (172) or centrally mediated abnormal pain sensitivity (173–175).

TABLE 6 Functional Cerebral Abnormalities in Fibromyalgia (Summary)

↓ Levels of rCBF in thalamus and caudate nucleus via single photon-emission
  tomography
Bilateral cerebral activation to unilateral painful stimulation, with increased rCBF
↓ Thalamic response to pain, via decreased rCBF

Abbreviation: rCBF, regional cerebral blood flow.

Psychological Abnormalities

Psychological or affective problems contribute to pain—both acute and chronic—regardless of the etiology of the pain. While acute pain may be seen more in conjunction with anxiety, chronic pain, which may induce psychological disturbances such as depression and anxiety disorders- these affective disorders may also aggravate pain in a vicious cycle. Because of the paucity of physiological/clinical findings in FMS, for many years clinicians have felt that FMS is primarily a somatoform disorder.

The frequencies of psychiatric disorders such as depression and anxiety in FMS have been found to be similar to other chronic pain-related disorders such as RA (176–179). Other studies (180,181) have demonstrated that FMS patients, as compared to RA patients, have a higher frequency of lifetime diagnoses of major depression and anxiety disorders as well as a higher familial incidence of major affective disorders. Unfortunately, the number of RA patients in the comparative studies was small, making the results less impressive.

Looking at cohorts of FMS patients compared to "nonpatients," or community members who meet the ACR criteria for FMS but are not seeking medical help, the psychiatric diagnoses were similar in both groups. It was noted that the FMS patients had a higher lifetime diagnosis of psychiatric illness than the community controls, but the diagnoses were similar in both groups. It was felt that although psychiatric disorders determined a patient's consultation with a clinician, they were not intrinsic to FMS (182,183).

Various studies note increased or similar levels of anxiety and depression in FMS patients as compared to RA patients or healthy controls (176,178,179,184,185).

Stress is of possibly greater import, as many studies show a greater degree of lifetime or daily stress/hassles in FMS patients compared to RA patients and controls (176,178,185). Recalling the changes in the HPA axis noted earlier, emotional or physical stress, possibly including an infectious illness, may contribute, in FMS patients, to enhanced abnormal pain sensitivity through their effects on abnormal neuroendocrine axes. CNS activation secondary to stress will stimulate the anterior pituitary to secrete prolactin and NGF (186). Prolactin enhances inflammatory processes, whereas NGF regulates SP expression in sensory nerves (see preceding text) and may also inhibit the antinociceptive effects of SP metabolites (187). Also associated with stress is increased production of proinflammatory cytokines such as IL-6 and tumor necrosis factor (188).

FMS patients, when compared to OA patients, note much greater increases in pain after half-hour long discussions of stressful events that are personally relevant (189).

Another study found FMS, lumbar pain, and lower extremity pain groups reporting increased physical/functional limitations, and the FMS and headache groups more psychosocial difficulties when compared to these groups and upper extremity pain, cervical pain, thoracic pain, and lower extremity pain groups (190).

It is possible that FMS patients, who may have impairments leading to blunted ACTH and epinephrine responses, may have inappropriate responses to daily stressors (191).

Depression and FMS have different psychophysiological and neuroendocrine responses. Functioning and abnormalities of the HPA axes and sleep EEG are different in FMS compared to depressed, pain-free patients (69,192). In depression, the HPA axis is hyperactive (10,193,194). The 24-hour urinary cortisol is increased in depression but not FMS (195). Essentially the HPA axis functioning in FMS is opposite to that seen in depression.

The number of positive TPs is associated with a history of past or present/ current psychological distress (196) along with abuse (197–199). Patients with depression have far fewer TPs than FMS patients (200).

Sexual assault has been associated with specific health problems including FMS, headache, chronic pelvic pain, and other pain syndromes (196,199). Depression alone does not account for poorer health in sexually assaulted women. A dose–response relationship has been postulated—more incidents of sexual or physical assault are associated with poorer health (201).

"Fibrofog" typically describes memory decline and mental confusion, neither of which is found on formal cognitive examination. It has been noted that these symptoms, along with higher levels of FMS symptom intensity and decreased mental well-being was more associated with dissociation, the separation of parts of experience from the full embodiment of consciousness (202).

Finally, it has been found that a patient given, or labeled, with the diagnosis of FMS does not show any significant adverse effects on long-term clinical outcome (203).

Genetic Factors

Pellegrino et al. (204) noted that over 50% of the first-degree relatives of a group of FMS patients had findings consistent with FMS, particularly lower pain thresholds in the female relatives (205) Buskila et al. (205) proposed that the findings were indicative of a sex-related autosomal dominant form of genetic transmission of FMS in which males showed lower penetrance.

Other work suggests a genetic impairment in a subgroup of FMS patients causing decreased ability to rapidly clear 5-HT in the synaptic cleft; the result would induce abnormal pain sensitivity secondary to changes in serotonergic neurotransmission, predominantly in women (206).

Fibromyalgia and Associated Disorders

FMS has been associated with a number of other disorders including CFS, interstitial cystitis, primary dysmenorrhea, MPS, temporomandibular myofascial dysfunction, migraine, tension-type headache, "transformed migraine" (207), IBS, periodic breathing during sleep (208), restless legs syndrome, periodic limb movement disorder, and multiple chemical sensitivity (10). Yunus has hypothesized that these syndromes are associated with each other, and were "hypersensitivity disorders" (209,210).

Rheumatological disorders with diffuse pain, which may mimic FMS include polymyalgia rheumatica, RA, SLE, inflammatory idiopathic myopathies, osteomalacia, and thyroid disease (211). FMS patients have been found to have thyroid autoimmunity with frequencies similar to RA patients and higher than controls. It was also noted that age and a postmenopausal state seemed to be associated with thyroid autoimmunity in FMS patients (212).

Associations have also been demonstrated between FMS and hepatitis C and Lyme disease (211).

Other rheumatic disorders that may overlap with or mimic FMS include OA and Sjogren's syndrome (213). The Chiari malformation (downward herniation of the cerebellar tonsils through the foramen magnum) may also present with clinical similarities to FMS (214,215). It is questioned as to whether this is a form of causality of FMS, or a concomitant disorder, like SLE, that is associated with FMS (216).

IBS has been identified in 20% to 23% of FMS patients (217). A significant association was noted between the presence of FMS and the severity of IBS (218). One study found the prevalence of IBS in FMS patients (n=105) to be 63% by Rome I criteria, and 81% by Rome II criteria (vs. placebo at 15% and 24%), showing the presence of IBS (and depressive symptoms) to be higher in FMS patients versus controls (219). IBS is also felt to be a common precipitant of CS (220).

Sjogren's syndrome is associated with the "sicca complex," or dry eyes and dry mouth. Fatigue and generalized arthralgias are also seen in this syndrome. There appears to be a moderate increase in FMS prevalence in this disorder (221,222).

FMS and Trauma
The question of the development of FMS after trauma is still unsettled.

Many of the initial reports describing post-traumatic FMS are case reports. Wolfe described a 37-year-old woman who was injured at work and then developed FMS and IBS (223). Greenfield et al. (224) reported that 14 of 127 patients self reported that their FMS began post-traumatically. Goldenberg et al. (227) reported that 33% of 332 patients diagnosed with FMS had initiating physical trauma, whereas 26% reported emotional trauma as an initiating factor and 46% had a gradual onset of FMS with no recognized initiating event.

A report indicated that 10% of a group of late whiplash syndrome patients had symptoms that conformed to the diagnosis of FMS (226).

A recent study found that whiplash injury and road accident trauma were not associated with FMS after more than 14.5 months of follow-up (227).

In 1996, a consensus report on FMS and disability indicated that the existing literature did not support a causal relationship between FMS and trauma (228).

Buskila et al. (229), in 1997, performed a controlled study comparing 102 patients who experienced cervical trauma (whiplash or industrial injury) with 59 patients who had lower extremity fractures, the majority from work-related injuries. They reported that 21.6% of the patients with neck injuries developed FMS versus 1.7% of the patients with lower extremity injuries.

Most recently, using questionnaires sent to 136 FMS patients and 152 age and sex-matched controls, it was concluded that physical trauma (in the 6 months prior to the onset of their disease) was significantly associated with the onset of FMS. Thirty-nine percent of FMS patients reported trauma compared to 24% of controls (230).

Of interest, in the publications, which appeared to be more slanted against the thought of such causation, the legal system, patients' psychological status, education, and motivation were given primary focus in causation (231,232).

Disability and Quality of Life
Patients with FMS have a significantly impaired quality of life (QOL) (233,234). One study found that the QOL of FMS patients when compared to patients with

OA, RA, chronic obstructive pulmonary disease, and insulin-dependent diabetes, was among the poorest (235). Another report indicated that FMS adversely affected work in 75% of patients, with more than 70% having familial relationships adversely affected (235).

Disability was found to be high in FMS, with more than 16% of patients receiving social security disability compared to 2.2% of the general population (236). In another study, disability in FMS patients assessed with the Health Assessment Questionnaire and simulated work tasks was found to be similar to RA patients (237).

A recent study looked at 643 female home-care workers. This study looked at the prevalence of TPs and FMS, relationships between the TP score and other signs and symptoms (including joint mobility, spinal posture and mobility, TPs, pain provocation at L4-S1, pain and pain intensity), if subgroups based on the TP score differed, and signs demonstrating the strongest correlations between disability and health. The prevalence of FMS in their cohort was 2%. They found that the TP score together with different symptoms showed strong correlation with disability (238).

Another study of working women with FMS found that the ability to remain working depended not only on work capacity limitations, but also on the capacity to adjust work environments and tasks (239).

Fibromyalgia Syndrome and Myofascial Pain Syndrome

Clinically, about 70% of FMS patients also have a local or regional MPS with associated myofascial trigger points (MTrPs) (240,241).

Initial trauma such as a slip-and-fall injury or a cervical strain/sprain from a motor vehicle injury ("whiplash") may induce a localized or regional MPS with associated MTrPs. The continuous barrage of nociceptive input from the peripherally located MTrPs centrally may induce CS with the concurrent spread of pain to other areas. CS with abnormal sensory processing may therefore play an initiating role in the onset of FMS. There may be a subgroup of patients who have a genetic susceptibility to these phenomena. There may also be a subgroup of patients who are particularly sensitive to stressors, life events, and traumas (physical and emotional) as predisposing factors in the development of FMS.

Psychosocial factors may also play a role in a subgroup of patients with the FMS/MPS complex. The idea of major life events (death of a parent or spouse, divorce, etc.) and repeated life stressors being precipitating events leading to hypervigilance and chronic activation of the ANS's "fight or flight" response may be reasonable (242). Looking at this group of factors, one author (243) felt that FMS could be a generalized form of CPRS/reflex sympathetic dystrophy. This might also lead to the possibility that in a subgroup of patients, sympathetically maintained pain may be an overlapping etiological factor in MPS and FMS.

It appears possible that MPS and FMS may overlap. Patients with multiregional MPS may be mistakenly diagnosed with FMS.

In at least one subgroup of patients, the development of an MTrP/s may be the first step in a final common pathway leading to the onset or pathoetiology of more generalized muscle pain syndromes including FMS.

These mechanisms may help to explain the frequently noted initial lack of significant physical peripheral damage being found that appears seemingly out of context in relation to the intensity of a patient's chronic pain.

It may help to note Bennett's view that chronic pain is a continuous spectrum ranging from transient local pain to widespread allodynia (242).

Finally, continuous muscle pain in fibromyalgia and in myofascial pain, post-traumatic pain, pain from muscle overload, and inflammatory pain in rheumatic disorders may be a consequence of generalized pain hypersensitivity (244). Other predisposing factors may be functioning, particularly in fibromyalgia (244).

It appears that tenderness and referred pain related to chronic musculoskeletal pain may well result from peripheral and central sensitization, which can then be instrumental in transitioning acute to chronic pain.

The fact that chronic musculoskeletal pain is associated with CS has been noted in several recent studies with regard to fibromyalgia (245–248).

Although there are no "gold standard" tests that can be performed to confirm the diagnosis of FMS, there are enough known abnormalities, in the neuroendocrine system, the ANS, and the neurotransmitter/neuropeptide systems, that this may not be so far in the future (Tables 3–5).

Pathoetiology—Hypotheses

As expressed earlier, at least some of the pathophysiological aspects of FMS are beginning to be understood. The trigger, or pathoetiology of the disorder remains unknown.

It would appear, as abnormal CNS processing does seem apparent, that there may be a number of different triggers. Some thoughts noted earlier, and some other possible triggers include the following:

1. Norepinephrine-evoked pain was found in FMS patients, which would support the hypothesis that FMS may be a form of sympathetically maintained pain syndrome (83).
2. FMS may be a neuroimmunoendocrine disorder in which there is increased release of CRH and SP from neurons found in specific muscle sites can trigger local mast cells to release proinflammatory and neurosensitizing chemicals (249).
3. FMS has been proposed to be considered a neuropathic pain syndrome. However, although there is evidence that widespread pain and tenderness in FMS is associated with chronic (central) sensitization of the CNS, there is no evidence of nerve dysfunction (the primary definition of a neuropathic pain disorder), just continuous nervous system dysfunction (250).
4. The pain in FMS, as has been discussed, may be maintained by tonic nociceptive input from deep soft tissue (muscle) as well as joints and may determine/ originate and/or maintain CS. It is also possible that the original nociceptive input is secondary to trauma or infection and the specific development of related hyperalgesia/allodynia and/or CS (251). The initiation and/or maintenance of CS secondary to nociception originating peripherally is appearing more likely. Continued, persistent peripheral nociception can induce neuroplastic changes in the spinal cord and the brain, leading to both CS and pain (252). After the development of pain associated with CS, only continued minimal nociceptive input is necessary to maintain it. Finally, although a great deal of importance has been given to CS, peripheral factors including average/maximal pain and the number of painful body areas do contribute to the variance of the overall FMS pain, making such peripheral nociception clinically relevant (253).
5. Early data shows a possible suppression of presynaptic dopaminergic activity with concurrent suppression of dopamine activity in the limbic system (254,255).

REFERENCES

1. Reynolds MD. The development of the concept of fibrositis. J Hist Med Allied Sci 1983; 38:5–35.
2. Simons DG. Muscle pain syndrome-Part 1. Am J Phys Med 1975; 54:289–311.
3. Gowers WR. Lumbago: its lessons and analogues. BMJ 1904; 1:117–121.
4. Traut EF. Fibrositis. J Am Geriatr Soc 1968; 16:531–538.
5. Yunus MB, Masi AT, Calabro JJ, et al. Primary fibromyalgia (fibrositis): clinical study of 50 patients with matched normal controls. Semin Arthritis Rheum 1981; 11:151–171.
6. Wolfe F, Smythe HA, Yunus MB, et al. The American College of Rheumatology 1990 criteria for the classification of fibromyalgia. Report of the Multicenter Criteria Committee. Arthritis Rheum 1990; 33:160–172.
7. Goldenberg DL. Fibromyalgia syndrome: An emerging but controversial condition. JAMA 1987; 257:2782–2787.
8. Bengtsson A, Henriksson KG, Jorfeldt L, et al. Primary fibromyalgia. A clinical and laboratory study of 55 patients. Scand J Rheumatol 1986; 40:340–347.
9. Wolfe F, Ross K, Anderson J, et al. The prevalence and characteristics of fibromyalgia in the general population. Arthritis Rheum 1995; 38:19–28.
10. Yunus MB, Inanici F. Fibromyalgia syndrome: Clinical features, diagnosis and biopatho-physiologic mechanisms. In: Rachlin ES, Rachlin IS, eds. Myofascial Pain and Fibromyalgia: Trigger point management. 2nd ed. St. Louis, Mo: Mosby, 2002:3–31.
11. Wolfe F. The fibromyalgia problem. J Rheumatol 1997; 24:1247–1249.
12. Barsky AJ, Borus JF. Functional somatic syndromes. Ann Intern Med 1999; 130:910–921.
13. Hadler NM. Fibromyalgia: la maladie est morte. Vive le malade! J Rheumatol 1997; 24:1250–1251.
14. Lawrence RC, Hochberg MC, Kelsey JL, et al. Estimates of prevalence of selected arthritic and musculoskeletal diseases in the United States. J Rheumatol 1989; 16:427–441.
15. Magni G, Marchetti M, Moreschi C, et al. Chronic musculoskeletal pain and depressive symptoms in the National Health and Nutrition Examination. I. Epidemiologic follow-up study. Pain 1993; 53:163–168.
16. Wolfe F, Ross K, Anderson J, et al. The prevalence and characteristics of fibromyalgia in the general population. Arthritis Rheum 1995; 38:19–28.
17. White KP, Harth M. The occurrence and impact of generalized pain. Baillieres Clin Rheumatol 1999; 13:379–389.
18. Croft P, Schollum J, Silman A. Population study of tender point counts and pain as evidence of fibromyalgia. BMJ 1994; 309:696–699.
19. White KP, Speechley M, Harth M, et al. Comparing self-reported function and work disability in 100 random community cases of fibromyalgia versus control in London, Ontario: the London Fibromyalgia Epidemiology Study. Arthritis Rheum 1999; 42:76–83.
20. White DP, Speechley M, Harth M, et al. The London Fibromyalgia Epidemiology Study: comparing the demographic and clinical characteristics in 100 random community cases of fibromyalgia versus controls. J Rheumatol 1999; 26:1577–1585.
21. White KP, Harth M, Speechley M, et al. A general population study of fibromyalgia tender points in non-institutionalized adults with chronic widespread pain. J Rheumatol 2000; 27:2677–2682.
22. White DP, Harth M. Classification, epidemiology and natural history of fibromyalgia. Curr Pain Headache Rep 2001; 5:320–329.
23. Russell IJ. Is fibromyalgia a distinct clinical entity? The clinical investigators evidence. Ballieres Best Pract Res Clin Rheumatol 1999; 13:445–454.
24. Roizenblatt S, Tufik S, Goldenberg J, et al. Juvenile fibromyalgia: clinical and polysom-nographic aspects. J Rheumatol 1997; 24:579–585.
25. Yunus MB, Masi AT. Juvenile primary fibromyalgia syndrome. Arthritis Rheum 1985; 28:138–144.
26. Yunus MB, Holt GS, Masi AT, et al. Fibromyalgia syndrome among the elderly: compar-ison with younger patients. J Am Geriatr Soc 1988; 35:987–995.

27. Wolfe F, Ross K, Anderson J, et al. The prevalence and characteristics of fibromyalgia in the general population. Arthritis Rheum 1995; 38:19–28.

28. Raphael KG, Janal MN, Nayak S, et al. Psychiatric comorbidities in a community sample of women with fibromyalgia. Pain 2006; 124(1–2):117–125.

29. White KP, Speechley M, Harth M, Ostbye T. The London Fibromyalgia Epidemiology Study: the prevalence of fibromyalgia syndrome in London, Ontario. J Rheumatol 1999; 26:1570–1576.

30. McNally JD, Matheson DA, Bakowsky VS. The epidemiology of self-reported fibromyalgia in Canada. Chronic Dis Can 2006; 27(1):9–16.

31. Weir PT, Harlan GA, Nkoy FL, et al. The incidence of fibromyalgia and its associated comorbidities: a population-based retrospective cohort study based on International Classification of Diseases, 9th Revision codes. J Clin Rheumatol 2006; 12(3):124–128.

32. Ifergane G, Buskila D, Simiseshvely N, et al. Prevalence of fibromyalgia syndrome in migraine patients. Cephalalgia 2006; 26(4):451–456.

33. Bennett RM. Fibromyalgia and the disability dilemma. A new era in understanding a complex, multidimensional pain syndrome. Arthritis Rheum 1996; 39(10):1627–1634.

34. Reilly PA, Littlejohn GO. Peripheral arthralgic presentation of fibrositis/fibromyalgia syndrome. J Rheumatol 1992; 19:281–283.

35. Yunus MB, Inanici F, Aldag JC, Mangold RF. Fibromyalgia in men: comparison of clinical features with women. J Rheumatol 2000; 27:485–490.

36. Moldofsky H. Chronobiological influences on fibromyalgia syndrome: theoretical and therapeutic implications. Baillieres Clin Rheumatol 1994; 8:801–810.

37. Tunks E, McCain GA, Hart LE, et al. The reliability of examination for tenderness in patients with myofascial pain, chronic fibromyalgia and controls. J Rheumatol 1995; 22:944–952.

38. Russell IJ, Vipraio GA, Morgan WW, Bowden CL. Is there a metabolic basis for the fibrositis syndrome? Am J Med 1986; 81:50–56.

39. Russell IJ. The reliability of algometry in the assessment of patients with fibromyalgia syndrome. J Musculoskel Pain 1998; 6:139–152.

40. Yunus MB. Gender differences in fibromyalgia and other related syndromes. J Gend Specif Med 2002; 5(2):42–47.

41. Buskila D, Neumann L, Alhoashle A, Abu-Shakra M. Fibromyalgia syndrome in men. Semin Arthritis Rheum 2000; 30:47–51.

42. Wolfe F, Ross K, Anderson J, Russell IJ. Aspects of fibromyalgia in the general population: sex, pain threshold and fibromyalgia symptoms. J Rheumatol 1995; 22(1):151–156.

43. Inanici F, Yunus MB, Aldag JC. Psychological features in men with fibromyalgia syndrome [abstr]. Ann Rheum Dis 2000; 59(suppl 1):62.

44. Celentano DD, Linet MS, Stewart WF. Gender differences in the experience of headache. Soc Sci Med 1990; 30:1289–1295.

45. Mehendale AW, Goldman MP. Fibromyalgia syndrome, idiopathic widespread persistent pain of syndrome of myalgic encephalomyelopathy (SME): what is its nature? Pain Practice 2002; 2(1):35-46.

46. Wigers SH. Fibromyalgia- an update. Tidsskr Nor Laegeforen 2002; 122:1300–1304.

47. Smitherman SR. Peripheral and central sensitization in fibromyalgia: pathogenetic role. Curr Pain Headache Rep 2002; 6(4):259–266.

48. Staud R. Evidence of involvement of central neural mechanisms in generating fibromyalgia pain. Curr Rheumatol Rep 2002; 4(4): 299–305.

49. Malt EA, Olafsson S, Lund A, Ursin H. Factors explaining variance in perceived pain in women with fibromyalgia. BMC Musculoskelet Disord 2002; 3:12–16.

50. Staud R, Domingo M. Evidence for abnormal pain processing in fibromyalgia syndrome. Pain Med 2001; 2(3):208–215.

51. Hurtig IM, Raak RI, Kendall SA, et al. Quantitative sensory testing in fibromyalgia patients and in healthy subjects: identification of subgroups. Clin J Pain 2001; 17(4): 316–322.

52. Granot M, Buskila D, Granovsky Y, et al. Simultaneous recording of late and ultra-late pain evoked potentials in fibromyalgia. Clin Neurophys 2001; 112(10):1881–1887.

53. Montoya P, Sitges C, Garcia-Herrera M, et al. Reduced brain habituation to somatosensory stimulation in patients with fibromyalgia. Arthritis Rheum 2006; 54(6):1995–2003.

54. Berglund B, Harju E, Kosek E, Lindblom U. Quantitative and qualitative perceptual analysis of cold dysesthesia and hyperalgesia in fibromyalgia. Pain 2002; 96:177–187.
55. Simms RW, Roy SH, Hrovat M, et al. Lack of association between fibromyalgia syndrome and abnormalities in muscle energy metabolism. Arthritis Rheum 1994; 37: 794–800.
56. De Stefano R, Selvi E, Villanova M, et al. Image analysis quantification of substance P immunoreactivity in the trapezius muscle of patients with fibromyalgia and myofascial pain syndrome. J Rheumatol 2000; 27:2906–2910.
57. Staud R, Smitherman ML. Peripheral and central sensitization in fibromyalgia: pathogenetic role. Curr Pain Headache Rep 2002; 6:259–266.
58. Kim SH, Jang TJ, Moon IS. Increased expression of N-methyl-D-aspartate receptor subunit 2D in the skin of patients with fibromyalgia. J Rheumatol 2006; 33(4): 785–788.
59. Woolf CJ, Thompson SW. The induction and maintenance of central sensitization is dependent on N-methyl-D-aspartic acid receptor activation; implications for the treatment of post-injury pain hypersensitivity states. Pain 1991; 44:293–299.
60. Stein C, Machelska H, Binder W, Schafer M. Peripheral opioid analgesia. Curr Opin Pharmacol 2001; 1:62–65.
61. Brenman JE, Bredt DS. Synaptic signaling by nitric oxide. Curr Opin Neurobiol 1997; 7:374–378.
62. Schuman EM, Madison DV. Nitric oxide and synaptic function. Ann Rev Neurosci 1994; 17:153–183.
63. Aimar P, Pasti L, Carmignoto G, Merighi A. Nitric oxide-producing islet cells modulate the release of sensory neuropeptides in the rat substantia gelatinosa. J Neurosci 1998; 18:10357–10388.
64. Price DD, Mao J, Frenk H, Mayer DJ. The N-methyl-D-aspartate receptor antagonist dextromethorphan selectively reduces temporal summation of second pain in man. Pain 1994; 59:165–174.
65. Price DD, Hu JW, Dubner R, Gracely RH. Peripheral suppression of first pain and central summation of second pain evoked by noxious heat pulses. Pain 1977; 3:57–68.
66. Price DD. Characteristics of second pain and flexion reflexes indicative of prolonged central summation. Exp Neurol 1972; 37:371–387.
67. Sorensen J, Bengtsson A, Backman E, et al. Pain analysis in patients with fibromyalgia. Effects of intravenous morphine, lidocaine, and ketamine. Scand J Rheumatol 1995; 24:360–365.
68. Graven-Nielsen T, Kendall SA, Henriksson KG, et al. Ketamine reduces muscle pain, temporal summation and referred pain in fibromyalgia patients. Pain 2000; 85: 483–491.
69. Yunus MB, Inanici F. Clinical characteristics and biopathophyisological mechanisms of fibromyalgia syndrome. In: Baldry PE, ed. Myofascial Pain and Fibromyalgia Syndrome. London, UK: Churchill Livingstone. 2001:351–378.
70. Elvin A, Siosteen AK, Nilsson A, Kosek E. Decreased muscle blood flow in fibromyalgia patients during standardized muscle exercise: a contrast media enhanced colour Doppler study. Eur J Pain 2006; 10(2):137–144.
71. Kasikcioglu E, Dinler M, Berker E. Reduced tolerance of exercise in fibromyalgia may be a consequence of impaired microcirculation initiated by deficient action of nitric oxide. Med Hypotheses 2006; 66(5):950–952.
72. Yunus MB, Kalyan-Raman UP, Masi AT, et al. Electron microscopic studies of muscle biopsy in primary fibromyalgia syndrome: a controlled and blinded study. J Rheumatol 1989; 16:97–101.
73. Bengtsson A, Henriksson KG, Larsson J. Muscle biopsy in primary fibromyalgia: light microscopical and histochemical findings. Scand J Rheumatol 1986; 15:106.
74. Drewes AM, Andreasen A, Schroder HD, et al. Muscle biopsy in fibromyalgia. Scand J Rheumatol 1992; 94(suppl):20.
75. Bengtsson A, Henriksson KG, Larsson J. Reduced high-energy phosphate levels in the painful muscles of patients with primary fibromyalgia. Arthritis Rheum 1986; 29:817–821.
76. Simms RW. Fibromyalgia is not a muscle disorder. Am J Med Sci 1998; 315:346–350.

77. Simms RW. Is there muscle pathology in fibromyalgia syndrome? Rheum Dis Clin North Am 1996; 22:245–266.
78. Martinez-Lavin M, Hermosillo AG, Mendoza C, et al. Orthostatic sympathetic derangement in subjects with fibromyalgia. J Rheumatol 1997; 24(4):714–718.
79. Martinez-Lavin M, Hermosillo AG, Rosas M, Soto ME. Circadian studies of autonomic nervous balance in patients with fibromyalgia: a heart rate variability analysis. Arthritis Rheum 1998; 41:1966–1971.
80. Clauw DJ, Radulovic D, Heshmat Y, Barbey JT. Heart rate variability as a measure of autonomic function in patients with fibromyalgia (FM) and chronic fatigue syndrome (CSF) [abstr]. J Musculoskel Pain 1995; 3(suppl 1):78.
81. Ozgocmen S, Yoldas T, Yigiter R, Kaya A, Ardicoglu O. R-R interval variation and sympathetic skin response in fibromyalgia. Arch Med Res 2006; 37(5):630–634.
82. Bou-Holaigah I, Calkins H, Flynn JA, et al. Provocation of hypotension and pain during upright tilt table testing in adults with fibromyalgia. Clin Exp Rheumatol 1997; 15: 239–246.
83. Martinez-Lavin M, Vidal M, Barbosa RE, et al. Norepinephrine-evoked pain in fibromyalgia. A randomized pilot study. BMC Musculoskelet Disord 2002; 3:2.
84. Marinus J, Van Hilten JJ. Clinical expression profiles of complex regional pain syndrome, fibromyalgia and a-specific repetitive strain injury: more common denominators than pain? Disabil Rehabil 2006; 28(6):351–362.
85. Maekawa K, Clark GT, Kuboki T. Intramuscular hypoperfusion, adrenergic receptors, and chronic muscle pain. J Pain 2002; 3(4):251–260.
86. Bonnet MH, Arand DL. Heart rate variability: sleep stage, time of night, and arousal influences. Electroencephalogr Clin Neurophysiol 1997; 102:390–396.
87. Naschitz JE, Mussafia-Priselac R, Kovalev Y, et al. Patterns of hypocapnia on tilt in patients with fibromyalgia, chronic fatigue syndrome, nonspecific dizziness, and neurally mediated syncope. Am J Med Sci 2006; 331(6):295–303.
88. Krieger DT, Rizzo F. Serotonin mediation of circadian periodicity of plasma 17-hydroxycorticosteroids. Am J Physiol 1969; 217:1703–1707.
89. Holms MC, Di Renzo G, Beckford U, et al. Role of serotonin in the control of secretion of corticotrophin releasing factor. J Endocrinol 1982; 93:151–160.
90. Wolfe F, Russell IJ, Vipraio G, et al. Serotonin levels, pain threshold and fibromyalgia symptoms in the general population. J Rheumatol 1997; 24:555–559.
91. Russell IJ, Michalek JE, Vipraio GA, et al. Serum amino acids in fibrositis/fibromyalgia syndrome. J Rheumatol 1989; 19(suppl):158–163.
92. Russell IJ, Michalek, Vipraio GA, et al. Platelet 3H-imipramine uptake receptor density and serum serotonin levels in patients with fibromyalgia/fibrositis syndrome. J Rheumatol 1992; 19:104–109.
93. Yunus MB, Dailey JW, Aldag JC, et al. Plasma tryptophan and other amino acids in primary fibromyalgia: a controlled study. J Rheumatol 1992; 19:90–94.
94. Yunus MB, Dailey JW, Aldag JC, et al. Plasma and urinary catecholamines in primary fibromyalgia: a controlled study. J Rheumatol 1992; 19:95–97.
95. Russell IJ, Vaeroy H, Javors M, Nyberg F. Cerebrospinal fluid biogenic amine metabolites in fibromyalgia/fibrositis syndrome and rheumatoid arthritis. Arthritis Rheum 1992; 35:550–556.
96. Russell IJ, Vipraio GA. Serotonin (5HT) in serum and platelets (PLT) from fibromyalgia patients (FS) and normal controls (NC) [abstr]. Arthritis Rheum 1994; 37(suppl):S214.
97. Kang Y-K, Russell IJ, Vipraio GA, Acworth IN. Low urinary 5-hydroxyindole acetic acid in fibromyalgia syndrome: evidence in support of a serotonin-deficiency pathogenesis. Myalgia 1998; 1:14–21.
98. Russell IJ, Vipraio GA, Acworth I. Abnormalities in the central nervous system (CNS) metabolism of tryptophan (TRY) to 3-hydroxy kynurenine (OHKY) in fibromyalgia syndrome (FS) [abstr]. Arthritis Rheum 1993; 36:S222.
99. Yunus MB, Denko CW, Masi AT. Serum beta-endorphin in primary fibromyalgia syndrome: a controlled study. J Rheum 1986; 13(1):183–186.
100. Vaeroy H, Helle R, Forre O, et al. Cerebrospinal fluid levels of B-endorphin in patients with fibromyalgia (fibrositis syndrome). J Rheum 1988; 15:1804–1806.

101. Panerai AE, Vecchiet J, Panzeri P, et al. Peripheral blood mononuclear cell B-endorphin concentration is decreased in chronic fatigue syndrome and fibromyalgia but not in depression: Preliminary report. Clin J Pain 2002; 18(4):270–273.

102. Sorensen J, Bengtsson A, Backman E, et al. Pain analysis in patients with fibromyalgia. Effects of intravenous morphine, lidocaine and ketamine. Scand J Rheumatol 1995; 24(6):360–365.

103. Han JS, Xie CW. Dynorphin: potent analgesic effect in spinal cord of the rat. Life Sci 1982; 31:1781–1784.

104. Vanderah T, Laughlin T, Lashbrook J, et al. Single intrathecal injections of dynorphin A or des-Tyr-dynorphins produce long lasting allodynia in rats: blockade by MK-801 but not naloxone. Pain 1996; 68:275–281.

105. Laughlin TM, Vanderah T, Lashbrook JM, et al. Spinally administered dynorphin A produces long lasing allodynia: involvement of NMDA but not opioid receptors. Pain 1997; 72:253–260.

106. Laughlin TM, Larson AA, Wilcox GL. Mechanisms of induction of persistent nociception by dynorphin. J Pharmacol Exp Ther 2001; 299(1):6–11.

107. Vaeroy H, Nyberg F, Terenius L. No evidence for endorphin deficiency in fibromyalgia following investigation of cerebrospinal fluid (CSF) dynorphin A and Met-enkephalin-Arg6-Phe7. Pain 1991; 46:139–143.

108. Coderre TJ, Katz J, Vaccarino AL, Melzack R. Contribution of central neuroplasticity to pathological pain: review of clinical and experimental evidence. Pain 1993; 52: 259–285.

109. Tsigos C, Diemel LT, White A, et al. Cerebrospinal fluid levels of substance P and calcitonin-gene-related peptide: correlation with sural nerve levels and neuropathic signs in sensory diabetic polyneuropathy. Clin Sci (Colch) 1993; 84:305–311.

110. Galeazza MT, Garry MG, Yost HJ, et al. Plasticity in the synthesis and storage of substance P and calcitonin gene-related peptide in primary afferent neurons during peripheral inflammation. Neuroscience 1995; 66:443–458.

111. Vaeroy H, Helle R, Forre O, et al. Elevated CSF levels of substance P and high incidence of Raynaud's phenomenon in patients with fibromyalgia: new features for diagnosis. Pain 1988; 32:21–26.

112. Russell IJ, Orr MD, Littman B, et al. Elevated cerebrospinal fluid levels of substance P in patients with the fibromyalgia syndrome. Arthritis Rheum 1994; 37:1593–1601.

113. Welin M, Bragee B, Nyberg F, Kristiansson M. Elevated substance P levels are contrasted by a decrease in met-enkephalin-arg-phe levels in CSF from fibromyalgia patients. J Musculoskel Pain 1995; 3:4.

114. Bradley LA, Alberts KR, Alarcon GS, et al. Abnormal brain regional cerebral blood flow (rCBF) and cerebrospinal fluid (CSF) levels of substance P (SP) in patients and non-patients with fibromyalgia (FM). Arthritis Rheum1996; 39(suppl 19):S212.

115. Russell IJ, Fletcher EM, Vipraio GA, et al. Cerebrospinal fluid (CSF) substance P (SP) in fibromyalgia: changes in CSF SP over time parallel changes in clinical activity [abstr]. J Musculoskel Pain 1998; 6(suppl 2):77.

116. Schwarz MJ, Spath M, Muller-Bardorff H, et al. Relationship of substance P, 5-hydroxyindole acetic acid and tryptophan in serum of fibromyalgia patients. Neurosci Lett 1999; 259:196–198.

117. Lindsay RM, Harmar AJ. Nerve growth factor regulates expression of neuropeptides genes in adult sensory neurons. Nature 1989; 337:362–364.

118. Petty BG, Cornblath DR, Adornato BT, et al. The effect of systemically administered recombinant human nerve growth factor in healthy human subjects. Ann Neurol 1994; 36:244–246.

119. Giovengo SL, Russell IJ, Larson AA. Increased concentrations of nerve growth factor in cerebrospinal fluid of patient with fibromyalgia. J Rheumatol 1999; 26:1564–1596.

120. Vaeroy H, Sakurada T, Forre O, et al. Modulation of pain in fibromyalgia (fibrositis syndrome): cerebrospinal fluid (CSF) investigation of pain related neuropeptides with special reference to calcitonin gene-related peptide (CGRP). J Rheumatol Suppl 1989; 19:94–97.

121. Crofford LJ, Pillemer SR, Kalogeras KT, et al. Hypothalamic-pituitary-adrenal axis perturbations in patients with fibromyalgia. Arthritis Rheum 1994; 37(11):1583–1592.

122. van Denderen JC, Boersma JW, Zeinstra P, et al. Physiological effects of exhaustive physical exercise in primary fibromyalgia syndrome (PFS): is PFS a disorder of neuroendocrine reactivity? Scand J Rheumatol 1992; 21(1):35–37.

123. Pillemer SR, Bradley LA, Crofford LJ, et al. The neuroscience and endocrinology of fibromyalgia. Arthritis Rheum 1997; 40:1928–1939.

124. Yunus MB, Aldag JC, Dailey JW, Jobe PC. Interrelationships of biochemical parameters in classification of fibromyalgia syndrome and healthy normal controls. J Musculoskel Pain 1995; 3(4):15–24.

125. Pall ML. Common etiology of posttraumatic stress disorder, fibromyalgia, chronic fatigue syndrome and multiple chemical sensitivity via elevated nitric oxide/peroxynitrite. Med Hypotheses 2001; 57(2):139–145.

126. Watkins LR, Milligan ED, Maier SF. Glial activation: a driving force for pathological pain. Trends Neurosci 2001; 24:450–455.

127. Kreutzberg GW. Microglia: a sensor for pathological events in the CNS. Trends Neurosci 1996; 19:312–318.

128. Raivich G, Bluethmann H, Kreutzberg GW. Signaling molecules and neuroglial activation in the injured central nervous system. Keio J Med 1996; 45:239–247.

129. Sarchielli P, ALberti A, Candeliere A, et al. Glial cell line-derived neurotrophic factor and somatostatin levels in cerebrospinal fluid of patients affected by chronic migraine and fibromyalgia. Cephalalgia 2006; 26(4):409–415.

130. Wallace DJ, Linker-Israeli M, Hallegua D, et al. Cytokines play an aetiopathogenetic role in fibromyalgia: a hypothesis and pilot study. Rheumatology 2001; 40:743–749.

131. Laske C, Stransky E, Eschweiler GW, et al. Increased BDNF serum concentration in fibromyalgia with or without depression or antidepressants. J Psychiatr Res 2007; 41(7):600–605.

132. Yaksh TL. Pharmacology and mechanisms of opioid analgesic activity. In: Yaksh TL, Lynch C III, Zapol WM, Maze M, et al., eds. Anesthesia: Biologic Foundations. Philadelphia, Pa: Lippincott-Raven, 1997:921–934.

133. Carter BD, Medzihradsky F. Go mediates the coupling of the mu opioid receptor to adenyl cyclase in cloned neural cells and brain. Proc Natl Acad Sci USA 1993; 90:4062–4066.

134. Galeotti N, Ghelardini C, Zoppi M, et al. A reduced functionality of Gi proteins as a possible cause of fibromyalgia. J Rheumatol 2001; 28:2298–2304.

135. Galeotti N, Ghelardini C, Zoppi M, et al. Hypofunctionality of Gi proteins as aetiopathogenic mechanism for migraine and cluster headache. Cephalalgia 2001; 21:38–45.

136. Lentjes EGWM, Griep EN, Boersma, JW, et al. Glucocorticoid receptors, fibromyalgia and low back pain. Psychoneuroendocrinology 1997; 22(8):603–614.

137. Crofford LJ, Demitrack MA. Evidence that abnormalities of central neurohormonal systems are key to understanding fibromyalgia and chronic fatigue syndrome. Rheum Dis Clin North Am 1996; 22:267–284.

138. Crofford LJ, Pillemer SR, Kalogeras KT, et al. Hypothalamic-pituitary-adrenal axis perturbations in patients with fibromyalgia. Arthritis Rheum 1994; 37:1583–1592.

139. Griep EN, Boersma JW, Lentjes EG, et al. Function of the hypothalamic-pituitary-adrenal axis in patients with fibromyalgia and low back pain. J Rheumatol 1998; 25(7):1374–1381.

140. McCain GA, Tilbe KS. Diurnal variation in fibromyalgia syndrome: a comparison with rheumatoid arthritis. J Rheumatol 1989; 19(suppl):154–157.

141. Riedel W, Kayka H, Neeck G. Secretory pattern of GH, TSH, thyroid hormones, ACTH, cortisol, FSH and LH in patients with fibromyalgia syndrome following systemic injection of the relevant hypothalamic-releasing hormones. Z Rheumatol 1998; 57(suppl 2):81–87.

142. Griep EN, Boersma JW, de Kloet ER. Altered reactivity of the hypothalamic-pituitary-adrenal axis in the primary fibromyalgia syndrome. J Rheumatol 1993; 20:469–474.

143. Torpy DJ, Papanicolaou DA, Lotsikas AJ, et al. Responses of the sympathetic nervous system and the hypothalamic-pituitary-adrenal axis to interleukin-6: a pilot study in fibromyalgia. Arthritis Rheum 2000; 43:872–880.

144. Leal-Cerro A, Povedano J, Astroga R, et al. The growth hormone (GH)-releasing hormone-GH-insulin-like growth factor-1 axis in patients with fibromyalgia syndrome. J Clin Endocrinol Metab 1999; 84:3378–3381.

145. Bagge E, Bengtsson BA, Carlsson L, Carlsson J. Low growth hormone secretion in patients with fibromyalgia- a preliminary report on 10 patients and 10 controls. J Rheumatol 1998; 25:145–148.
146. Adler GK, Manfredsdottir VF, Creskoff KW. Neuroendocrine abnormalities in fibromyalgia. Curr Pain Headache Rep 2002; 6:289–298.
147. Bennett RM, Clark SR, Burckhardt CS, Campbell SM. Hypothalamic-pituitary-insulin-like growth factor-1 axis dysfunction in patients with fibromyalgia. J Rheumatol 1997; 24(7):1384–1389.
148. Van Cauter E, Plat L, Copinschi G. Interrelations between sleep and the somatotopic axis. Sleep 1998; 21(6):553–566.
149. Moldofsky H, Scarisbrick P, England R, et al. Musculoskeletal symptoms and non-REM sleep disturbance in patients with "fibrositis" syndrome and healthy subjects. Psychosom Med 1975; 37:341–351.
150. Kato Y, Murakami Y, Sohmiya M, Nishiki M. Regulation of human growth hormone secretion and its disorders. Intern Med 2002; 41(1):7–13.
151. Anderson SM, Shah N, Evans WS, et al. Short-term estradiol supplementation augments growth hormone (GH) secretory responsiveness to dose-varying GH-releasing peptide infusions in healthy post-menopausal women. J Clin Endocrinol Metab 2001; 86(2):551–560.
152. Cordido F, Dieguez C, Casanueva FF. Effect of central cholinergic neurotransmission enhancement by pyridostigmine on the growth hormone secretion elicited by clonidine, arginine or hypoglycemia in normal and obese subjects. J Clin Endocrinol Metab 1990; 70(5):1361–1370.
153. Bennett RM, Cook DM, Clark SR, et al. Hypothalamic-pituitary-insulin-like growth factor-1 axis dysfunction in patients with fibromyalgia. J Rheumatol 1997; 24:1384–1389.
154. Neeck G, Riedel W. Thyroid function in patients with fibromyalgia syndrome. J Rheumatol 1992; 19:1120–1122.
155. Press J, Phillip M, Neumann L, et al. Normal melatonin levels in patients with fibromyalgia syndrome. J Rheumatol 1998; 25:551–555.
156. Korszun A, Sackett-Lundeen L, Papadopoulos E, et al. Melatonin levels in women with fibromyalgia and chronic fatigue syndrome. J Rheumatol 1999; 26:2675–2680.
157. Wikner J, Hirsch U, Wetterberg L, Rodjmark S. Fibromyalgia: a syndrome associated with decreased nocturnal melatonin secretion. Clin Endocrinol 1998; 49(2):179–183.
158. Branco JC, Atalaia A, Paiva T. Sleep cycles and alpha-delta sleep in fibromyalgia syndrome. J Rheumatol 1994; 21:1113–1117.
159. Drewes AM, Gade J, Nielsen KD, et al. Clustering of sleep electroencephalopathic patterns in patients with the fibromyalgia syndrome. Br J Rheumatol 1995; 34:1151–1156.
160. Perlis ML, Giles DE, Bootzin RR, et al. Alpha sleep and information processing, perception of sleep, pain and arousability in fibromyalgia. Int J Neurosci 1997; 89:265–280.
161. Moldofsky H, Lue FA, Smythe HA. Alpha EEG sleep and morning symptoms in rheumatoid arthritis. J Rheumatol 1983; 10:373–379.
162. Moldofsky H, Saskin P, Lue FA. Sleep symptoms in fibrositis syndrome after a febrile illness. J Rheumatol 1988; 15:1701–1704.
163. Moldofsky H. Sleep and pain. Sleep Med Rev 2001; 5(5):385–396.
164. Binder JR, Swanson SJ, Hammeke TE, et al. Determination of language dominance using functional MRI: a comparison with the Wada test. Neurology 1996; 46:978–984.
165. Mountz JM, Bradley LA, Modell JG, et al. Fibromyalgia in women. Abnormalities of regional cerebral blood flow in the thalamus and the caudate nucleus are associated with low pain threshold levels. Arthritis Rheum 1995; 38:926–938.
166. Lineberry CG, Vierck CJ. Attenuation of pain reactivity by caudate nucleus stimulation in monkeys. Brain Res 1975; 98:119–134.
167. Bradley LA, Sotolongo A, Alberts KR, et al. Abnormal regional cerebral blood flow in the caudate nucleus among fibromyalgia patients and non-patients is associated with insidious symptom onset. J Musculoskel Pain 1999; 7:285–292.
168. Coghill RC, Talbot JD, Evans AC, et al. Distributed processing of pain and vibration by the human brain. J Neurosci 1994; 14:4095–4108.
169. Coghill RC, Sang CN, Maisog JM, Iadarola MJ. Pain intensity processing within the human brain: a bilateral, distributed mechanism. J Neurophysiol 1999; 82:1934–1943.

170. Cianfrini LR, McKendree-Smith NL, Bradley LA, et al. Pain sensitivity and bilateral activation of brain structures during pressure stimulation of patients with fibromyalgia (FM) is not mediated by major depression (DEP). Arthritis Rheum 2001; 44:S395.
171. Mountz JM, Bradley LA, Alarcon GS. Abnormal functional activity of the central nervous system in fibromyalgia syndrome. Am J Med Sci 1998; 315:385–396.
172. Gracely RH, Petzke F, Wolf JM, Clauw DJ. Functional magnetic resonance imaging evidence of augmented pain processing in fibromyalgia. Arthritis Rheum 2002; 46(5):1333–1344.
173. Pillemer SR, Bradley LA, Crofford LJ, et al. The neuroscience and endocrinology of fibromyalgia. Arthritis Rheum 1997; 40:1928–1939.
174. Weigent DA, Bradley LA, Blalock JE, Alarcon GS. Current concepts in the pathophysiology of abnormal pain perception in fibromyalgia. Am J Med Sci 1998; 315:405–412.
175. Pauli P, Wiedemann G, Nickola M. Pain sensitivity, cerebral laterality, and negative affect. Pain 1999; 80:359–364.
176. Ahles TA, Yunus MB, Masi AT. Is chronic pain a variant of depressive disease? The case of primary fibromyalgia syndrome. Pain 1987; 29:105–111.
177. Ahles TA, Khan SA, Yunus MB, et al. Psychiatric status of patients with primary fibromyalgia, patients with rheumatoid arthritis and subjects without pain: a blind comparison of DSM-III diagnoses. Am J Psychiatry 1991; 148:1721–1726.
178. Clark S, Campbell SM, Forehand ME, et al. Clinical characteristics of fibrositis. II. A "blinded," controlled study using standard psychological tests. Arthritis Rheum 1985; 28:132–137.
179. Kirmayer LJ, Robbins JM, Kapusta MA. Somatization and depression in fibromyalgia syndrome. Am J Psychiatry 1988; 145:950–954.
180. Hudson JI, Hudson MS, Pliner LF, et al. Fibromyalgia and major affective disorder: a controlled phenomenology and family history study. Am J Psychiatry 1985; 142:441–446.
181. Hudson JI, Goldenberg DL, Pope HG Jr, et al. Comorbidity of fibromyalgia with medical and psychiatric disorders. J Rheumatol Suppl 1992; 92:363–367.
182. Aaron LA, Bradley LA, Alarcon GS, et al. Psychiatric diagnoses in patients with fibromyalgia are related to health care-seeking behavior rather than to illness. Arthritis Rheum 1996; 39:436–445.
183. White KP, Nielson WR, Harth M, et al. Chronic widespread musculoskeletal pain with or without fibromyalgia: psychological distress in a representative community adult sample. J Rheumatol 2002; 29:588–594.
184. Ahles TA, Yunus MB, Riley SD, et al. Psychological factors associated with primary fibromyalgia syndrome. Arthritis Rheum 1984; 27:1101–1106.
185. Dailey PA, Bishop GD, Russell IJ, Fletcher EM. Psychological stress and the fibrositis/fibromyalgia syndrome. J Rheumatol 1990; 17:1380–1385.
186. Missole C, Toroni F, Sigala S, et al. Nerve growth factor in the anterior pituitary: localization in mammotroph cells and cosecretion with prolactin by a dopamine-regulated mechanism. Proc Natl Acad Sci U S A 1996; 93:4240–4245.
187. Lindsay RM, Lockett C, Sternberg J, Winter J. Neuropeptide expression in cultures of adult sensory neurons: modulation of substance P and calcitonin gene-related peptide levels by nerve growth factor. Neuroscience 1989; 33:53–65.
188. Goebel MU, Mills PJ, Irwin MR, Ziegler MG. Interleukin-6 and tumor necrosis factor-alpha production after acute psychological stress, exercise and infused isoproterenol: differential effects and pathways. Psychosom Med 2000; 62:591–598.
189. Davis MC, Zautra AJ, Reich JW. Vulnerability to stress among women in chronic pain from fibromyalgia and osteoarthritis. Ann Behav Med 2001; 23:215–226.
190. Porter-Moffitt S, Gatchel RJ, Robinson RC, et al. Biopsychosocial profiles of different pain diagnostic groups. J Pain 2006; 7(5):308–318.
191. Adler GK, Kinsley BT, Hurwitz S, et al. Reduced hypothalamic-pituitary and sympathoadrenal responses to hypoglycemia in women with fibromyalgia syndrome. Am J Med 1999; 106:534–543.
192. Lentjes EG, Griep EN, Boersma JW, et al. Glucocorticoid receptors, fibromyalgia and low back pain. Psychoneuroendocrinology 1997; 22:603–614.

193. Schatzberg AF, Rothschild AJ, Stahl JB, et al. The dexamethasone suppression test: identification of subtypes of depression. Am J Psychiatry 1983; 140:88–91.

194. Banki CM, Bissette G, Arato M, et al. CSF corticotropin-releasing factor-like immunore-activity in depression and schizophrenia. Am J Psychiatry 1987; 144:873–877.

195. Maes M, Lin A, Bonaccorso S, et al. Increased 24-hour urinary cortisol excretion in patients with post-traumatic stress disorder and patients with major depression, but not in patients with fibromyalgia. Acta Psychiatr Scand 1998; 98:328–335.

196. Alexander RW, Bradley LA, Alarcon GS, et al. Sexual and physical abuse in women with fibromyalgia: association with outpatients health care utilization and pain medication usage. Arthritis Care Res 1998; 11:102–115.

197. Goldberg RT, Pachas WN, Keith D. Relationship between traumatic events in childhood and chronic pain. Disabil Rehabil 1999; 21:23–30.

198. McBeth J, Macfarlane GJ, Benjamin S, et al. The association between tender points, psychological distress, and adverse childhood experiences: a community based study. Arthritis Rheum 1999; 42:1397–1404.

199. Boisset-Pioro MH, Esdaile JM, Fitzcharles MA. Sexual and physical abuse in women with fibromyalgia syndrome. Arthritis Rheum 1995; 38:235–241.

200. Fassbender K, Samborsky W, Kellner M, et al. Tender points, depressive and functional symptoms: comparison between fibromyalgia and major depression. Clin Rheumatol 1997; 16:76–79.

201. Golding JM. Sexual-assault history and long-term physical health problems: evidence from clinical and population epidemiology. Curr Dir Psychol Sci 1999; 8(6):191–194.

202. Leavitt F, Katz RS, Mills M, Heard AR. Cognitive and dissociative manifestations in fibromyalgia. J Clin Rheumatol 2002; 8:77–84.

203. White KP, Nielson WR, Harth M, et al. Does the label "fibromyalgia" alter health status, function, and health service utilization? A prospective, within-group comparison in a community cohort of adults with chronic widespread pain. Arthritis Care Res 2002; 47(3):260–265.

204. Pelligrino MJ, Waylonis GW, Sommer A. Familial occurrence of primary fibromyalgia. Arch Phys Med Rehabil 1989; 70:61–63.

205. Buskila D, Neumann L. Fibromyalgia syndrome (FM) and nonarticular tenderness in relatives of patients with FM. J Rheumatol 1997; 24:941–944.

206. Offenbaecher M, Bondy B, de Jonge S, et al. Possible association of fibromyalgia with a polymorphism in the serotonin transporter gene regulatory region. Arthritis Rheum 1999; 42:2482–2488.

207. Peres MFP, Young WB, Kaup AO, et al. Fibromyalgia is common in patients with transformed migraine. Neurology 2001; 57:1326–1328.

208. Sergi M, Rizzi M, Braghiroli A, et al. Periodic breathing during sleep in patients affected by fibromyalgia syndrome. Eur Resp J 1999; 14(1):203.

209. Yunus MB. Central sensitivity syndrome: a unified concept for fibromyalgia and other similar maladies. J Indian Rheum Assoc 2000; 8:27–33.

210. Yunus MB. Psychological aspects of fibromyalgia syndrome: a component of the dysfunctional spectrum syndrome. Baillieres Clin Rheumatol 1994; 8:811–837.

211. Daoud KF, Barkhuizen A. Rheumatic mimics and selected triggers of fibromyalgia. Curr Pain Headache Rep 2002; 6:284–288.

212. Pamuk ON, Cakir N. The frequency of thyroid antibodies in fibromyalgia patients and their relationship with symptoms. Clin Rheumatol 2006 [Epub ahead of print].

213. Martinez-Lavin M. Overlap of fibromyalgia with other medical conditions. Curr Pain Headache Rep 2001; 5:347–350.

214. Milhorat TH, Chou MW, Trinidad EM, et al. Chiari I malformation redefined: clinical and radiographic findings for 364 symptomatic patients. Neurosurgery 1999; 44:1005–1017.

215. Thimineur M, Kitaj M, Kravitz E, et al. Functional abnormalities of the cervical cord and lower medulla and their effect on pain: observations in chronic pain patients with incidental mild Chiari I malformation and moderate to severe cervical cord compression. Clin J Pain 2002; 18:171–179.

216. Heffez DS, Ross RE, Shade-Zeldow Y, et al. Clinical evidence for cervical myelopathy due to Chiari malformation and spinal stenosis in a non-randomized group of patients with the diagnosis of fibromyalgia. Eur Spine J 2004; 13(6):516–523.
217. Abdullah C, Yuksel G, Abdullah E, Salih C. Prevalence of fibromyalgia in patients with irritable bowel syndrome. Turk J Gastroenterol 2001; 12:141–144.
218. Whitehead WE, Palsson O, Jones KR. Systematic review of the comorbidity of irritable bowel syndrome with other disorders: what are the causes and implications? Gastroenterology 2002; 122:1140–1156.
219. Kurland JE, Coyle WJ, Winkler A, Zable E. Prevalence of irritable bowel syndrome and depression in fibromyalgia. Dig Dis Sci 2006; 51(3):454–460.
220. Verne GN, Price DD. Irritable bowel syndrome as a common precipitant of central sensitization. Curr Rheumatol Rep 2002; 4(4):322–328.
221. Ostuni P, Botsios C, Sfriso P, et al. Fibromyalgia in Italian patients with primary Sjogren's syndrome. Joint Bone Spine 2002; 69:51–57.
222. Lindvall B, Bengtsson A, Ernerudh J, Eriksson P. Subclinical myositis is common in primary Sjogren's syndrome and is not related to muscle pain. J Rheumatol 2002; 29:717–725.
223. Wolfe F. Post-traumatic fibromyalgia: a case report narrated by the patient. Arthritis Care Res 1994; 7:161–165.
224. Greenfield S, Fitzcharles MA, Esdaile JM. Reactive fibromyalgia syndrome. Arthritis Rheum 1992; 35:678–681.
225. Goldenberg DL, Mossey CJ, Schmid CH. A model to assess severity and impact of fibromyalgia. J Rheumatol 1995; 22:2313–2318.
226. Magnusson R. Extracervical symptoms after whiplash trauma. Cephalalgia 1994; 14(3):223.
227. Tishler M, Levy O, Maslakov I, et al. Neck injury and fibromyalgia—are they really associated? J Rheumatol 2006; 33(6):1183–1185.
228. Wolfe F. The fibromyalgia syndrome: a consensus report on fibromyalgia and disability. J Rheumatol 1996; 23:534–539.
229. Buskila D, Neumann L, Vaisberg G, et al. Increased rates of fibromyalgia following cervical spine injury. Arthritis Rheum 1997; 40:446–451.
230. Al-Allaf AW, Dunbar KL, Hallum NS, et al. A case-control study examining the role of physical trauma in the onset of fibromyalgia syndrome. Rheumatology 2002; 41:450–453.
231. Gardner GC. Fibromyalgia following trauma: psychology or biology? Curr Rev Pain 2000; 4:295–300.
232. Ferrari R. Fibromyalgia and motor vehicle collisions- Oh, the pain! BC Med J 2002; 44(5):257–260.
233. Martinez JE, Ferraz MB, Sato EI, Atra E. Fibromyalgia versus rheumatoid arthritis: a longitudinal comparison of the quality of life. J Rheumatol 1995; 22:270–274.
234. Henriksson CM. Longterm effects of fibromyalgia on everyday life. A study of 56 patients. Scand J Rheumatol 1994; 23:36–41.
235. Burckhardt CS, Clark SR, Bennett RM. Fibromyalgia and quality of life: a comparative analysis. J Rheumatol 1993; 20:475–479.
236. Wolfe F, Anderson J, Harkness D, et al. Work and disability status of persons with fibromyalgia. J Rheumatol 1997; 24:1171–1178.
237. Cathey MA, Wolfe F, Kleinheksel SM. Functional ability and work status in patients with fibromyalgia. Arthritis Care Res 1988; 1:25–33.
238. Lundberg G, Gerdle B. Tender point scores and their relations to signs of mobility, symptoms, and disability in female home care personnel and the prevalence of fibromyalgia syndrome. J Rheumatol 2002; 29:603–613.
239. Leidberg GM, Henriksson CM. Factors of importance for work disability in women with fibromyalgia: an interview study. Arthritis care Res 2002; 47:266–274.
240. Granges G, Littlejohn G. Prevalence of myofascial pain syndrome in fibromyalgia syndrome and regional pain syndrome: a comparative study. J Musculoskel Pain 1993; 1(2):19–35.
241. Gerwin RD. A study of 96 subjects examined both for fibromyalgia and myofascial pain [abstr]. J Musculoskel Pain 1995; 3(suppl 1):21.

242. Bennett RM. Emerging concepts in the neurobiology of chronic pain: evidence of abnormal sensory processing in fibromyalgia. Mayo Clin Proc 1999; 74:385–398.
243. Martinez-Lavin M. Is fibromyalgia a generalized reflex sympathetic dystrophy? Clin Exp Rheumatol 2001; 19:1–3.
244. Henriksson KG. Hypersensitivity in muscle pain syndromes. Curr Pain Headache Rep 2003; 7:426–432.
245. Sorensen J, Graven-Nielsen T, Hendriksson KG, et al. Hyperexcitability in fibromyalgia. J Rheumatol 1998; 25:152–155.
246. Wright A, Graven-Nielsen T, Davies, Arendt-Nielsen L. Temporal summation of pain from skin, muscle and joint following nociceptive ultrasonic stimulation in humans. Exp Brain Res 2002; 144:475–482.
247. Staud R, Vierck CJ, Cannon RI, et al. Abnormal sensitization and temporal summation of second pain (wind-up) in patients with fibromyalgia syndrome. Pain 2001; 91:165–175.
248. Graven-Nielsen T, Kendall SA, Henriksson KG, et al. Ketamine reduces muscle pain, temporal summation and referred pain in fibromyalgia patients. Pain 2000; 85:483–491.
249. Lucas HJ, Brauch CM, Settas L, Theoharides TC. Fibromyalgia—new concepts of pathogenesis and treatment. Int J Immunopathol Pharmacol 2006;19(1):5–10.
250. Rowbotham MC. Is fibromyalgia a neuropathic pain syndrome? J Rheumatol Suppl 2005; 75:38–40.
251. Price DD, Staud R. Neurobiology of fibromyalgia syndrome. J Rheumatol Suppl 2005; 75:22–28.
252. Staud R. Biology and therapy of fibromyalgia: pain in fibromyalgia syndrome. Arthritis Res Ther 2006; 8(3):208.
253. Staud R, Vierck CJ, Robinson ME, Price DD. Overall fibromyalgia pain is predicted by ratings of local pain and pain-related negative affect—possible role of peripheral tissues. Rheumatology 2006; 45(11):1409–1415.
254. Wood PB. A reconsideration of the relevance of systemic low-dose ketamine to the pathophysiology of fibromyalgia. J Pain 2006; 7(9):611–614.
255. Wood PB, Patterson JC 2nd, Sunderland JJ, et al. Reduced presynaptic dopamine activity in fibromyalgia syndrome demonstrated with positron emission tomography: a pilot study. J Pain 2007; 8(1):51–58.

9

Fibromyalgia: Clinical Evaluation and Medical Management

Although the fibromyalgia syndrome (FMS) is NOT a diagnosis of exclusion, there appears to be a disconnect between physicians and patients with this pain problem. Many FMS patients have a five- to seven-year history of symptoms prior to even seeing a physician (1). Misdiagnosis is common. One study indicates that the typical patient reports seeing an average of 15 physicians over approximately five years prior to obtaining a correct diagnosis (2).

As there is no widely available "gold standard" diagnostic test to confirm the diagnosis of FMS; a careful history along with a very thorough examination remain the bottom-line procedure for accurate diagnosis and better treatment of FMS.

HISTORY

A thorough history must be taken. As with the headache history, the clinician must know what specific questions to ask. Just chasing the concerns of a "chief complaint" will not prove helpful.

The history of pain, for example, should be evaluated to determine the presence or absence of widespread pain, pain on both sides of the body, pain above and below the waist, pain along the axial skeleton, and pain that has been constant and that has lasted for at least three months. These pain criteria were developed by the American College of Rheumatology (ACR) in their determination of the diagnostic classification of FMS (3). Other pertinent questions should deal with the onset of pain—sudden or gradual—any associated history of trauma? What are the pain attributes or descriptors—aching, sharp, radiating, burning, tender, sore?

The clinician should inquire about other associated symptoms such as sleep habits, fatigue, gastrointestinal (GI) problems, genitourinary problems, and more. Other, possibly coexisting conditions, should be identified through thorough historical questioning.

PHYSICAL EXAMINATION

Neurological examination typically is within normal limits. General physical examination may be pertinent to finding coexisting medical problems.

Musculoskeletal examination will reveal no signs of inflammation (redness, swelling, and heat). Tender points (TPs) may be found in multiple muscles, but the ACR has selected 18 symmetric sites now considered characteristic of FMS (3). (Table 1 in Chapter 8). Although the definitive diagnosis of FMS is made by finding tenderness to palpation (enough pressure to cause the fingernail to blanch—typically 4 kg/cm^2) of 11 or more out of the 18 specific TPs, patients with fewer than 11 sites may also have FMS. The number of acute TP sites changes over time.

Trigger points are found in palpable taut bands of muscle and frequently have associated local twitch responses; they are palpable and palpation will induce referred pain. TPs are not individually palpable, do not refer pain, and share no other similarities to myofascial trigger points (MTrPs).

An important consideration is that over 70% of FMS patients with typical TPs on examination also have MTrPs and other elements of a myofascial pain syndrome (MPS).

Again, clinical expertise in making the physical diagnosis of FMS, and of MPS, is necessary.

LABORATORY TESTING

The diagnosis of FMS is typically made, based on the ACR criteria or on the presence of the characteristic syndrome, or both.

There are no laboratory tests that would confirm a diagnosis of FMS. Thyroid studies are frequently done because hypothyroidism can mimic FMS.

There are laboratory abnormalities, but these are not found in routine testing: decreased serum serotonin (5-HT) (4), decreased serum tryptophan (5), increased cerebrospinal fluid substance P (5), increased serum interleukin-8 (6), thyroid hormone and thyroid stimulating hormone that may be low (7), decreased calcium levels (7), and decreased growth hormone secretion (8) (see Chapter 8).

Laboratory tests are most useful in determining the presence of or ruling out coexisting conditions.

EDUCATION

Before FMS patients can even be in a psychological place to learn, they must feel that the physician and his/her clinical associates are empathic, and affirm the patients' pain. Once the patient's symptoms have been validated, they may be able to better understand the nature of FMS: while not benign, it will not kill them, and they can help themselves! Educational emphasis should continue on improving and maintaining function, mind–body therapies (MBTs), the need for the patient to be an active member of the treatment team, and full information regarding all medications used and nondrug treatment options should be shared with patients. Clinically, a significant degree of effectiveness may be noted when patients are taught in groups. It is the author's practice to have previously educated FMS patients work, if possible, with the clinical treatment team; many patients appear to find it easier to accept/learn coping strategies and self-treatment techniques from other patients.

Published studies have emphasized the importance of education to FMS patients (9–11).

GENERAL COMMENTS

It is worthy to evaluate the general treatment of FMS patients with an important caveat noted by Turk (12). He suggests that the myth of patient homogeneity—the thought that all patients with the same chronic pain syndrome are also similar in all associated variables—may be a reason for the lack of satisfactory treatment outcomes. He believes that patients should be split into subgroups that may have more meaningful outcomes, and indicates that it may be appropriate to divide patients into subgroups based on their psychosocial and behavioral characteristics.

Goldenberg et al. (13) note that the optimal treatment of FMS remains unclear; evidence-based medicine guidelines have not been espoused. After a review of the literature, they note that many of the published treatment trials have not been optimal, as they have short durations and no blinding. They note that there have been no medications approved by the FDA specifically for the treatment of FMS. They do note that education, specific medications, exercise, and cognitive therapy, individually or all four treatments together have been clinically beneficial.

There have been no pharmacoeconomic evaluations for treatment of FMS (14). This information would be considered both important and overdue.

Another important aspect of dealing with FMS is the problem of adherence to treatment. A recent study found that treatment adherence is influenced by patient–physician discordance as well as pain (clinical) and by distress (psychological factors) in women with FMS (15). If these issues could be improved, as a part of treatment or prior to treatment, it may improve adherence to FMS treatment.

PHARMACOLOGICAL TREATMENT

The goal of pharmacological treatment is symptom amelioration, as it would rarely, if ever totally, obviate a symptom. Another important aspect is the importance of appropriate pharmacological treatment as a part of interdisciplinary treatment, as the medications alone do not, clinically, provide the fullest form of relief (16,17). Unfortunately, overmedication and indiscriminant polypharmacy frequently occurs. Physicians must be very familiar with all the pharmacological aspects of medications, particularly the side effects, as many FMS patients are very sensitive to medication effects and especially their side effects, particularly those dealing with fatigue, sedation, and cognitive decrement.

In general, medications should be started "low and slow," with small doses increased gradually. It is not unusual to find that effective medication dosages are lower than those noted in general medication textbooks. Some FMS patients are seemingly intolerant to almost all medications, making them very resistant to pharmacological treatment. Nonpharmacological treatment should be encouraged for these patients. Anther frequently seen problem is stopping a medication before it has had a pharmacological chance to help the patient.

Pharmacological treatment is utilized to help address the major FMS symptoms.

Analgesics

Pain is the most significant feature of FMS. Although analgesic medications are not expected to totally eradicate FMS pain, they are palliative, used to decrease pain enough to help patients improve with functional restoration.

In spite of the lack of peripheral or central inflammation, nonsteroidal anti-inflammatory (NSAIDs) medications are the most common analgesics utilized, in about 90% of FMS patients, with corticosteroids used in 24% of patients (18); this is in spite of the noted lack of efficacy of these medications (19–21). Acetaminophen and NSAIDs may be clinically effective when they are combined with centrally acting medications such as amitriptyline (AMI) (22). Some patients have found some relief with the use of these medications (23), although NSAIDs have not been found to be superior to placebo (19,24). The efficacy of cyclooxygenase-2 inhibitors (Cox-2) has not been established in FMS (25). Only Celecoxib remains on the market at this time, in this drug classification. The use of these medications does make surveillance for GI symptoms imperative.

Tramadol appears to inhibit ascending pain pathways; it inhibits reuptake of norepinephrine and 5-HT and it is also a mu-receptor agonist. In randomized controlled trials (RCTs), tramadol does provide pain relief that is superior to placebo (26). It has been noted to be as effective as acetaminophen and codeine (27). Another RCT and other reports also indicate tramadol's efficacy (28,29); at high dosages nausea, dizziness, and seizures, have been noted (30).

The apparent pathophysiological aspects of peripheral and central sensitization and allodynia make the use of opioids appropriate in select patients with pain-limited functionality.

There is no clinical evidence of the efficacy of opioids for the treatment of FMS (31). Short-acting opioids may be useful when taken 30 to 60 minutes prior to exercise or physical therapy for patients in whom pain prevents the treatment. Chronic, moderate-to-high dose opioid usage may induce problems with deep sleep and with the immune system (32). However, chronic opioid analgesic therapy (COAT) for select patients who need significant help to become functional and maintain their functionality, may be indicated. Extended time-release opioids such as Oxycontin, Durgesic patches, or extended release morphine may be used. An opiate agreement must be used, and the patients told of the possibility of dependence. They should be monitored regularly to evaluate the patients' function and their appropriate use of the medication (33).

There are physician, patient, payer, and societal barriers to the appropriate utilization of opioids, including outmoded concerns about abuse, dependency, and tolerance, as well as underutilization, all secondary to poor education (34,35).

Muscle relaxants (see Chapter 6) are useful, along with analgesics, to help deconditioned patients get through appropriate early and later exercise and rehabilitation. Tizanidine, a chronic muscle relaxant, an alpha$_2$-adrenergic agonist, has been reported to help decrease pain in FMS patients (36).

Lidocaine injections to TPs have been noted in several studies to benefit the FMS patient (37,38). Postinjection soreness is frequently great. Intravenous lidocaine appears to decrease pain and increase quality of life (39). A recent study indicates that injection therapy for FMS may be more effective if it focused less on TPs and more on trigger points found in association with MPS associated with FMS (40).

The use of N-Methyl-D-aspartate (NMDA) receptor antagonists (see Chapters 2 and 11), including ketamine (41) and dextromethorphan in the treatment of FMS needs more research (42). A recent study (43) found that patients with FMS showed abnormal windup during thermal and mechanical stimulation as compared with normal controls. Dextromethorphan reduced both thermal and mechanical windup and decreased stimulus intensity in both FMS patients and normal controls. Another study found that response to intravenous (IV) ketamine infusions were predictive of a response to oral dextromethorphan (44).

Methadone, a narcotic with a long half-life, has a modest amount of NMDA receptor antagonism.

Antidepressants

New classes of antidepressants (ADMs) and antiepileptic drugs (ACMs) have created new opportunities for the treatment of chronic nonmalignant pain. These drugs modulate pain by interacting with specific neurotransmitters and different ion channels. Newer antidepressants have been found to have varying degrees of effectiveness in the treatment of neuropathic pain (bupropion, venlafaxine, duloxetine). Older tricyclic antidepressants (TCAs) including amitriptyline, nortriptyline, and desipramine are also used for the treatment of neuropathic pain. The first-generation anticonvulsants (carbamazepine, valproic acid, and phenytoin) and newer ACMs (gabapentin, pregabalin) are also effective in the treatment of neuropathic pain (45).

TCAs have documented efficacy in the treatment of FMS. Duloxetine, an ADM, and pregabalin appear to have modest efficacy in patients with FMS (45).

5-HT is involved in moderating pain, sleep, depression, and hypothalamic hormone release. The majority of the various types of ADMs deal, at least partially, with 5-HT reuptake.

Tricyclic Antidepressants

TCAs, particularly AMI, are known to be beneficial to the treatment of FMS as found in RCTs (19,46–48). AMI is known to inhibit reuptake of both 5-HT and norepinephrine. It is the most frequently prescribed medication for the treatment of FMS (49). One report indicates that only about a third of patients find significant clinical improvement with AMI (50). AMI is felt to have both central and peripheral analgesic effectiveness, as noted before. Common side effects include weight gain, constipation, dry mouth, sedation, and, in a small percentage (up to 20%) of patients, agitation (51). Patients note decreased morning stiffness, better sleep, and increased energy with AMI (32).

As already noted, treatment with a TCA should be started with a low dosage— 10 mg of AMI, for example, and be increased slowly. ADM dosages (75—100 mg/ day to 300 mg/day) are frequently too high for the FMS patient to tolerate. Nortriptyline (52), doxepin, and cyclobenzaprine may be used if patients do not respond to AMI (52). Imipramine has been noted to be ineffective (53).

Cyclobenzaprine (CBP), a tricyclic agent, although not decreasing pain in all studies, does help improve sleep and fatigue in other RCTs (54–56). Another study, a double-blind crossover study of CBP at two different strengths, finds improvements in the quality of sleep, anxiety, fatigue, stiffness, the number of TPs, and irritable bowel syndrome (57).

Selective Serotonin Reuptake Inhibitors

Selective serotonin reuptake inhibitors (SSRIs), in general, have little analgesic effectiveness in FMS patients but do help with depression and sleep disorders (31,58). RCTs have found a diminution of pain with fluoxetine (59) and citalopram (60). Sertraline has been found to both decrease pain and have no effect on pain (61). A recent study shows that FMS patients treated with sertraline had a better outcome in terms of pain, improved sleep, and decreased morning stiffness when compared to a group of FMS patients treated with physical therapy (62). Studies have found the combination of fluoxetine and AMI to be more effective than either medication alone or placebo (59,63).

It must also be noted that the nonselective 5-HT reuptake inhibitors (especially if there is a noradrenergic component) such as venlafaxine, nefazodone, and bupropion appear to be effective in FMS particularly in decreasing pain (venlafaxine) (64). Other, newer prominent noradrenergic or dopaminergic system effects may be more effective in reducing pain (65).

Duloxetine, a specific serotonin and norepinephrine reuptake inhibitor (SNRI)—as is venlafaxine—has been found in a randomized, controlled placebo lead-in phase, to be effective and safe in the treatment of symptoms of FMS in subjects with or without a major depressive disorder, particularly for women (66,67).

Milnacipran, a norepinephrine serotonin reuptake inhibitor (NSRI) was shown to have better analgesic properties, reportedly, than the SSRIs (68). It was also found that milnacipran can relieve not only pain, but other symptoms of FMS, including fatigue, sleep, and depression (69,71).

Mirtazapine (which selectively blocks 5-HT2 and 5-HT3 receptors) is a novel ADM. In an open label study, it was found to be effective in diminishing the pain of FMS (72).

Two evidence-based medicine (EBM) articles deal with the treatment of FMS with ADMs (73,74). The general consensus of both articles is that ADMs were efficacious in treating various symptoms of FMS, but one questioned if this action was independent of depression. More studies were felt to be needed.

Another study evaluated the RCT data for the use of ADMs and cognitive behavioral therapy to be, for some of 11 somatic syndromes (including irritable bowel syndrome, chronic back pain, headache, FMS, chronic fatigue syndrome, tinnitus, menopausal symptoms, chronic facial pain, noncardiac chest pain, interstitial cystitis, and chronic pelvic pain) to be either robust or too scanty to be useful (75).

Anticonvulsant Medications

It would make teleological sense that these medications may decrease pain from peripheral and/or central sensitization (76). One recent RCT demonstrates that pregabalin was effective in FMS patients in the reduction of pain, sleep disturbance, and fatigue when compared to controls (77).

5-HT3 Receptor Antagonists

Ondansetron has been compared to paracetamol in a double-blind, crossover trial and was found to decrease pain in FMS patients (78). Tropisetron was also found to decrease pain and tenderness over TPs, with GI distress being the major side effect (79,80).

Other studies also find tropisetron, a 5-HT3 receptor antagonist, able to provide significant pain relief for FMS patients (81). Serum substance P levels were decreased in FMS patients who responded to tropisetron, with corresponding decrement of pain (82).

Benzodiazepines

An RCT found that alprazolam, either alone or in combination with ibuprofen had good efficacy in FMS pain amelioration, but a high dropout rate was found (83). Temazepam, in an RCT, was also noted to decrease pain and improve sleep (84).

In general, however, benzodiazepines are not recommended for FMS because they can decrease the efficacy of deep sleep.

Atypical Antipsychotics

Olanzapine, an atypical antipsychotic, was used as an adjunctive medication in 25 FMS patients. A subgroup of responders did well, with decreased pain and good sense of well-being; the major adverse event causing patients to stop the drug was weight gain (85).

Sedatives/Hypnotics

Nonrefreshing sleep, along with initial insomnia and frequent nocturnal awakenings, are almost universal in FMS (86–90). In general, after dealing with elements of sleep hygiene, pharmacological treatment includes sedatives that act on benzodiazepine receptors, sedating antidepressants, and sedating antihistamines. Zolpidem and Zopiclone (91–93) show no efficacy on pain relief, but improvement of sleep disorder complaints and daytime energy is seen.

Interestingly, chlorpromazine (100 mg) with L-tryptophan (5 g) given at night, in a controlled, double-blind study of 15 patients, significantly increased stage four sleep time (94). While chlorpromazine improved pain scores and decreased TP-related pain, it is not recommended in FMS secondary to its possible neurological side effects.

Other Agents

A case report indicates that ribose was helpful in a woman with FMS, possibly as it acted on the known energy depletion (95).

DHEA (dehydroepiandrosterone) did not improve pain, fatigue, cognition, mood, or quality of life in an RCT (96).

S-adenosylmethionine (SAMe), an active derivative of methionine has been noted in two RCTs to improve pain and depression (97,98).

L-tryptophan usage demonstrated a decreased number of TPs and decrease in patient pain ratings (at 100 mg tid x 30 days) (99).

Calcitonin was not found to be helpful in decreasing pain (100).

As noted in Chapter 8, FMS patients with low levels of insulin-like growth factor-1 who received daily injections of growth hormone (over nine months) had significant improvements in symptoms when compared to placebo (101). The injections are extremely, prohibitively, expensive.

Dopaminergics

This drug group may become more important over time, as the rationale for its use is becoming more distinct.

It has been noted before that there are autonomic nervous system (ANS) abnormalities associated with FMS, possibly including increased arousal, as shown by Moldofsky (71,87,102).

Norepinephrine, the precursor of which is dopamine, evokes pain in FMS patients, supporting the hypothesis that FMS may be a form of sympathetically maintained pain syndrome (103).

It is felt that dopamine and dopamine subreceptors control a variety of important limbic system functions regarding the stress response (104). Although there are no D_3 receptors in the brain stem where autonomic arousal is generated, the limbic system is rich with dopamine receptors, including D_3.

Studies with another D_3 agonist, pramipexole, indicate that low doses of this drug would cause the limbic neurons to become less functional; as this is a gate for brain stem arousal, it would therefore be left "wide open," with arousal allowed to go unchecked (105). Excessive autonomic stimulation would induce sleep problems and other ANS problems. As doses of the drug increase, the neuronal concentration increases leading to postsynaptic neurotransmission becoming more significant than presynaptic transmission. A higher concentration of a D_3 agonist would increase limbic function to block the brain stem arousals. This central limbic control might help reverse other autonomic problems such as sleep problems.

This may also help with induction of a decrement in pain perception secondary to a decrement in central hypersensitivity and decreased ANS arousal.

Both pramipexole and ropinirole have been found to be useful in the treatment of FMS (106,107).

Botulinum Toxin
Botulinum toxin was noted to be a poor therapy for FMS (108).

Serum
Human pooled immunoglobulin was thought to have potential treatment efficacy in chronic pain disorders with neuroimmune interactions (109). In an RCT, an anti-diencephalon immune serum (SER 282), as compared to amitriptyline and placebo, was found to promote stage four sleep (110).

Blocks
Sphenopalatine blocks were ineffective in FMS and MPS patients (111). One study (112) reported beneficial effects of regional sympathetic blockade in FMS patients. Epidural opioid blockade at rest and after exercise was helpful (25).

Pharmacological Treatment of Associated Syndromes
Restless Legs Syndrome
Restless legs syndrome (RLS) is typified by the perception of crawling sensations of the legs and strong urges to stretch noted early in the sleep cycle (113). This might also be associated with nocturnal myoclonus. RLS may respond to clonazepam (0.5–1.0 mg at bedtime), L-dopa/carbidopa (10/100 mg at suppertime), or low-dose narcotics at bedtime (114,115). Other dopamine agonists (pergolide, pramipexole) may also be effective (116,117).

Fatigue
Fatigue, a very common problem with FMS, may be treated with antidepressant medications if it is secondary to depression. Tropisetron, a 5-HT3 receptor antagonist reportedly helps in FMS-related fatigue and chronic fatigue syndrome (79,118,119). Amphetamines, methylphenidate, and modafinil have been used to benefit some patients with severe fatigue. Dopaminergic agents amantadine and pemoline in addition to protryptyline and SSRIs may also prove beneficial.

Dysautonomia
ANS abnormalities have been discussed in Chapter 5. The most common manifestation in FMS patients is neurally mediated hypotension in about 33% of patients (120–124). This is frequently associated with severe fatigue (121). Treatment includes increasing plasma volume (more fluids), increased salt intake, florinef, a mineralocorticoid, avoidance of medications that increase hypotension (TCAs, antihypertensives), prevention of the ventricle-baroreceptor reflex (B-adrenergic

antagonists or desopyramide), and minimizing the efferent limb of the barore-ceptor reflex (alpha-adrenergic agonists or anticholinergic agents) (125).

Cold Intolerance
Many FMS patients have cold-induced vasospasm (126). Low-grade aerobic exercise helps, as does treatment of dysautonomias and the use of vasodilators (calcium channel blockers), but these can potentially aggravate hypotension (125).

Cognitive Dysfunction
This is a common problem for FMS patients (127,128). It may be associated with poor memory and concentration and lead to problems with employment. It appears to be related to the effects of chronic pain, depression, mental fatigue, and sleep disorder. Treatment of these various problems is needed. In some patients medica-tion treatment of fatigue may be helpful with this problem, which appears to be the result of one or more other FMS-associated problem(s).

Complementary and Alternative Medical Therapies
A study from the Mayo clinic found, via a survey of 289 patients, that the ten most common complementary and alternative medical (CAM) therapies included exercise, spiritual healing (prayers), massage therapy, chiropractic therapy, vitamin C, vitamin E, magnesium, vitamin B complex, green tea, and weight loss programs (129).

NONPHARMACOLOGICAL TREATMENT

Generally speaking, some FMS patients may not wish to use pharmacological treat-ment, secondary to its possible lack of effectiveness, side effects, or just a worldview that traditional drug therapies are not for them. The use of all aspects of therapy in a multidisciplinary pain management center is discussed in Chapter 17.

The management of FMS patients is mostly based on empirical research, with only a few controlled studies (130). In a systematic review of MBTs for the treatment of FMS, MBT is more effective for some clinical outcomes as compared to being on a waiting list, treatment as usual, or placebo (131). However, when compared to active treatment, the results are largely inconclusive. Another study looked at complemen-tary medical treatment for FMS (132). This report indicated that the strongest data was found for MBT (biofeedback and cognitive behavioral therapy), especially when part of a multidisciplinary approach. The weakest data was for manipulative tech-niques (chiropractic and massage).

A 1996 report reviewed 24 controlled clinical trials for the treatment of FMS (133). The authors noted a large diversity of outcome measures and measurement instruments used to detect differences between treatment and placebo in FMS man-agement. Functionality and psychological status were infrequently included in data collection. Multiple experimental design errors were also noted.

A meta-analysis of FMS treatment interventions found that the optimal inter-vention for FMS involved both medication management and nonpharmacological treatments (especially exercise and cognitive behavioral therapy) to help sleep and pain symptoms (134).

Finally, a symptomatic review of RCTs of nonpharmacological FMS treatment interventions revealed the great difficulty noted and wide range of outcome measures, making conclusions across the studies very impractical (135). There was no strong evidence for any single intervention, although preliminary support of moderate evidence strength was noted for aerobic exercise.

Physical Therapy
Physical therapy (PT) is a source of excellent adjunctive therapies for FMS patients. The most commonly used are the hands-on treatments: massage, mobilization, stretching, and modalities (heat, ultrasound, electrical stimulation) (136). Most important are the various aspects of the home exercise program (HEP).

No controlled studies with appropriate construction (number of patients, methodology) have confirmed efficacy of PT in FMS patients.

Another study documented the reduction of FMS-induced pain and substance P along with improvements in sleep after massage therapy (137).

In a double-blind, placebo-controlled study, low-intensity infrared diode laser therapy was found to improve the number of TPs and global assessment scores (138).

In an open study, transcutaneous electrical nerve stimulation (TENS) was found to provide transient benefit in 70% of 40 patients (139).

Balneotherapy (warm, mineralized bath) was found to show improved pain and algometer scores when compared in an RCT, with relaxation exercises (140).

Exercise/Fitness Training
The majority of FMS patients show poor strength, flexibility, and aerobic fitness. Research has noted the benefits of exercise, including decreased perception of pain and lowered pain threshold (141,142). The benefits of exercise for FMS patients, and in general, are based on reasonable scientific evidence (143,144). The question is whether exercise may also have negative consequences. FMS introduces postexertional pain into the situation, secondary to central sensitization. Because of the elements of FMS pathophysiology, exercise may be both good and bad for FMS patients, as they would experience more postexertional pain than non-FMS patients (145–147). This is important to note, as it may be this problem and not a patient's lack of adherence to a too rigorous exercise program that causes FMS patients to have not be able to endure long-term follow up with exercise programs.

Deconditioning is very common in FMS patients and it is associated with many FMS symptoms (31). Various types of exercise including stationary cycling, aerobic walking, and aerobic dance have been evaluated (148–152), and it has been determined that aerobic exercise three times a week can reduce TP tenderness (31,153,154). Strength training and aerobic exercise is associated with improvements in pain, TP counts, and disturbed sleep (151,152,155). As indicated, maintenance of exercise programs in FMS tends to be poor (151,152).

Studies have shown the exercise-related improvement of objective and subjective pain measurements in primary fibromyalgia patients (148,150,152,156–158,159).

Another study shows an interesting corollary to exercise in FMS patients. In this study, 18 normal patients who regularly exercised ≥4 hours/week refrained from exercise for one week. Eight of these subjects reported an increase in pain, fatigue, and mood. They also had lower hypothalamic–pituitary–adrenal (HPA) axis, immune and autonomic function at baseline, when compared to the subjects who did not develop symptoms (160).

A systematic review (161) indicates that supervised aerobic exercise training will have beneficial effects on physical capacity and FMS symptoms. Strength training may also be beneficial. More research, per the authors, is needed.

Although positive RCTs have been reported (162), another study has shown that exercise is not helpful (163).

Acupuncture

A published meta-analysis of acupuncture in the treatment of FMS found that this treatment modality is a useful adjunctive treatment for FMS on a short-term basis (164). Another study looked at FMS patients' treatment with acupuncture for six weeks and found decreased pain levels and number of TPs associated with increased serum serotonin and substance P levels (165).

The results of another study (166) indicated that use of traditional acupuncture led to positive improvement in the visual analogue scale (VAS), myalgia index, number of TPs, and improvements in quality of life.

A more recent study found that acupuncture was no better than sham acupuncture in relieving the pain of FMS (167).

Martin et al. (168) used the Fibromyalgia Impact Questionnaire (FIQ) in patients given acupuncture and in control groups and found that the fatigue and anxiety scores of the FIQ were most improved. The activity and physical function scores did not change.

A controlled trial of electroacupuncture in FMS was found to be effective in decreasing the symptoms of FMS (169).

The National Institutes of Health consensus statement on acupuncture indicated that in some situations, including FMS, "acupuncture may be useful as an adjunct treatment or an acceptable alternative or may be included in a comprehensive management program" (170).

It is worth remembering that if acupuncture works by stimulating the endogenous opiate system, it may not work as well in patients taking chronic daily narcotics.

Manual Medicine

Two studies with limited statistical/medical outcome measures indicated a possible role for chiropractic care in the management of FMS (171,172).

Biofeedback

One controlled electromyography (EMG) biofeedback (vs. sham biofeedback) study found a decrease in plasma adrenocorticotropic hormone and beta-endorphin levels during EMG biofeedback training (173). Other studies showed improvements in pain in FMS patients (174), whereas another showed the opposite (175). Another study found that the addition of exercise to biofeedback and relaxation training led to significantly greater and longer lasting improvements than either treatment alone (176).

Hypnotherapy

Only one study of hypnotherapy in the management of FMS is found (177). This study indicated that hypnotherapy was useful in patients with FMS who were refractory to physical therapy. This, of course, may result in selection bias in favor of hypnotherapy.

Cognitive Behavioral Therapy

The primary goal of a cognitive behavioral therapy (CBT) program is to help patients develop an active self-management approach to coping with their FMS. Typically, the CBT program includes some or all of the following modalities: relaxation training, cognitive restructuring, meditation, aerobic exercise, stretching, pacing of activities, and patient and family education. The majority of published studies showed CBT to have some benefit (178–182). Some of the studies took place in interdisciplinary pain programs (183,184). Finally, improvement was noted after periods of six months (183) to 30 months (181).

CBT appears to be a very useful adjunctive modality in the treatment, particularly the multidisciplinary treatment, of FMS.

Support Groups and Online Chat Rooms

Many patients learn more from speaking with other patients with similar problems than with physicians. This can be done person-to-person at local FMS support groups (to find one, look at http://www.arthritis.org) or online in less personable chat rooms. Unless "bad medicine" is being touted, these are typically helpful; "self-help" groups that have patients who only complain about everything tend to "turn off" many patients who need a more supportive environment.

Multidisciplinary Treatment Programs

One RCT shows the effectiveness of multidisciplinary rehabilitation in the treatment of FMS (185). Another study shows that although a relatively brief multidisciplinary pain program may be helpful for some FMS patients, a subgroup of patients needs a more comprehensive program because of the patients' very poor level of functioning (186).

Other Potential Treatments

Shupak et al. found some support for the use of specific pulsed electromagnetic fields to reduce pain in both FMS and rheumatoid arthritis patients (187).

Usui et al. (188) found that the pain of FMS was reduced after electroconvulsive shock therapy (via VAS for pain and evaluation of TPs), which coincided with an improvement of thalamic blood flow.

REFERENCES

1. Goldenberg DL. Fibromyalgia syndrome a decade later. What we have learned. Arch Intern Med 1999; 159(8):777–785.
2. Gilliland RP. Fibromyalgia. emedicine.com/pmr/topic47.htm, 2001.
3. Wolfe F, Smythe HA, Yunus MB, et al. The American college of rheumatology 1990 criteria for the classification of fibromyalgia. Report of the Multicenter Criteria Committee. Arthritis Rheum 1990; 33(2):160–172.
4. Woolfe F, Russell IJ, Vipraio G, et al. Serotonin levels, pain threshold and fibromyalgia symptoms in the general population. J Rheumatol 1997; 24:555–559.
5. Schwarz MJ, Spath M, Muller-Bardorff H, et al. Relationship of substance P, 5-hydroxyindole acetic acid and tryptophan in serum of fibromyalgia patients. Neurosci Lett 1999; 259(3):196–198.
6. Gur A, Karakoc M, Nas K, et al. Cytokines and depression in cases with fibromyalgia. J Rheumatol, 2002; 29(2):358–361.
7. Neeck G, Riedel W. Thyroid function in patients with fibromyalgia syndrome. J Rheumatol 1992; 19:1120–1122.
8. Bagge E, Bengtsson BA, Carlsson L, Carlsson J. Low growth hormone secretion in patients with fibromyalgia—a preliminary report on 10 patients and 10 controls. J Rheumatol 1998; 25:145–148.

9. Vlaeyen JW, Teeken-Gruben NJ, Goossens ME, et al. Cognitive-educational treatment of fibromyalgia: a randomized clinical trial. I. Clinical Effects. J Rheumatol 1996; 23:1237–1245.

10. Burckhardt CS, Bjelle A. Education programmes for fibromyalgia patients: description and evaluation. Baillieres Clin Rheumatol 1994; 8:935–955.

11. Gowens SE, de Hueck A, Voss S, Richardson M. A randomized controlled trial of exercise and education for individuals with fibromyalgia. Arthritis Care Res 1999; 12:120–128.

12. Turk DC. The potential of treatment matching for subgroups of patients with chronic pain: lumping versus splitting. Clin J Pain 2005; 21(1):44–55.

13. Goldenberg DL, Burckhardt C, Crofford L. Management of fibromyalgia syndrome. JAMA 2004; 292(19):2388–2385.

14. Robinson RL, Jones ML. In search of pharmacoeconomic evaluations for fibromyalgia treatments: a review. ExStaud R. Are tender point injections beneficial: the role of tonic nociception in fibromyalgia. Curr Pharm Des 2006; 12(1):23–27.

15. Dobkin PL, Sita A, Sewitch MJ. Predictors of adherence to treatment in women with fibromyalgia. Clin J Pain 2006; 22(3):286–294.

16. Melillo N, Corrado A, Quarta L, et al. Fibromyalgic syndrome: new perspectives in rehabilitation and management. A review. Minerva Med 2005; 96(6):417–423.

17. Arnold LM. Biology and therapy of fibromyalgia. New therapies in fibromyalgia. Arthritis Res Ther 2006; 8(4):212.

18. Wolfe F, Anderson J, Harkness D, et al. A prospective, longitudinal, multicenter study of service utilization and costs in fibromyalgia. Arthritis Rheum 1997; 40:1560–1570.

19. Goldenberg DL, Felson DT, Dinerman H. A randomized, controlled trial of amitriptyline and naproxen in the treatment of patients with fibromyalgia. Arthritis Rheum 1986; 29:1371–1377.

20. Yunus MB, Masi AT, Aldag JC. Short term effects of ibuprofen in primary fibromyalgia syndrome; a double blind, placebo controlled trial. J Rheumatol 1989; 16:527–532.

21. Clark S, Tindall E, Bennett RM. A double blind crossover trial of prednisone versus placebo in the treatment of fibrositis. J Rheumatol 1985; 12:980–983.

22. Ang D, Wilke WS. Diagnosis, etiology and therapy of fibromyalgia. Compr Ther 1999; 25:221–227.

23. Krsnich-Shriwise S. Fibromyalgia syndrome: an overview. Phys Ther 1997; 77:68–75.

24. Yunus MB, Masi AT, Aldag JC. Short term effects of ibuprofen in primary fibromyalgia syndrome: A double blind placebo controlled trial. J Rheumatol 1989; 16:527–532.

25. Buskila D. Drug Therapy. Baillieres Best Pract Res Clin Rheumatol 1999; 13:479–485.

26. Russell IJ, Kamin M, Sager D, et al. Efficacy of Ultram (tramadol HCl) treatment of fibromyalgia syndrome: preliminary analysis of a multi-center, randomized, placebo-controlled study. Arthritis Rheum 1997; 40(suppl 9):S117.

27. Rauck RL, Ruoff GE, McMillen JI. Comparison of tramadol and acetaminophen with codeine for long-term pain management in elderly patients. Curr Ther Res 1994; 55:1417–1431.

28. Biasi G, Manca S, Manganelli S, Marcolongo R. Tramadol in the fibromyalgia syndrome: a controlled clinical trial versus placebo. Int J Clin Pharmacol Res 1998; 18:13–19.

29. Russell IJ. Efficacy of ULTRAM (tramadol Hcl) treatment of fibromyalgia syndrome (FMS): secondary outcomes report. TPS-FM Study Group [abstr]. J Musculoskel Pain 1998; 6(suppl 2):147.

30. Gasse C, Derby L, Vasilakis-Scaramozza C, et al. Incidence of first-time idiopathic seizures in users of tramadol. Pharmacotherapy 2000; 20:629-634.

31. Leventhal LG. Management of fibromyalgia. Ann Intern Med 1999; 131:850–858.

32. Rospond RM, Spellman J. Fibromyalgia and the role of the pharmacist. U.S. Pharmacist 1997; 22:41–52.

33. Brown RL, Fleming MF, Patterson JJ. Chronic opiod analgesic therapy for chronic low back pain. J Am Board Fam Pract 1996; 9:191–204.

34. American Academy of Pain Medicine and the American Pain Society consensus statement. The use of opioids for the treatment of chronic pain. Clin J Pain 1997; 13:6–8.

35. Portenoy RK. Opioid therapy for chronic nonmalignant pain: a review of the critical issues. J Pain Symptom Manage 1996; 11:203–217.

36. McClain DA. The effects of tizanidine HCl (Zanaflex®) in patients with fibromyalgia. In: Jay GW, Krusz JC, Longmire DR, McLain DA: Current trends in the diagnosis and treatment of chronic neuromuscular pain syndrome. Am Academy of Pain Management. Procom International, August 2000.

37. Hong CZ, Hsueh TC. Difference in pain relief after trigger point injections in myofascial pain patients with and without fibromyalgia. Arch Phys Med Rehabil 1996; 77:1161–1166.

38. Yunus MB. Fibromyalgia syndrome: is there any effective therapy? Consultant 1996; 36:1279–1286.

39. Raphael JH, Southall JL, Treharne GJ, Kitas GD. Efficacy and adverse effects of intravenous lignocaine therapy in fibromyalgia syndrome. BMC Musculoskelet Disord 2002; 3(1):21.

40. Staud R. Are tender point injections beneficial: the role of tonic nociception in fibromyalgia. Curr Pharm Des 2006; 12(1):23–27.

41. Sorensen J, Bengtsson A, Ahlner J, et al. Fibromyalgia- are there different mechanisms in the processing of pain? A double blind crossover comparison of analgesic drugs. J Rheumatol 1996; 24:1615–1621.

42. Henriksson KG, Sorensen J. The promise of N-methyl-D-aspartate receptor antagonists in fibromyalgia. Rheum Dis Clin North Am 2002; 28(2):1–7.

43. Stuad R, Vierck CJ, Robinson ME, Price DD. Effects of the N-methyl-D-aspartate receptor antagonist dextromethorphan on temporal summation of pain are similar in fibromyalgia patients and normal controls subjects. J Pain 2005; 6(5):323–332.

44. Cohen SP, Verdolin MH, Chang AS, et al. The intravenous ketamine test predicts subsequent response to an oral dextromethorphan treatment regimen in fibromyalgia patients. J Pain 2006; 7(6):391–399.

45. Maizels M, McCarberg B. Antidepressants and antiepileptic drugs for chronic non-cancer pain. Am Fam Physician. 2005; 71(3):483–490.

46. Scudds RA, McCain GA, Rollman GB, Harth M. Improvements in pain responsiveness in patients with fibrositis after successful treatment with amitriptyline. J Rheumatol 1989; 19(suppl):98–103.

47. Carette S, McCain GA, Bell DA, Fam AG. Evaluation of amitriptyline in primary fibrositis. A double blind, placebo-controlled study. Arthritis Rheum 1986; 29(5):655–659.

48. Jaeschke R, Adachi J, Guyatt G, et al. Clinical usefulness of amitriptyline in fibromyalgia: The results of 23 N-of-1 randomized controlled trials. J Rheumatol 1991; 18(3):447–451.

49. Maurizio SJ, Rogers JL. Recognizing and treating fibromyalgia. Nurse Pract 1997; 22:18–33.

50. Simms RW. Fibromyalgia syndrome: current concepts in pathophysiology, clinical features, and management. Arthritis Care Res 1996; 9:315–328.

51. Wallace DJ. The fibromyalgia syndrome. Ann Med 1997; 29:9–21.

52. Creamer P. Effective management of fibromyalgia. J Musculoskel Med 1999; 16:622.

53. Wysenbeek AJ, Mor F, Lurie Y, et al. Imipramine for the treatment of fibrositis: a therapeutic trial. Ann Rheum Dis; 1985, 44:752–753.

54. Reynolds WJ, Moldofsky H, Saskin P, Lue FA. The effects of cyclobenzaprine on sleep physiology and symptoms in patients with fibromyalgia. J Rheumatol 1991; 18(3): 452–454.

55. Bennett RM, Gatter RA, Campbell SM, et al. A comparison of cyclobenzaprine and placebo in the management of fibrositis. A double blind controlled study. Arthritis Rheum 1988; 31(12):1535–1542.

56. Carrette S, Bell MJ, Reynolds WJ, et al. Comparison of amitriptyline, cyclobenzaprine and placebo in the treatment of fibromyalgia. Arthritis Thrum 1994; 37(1):32–40.

57. Santandrea S, Montrone F, Sarzi-Puttini P, et al. A double-blind crossover study of two cyclobenzaprine regimens in primary fibromyalgia syndrome. J Int Med Res 1993; 21:74–80.

58. McCain GA. A cost-effective approach to the diagnosis and treatment of fibromyalgia. Rheum Dis Clin North Am 1996; 22:323–349.

59. Goldenberg D, Mayskiy M, Mossey C, et al. A randomized, double blind crossover trial of Fluoxetine and amitriptyline in the treatment of fibromyalgia. Arthritis Rheum 1996; 39(11):1852–1859.

60. Anderberg UM, Marteinsdottir I, von Knorring L. Citalopram in patients with fibromyalgia- a randomized, double-blind, placebo controlled study. Eur J Pain 2000; 4(1):27–35.
61. Alberts K, Bradley L, Alarcon G, et al. Sertraline hydrochloride alters pain threshold, sensory discrimination ability and functional brain activity in patients with fibromyalgia (FM): a randomized controlled trial. Arthritis Rheum 1998; 41(suppl):S259.
62. Gonzalez-Viejo MA, Avellanet M, Henrandez-Morcuende MI. A comparative study of fibromyalgia treatment: ultrasonography and physiotherapy versus sertraline treatment. Ann Readapt Med Phys 2005; 48(8):610–615. (Epub ahead of print: abstr. www.ncbi.nlm. nih.gov/entrez).
63. Wolfe F, Cathey MA, Hawlet DJ. A double blind placebo controlled trial of fluoxetine in fibromyalgia. Scand J Rheumatol 1994; 23:255–259.
64. Dwight MM, Arnold LM, O'Brien H, et al. An open clinical trial of venlafaxine treatment of fibromyalgia. Psychosomatics 1998; 39:14–17.
65. Claw DJ. Treating fibromyalgia: science vs. art. Am Fam Physician 2000; 62:1492–1494.
66. Arnold LM, Lu Y, Crofford LJ, et al. A double-blind, multicenter trial comparing duloxetine with placebo in the treatment of fibromyalgia patients with or without major depressive disorder. Arthritis Rheum 2004; 50(9):2974–2984.
67. Arnold LM, Rosen A, Pritchett YL, et al. A randomized, double-blind, placebo-controlled trial of duloxetine in the treatment of women with fibromyalgia with or without major depressive disorder. Pain 2005; 119(1–3):5–15.
68. Rao SG, King T, Porreca F. Elucidation of the analgesic efficacy of Milnacipran in chronic pain. Presented at the International Association for the Study of Pain's Tenth World Congress on Pain, San Diego, California, Aug 17–22, 2002.
69. Vitton O, Gendreau M, Gendreau J, et al. A double-blind placebo-controlled trial of milnacipran in the treatment of fibromyalgia. Hum Psychopharmacol 2004; 19(suppl 1): S27–S35.
70. Gendreau RM, Thorn MD, Gendreau JF, et al. Efficacy of milnacipran in patients with fibromyalgia. J Rheumatol 2005; 2(10):1975–1985.
71. Martinez-Lavin M, Hermosillo AG, Rosas M, Soto ME. Circadian studies of autonomic nervous balance in patients with fibromyalgia: a heart rate variability analysis. Arthritis Rheum 1998; 41(11):1966–1971.
72. Samborski W, Sezanska-Szpera M, Rybakowski JK. Open trial of Mirtazapine in patients with fibromyalgia. Pharacopsychiatry 2004; 37(4):168–170.
73. Arnold LM, Keck PE, Welge JA. Antidepressant treatment of fibromyalgia. A meta-analysis and review. Psychosomatics 2000; 41(2):104–113.
74. O'Malley PG, Balden E, Tomkins G, et al. Treatment of fibromyalgia with antidepressants: a meta-analysis. J Gen Int Med 2000; 15(9):659–666. The Cochrane Database Syst Rev 2002; 4:05463.
75. Jackson JL, O'Malley PG, Kroenke K. Antidepressants and cognitive-behavioral therapy for symptom syndromes. CNS Spectr 2006; 11(3):121–122.
76. Wiffen P, Collins S, McQuay H, et al. Anticonvulsant drugs for acute and chronic pain (Cochrane Review). In: The Cochrane Library, Issue 4, Oxford: Update Software, 2002.
77. Crofford LJ, Rowbotham MC, Mease PJ, et al. Pregabalin for the treatment of fibromyalgia syndrome: results of a randomized, double-blind, placebo-controlled trial. Arthritis Rheum 2005; 52(4):1264–1273.
78. Hrycaj P, Stratz T, Mennet P, Muller W. Pathogenic aspects of responsiveness to Ondansetron (5-hydroxytryptamine type 3 receptor antagonist) in patients with primary fibromyalgia syndrome- a preliminary study. J Rheumatol 1996; 23:1418–1423.
79. Farber L, Stratz T, Bruckle W, et al. Efficacy and tolerability of Tropisetron in primary fibromyalgia- a highly selective and competitive 5-HT3 receptor antagonist. German Fibromyalgia Study Group. Scand J Rheumatol 2000; 113(suppl):49–54.
80. Samborski W, Stratz T, Lacki JK, et al. The 5-HT3 blockers in the treatment of the primary fibromyalgia syndrome: A 10 day open study with tropisetron at a low dose. Mater Med Pol 1996; 28:17–19.
81. Spath M, Stratz T, Neeck G, et al. Efficacy and tolerability of intravenous tropisetron in the treatment of fibromyalgia. Scand J Rheumatol 2004; 33(4):267–270.

82. Stratz T, Feibich B, Haus U, Muller W. Influence of tropisetron on the serum substance P levels in fibromyalgia patients. Scand J Rheumatol Suppl 2004; 33(119):41–43.
83. Russell IJ, Fletcher EM, Michalek JE, et al. Treatment of primary fibrositis/fibromyalgia syndrome with ibuprofen and alprazolam: a double blind, placebo-controlled study. Arthritis Rheum 1991; 34:552–560.
84. Hench PK, Cohen R, Mitler MM. Fibromyalgia: Effects of amitriptyline, Temazepam and placebo on pain and sleep [abstr]. Arthritis Rheum 1989; 32(suppl):S47.
85. Rico-Villademoros F, Hidalgo J, Dominguez I, et al. Atypical antipsychotics in the treatment of fi bromyalgia: a case series with olanzapine. Prog Neuropsychopharmacol Biol Psychiatry 2005; 29(1):161–164.
86. Moldofsky H, Scarisbrick P, England R, Smythe H. Musculoskeletal symptoms and non-REM sleep disturbances in patients with "fibrositis syndrome" and healthy subjects. Psychosom Med 1975; 37:341–351.
87. Moldofsky H, Scarisbrick P. Induction of neurasthenic musculoskeletal pain syndrome by selective sleep stage deprivation. Psychosom Med 1976; 38:35–44.
88. Moldofsky H. Sleep and musculoskeletal pain. Am J Med 1986; 81(suppl 3A):85–89.
89. Cote KA, Moldofsky H. Sleep daytime symptoms, and cognitive performance in patients with fibromyalgia. J Rheumatol 1997; 24:2014–2023.
90. Drewes AM, Nielsen KD, Taagholt SJ, et al. Sleep intensity in fibromyalgia: focus on the microstructure of the sleep process. Br J Rheum 1995; 34:629–635.
91. Moldofsky H, Lue FA, Mously C, et al. The effect of Zolpidem in patients with fibromyalgia: a dose ranging, double blind placebo controlled, modified crossover study. J Rheumatol 1996; 23(3):529–533.
92. Drewes AM, Andreasen A, Jennum P, Nielsen KD. Zopiclone the treatment of sleep abnormalities in fibromyalgia. Scand J Rheumatol 1991; 20(4):288–293.
93. Gronblad M, Nykanen J, Konttinen Y, et al. Effect of Zopiclone on sleep quality, morning stiffness, widespread tenderness and pain and general discomfort in primary fibromyalgia patients. A double blind randomized trial. Clin Rheumatol 1993; 12(2):186–191.
94. Moldofsky H, Benz B, Luc F, et al. Comparison of chlorpromazine and L-tryptophan on sleep, musculoskeletal pain, and mood in fibrositis syndrome. Sleep Research 1976; 5:76.
95. Gebhart B, Jorgenson JA. Benefit of ribose in a patient with fibromyalgia. Pharmacotherapy. 2004; 24(11):1646–1648.
96. Finckh A, Berner IC, Aubry-Rozier B, So AK. A randomized controlled trial of dehydroepiandrosterone in postmenopausal women with fibromyalgia. J Rheumatol 2005; 32(7):1336–1340.
97. Tavoni A, Vitali C, Bombardieri S, Pasero G. Evaluation of S-adenosylmethionine in primary fibromyalgia. A double blind crossover study. Am J Med 1987; 83(5A):107–110.
98. Tavoni A, Jeracitano G, Cirigloiano G. Evaluation of S-adenosylmethionine in secondary fibromyalgia: a double blind study [letter]. Clin Exp Rheumatol 1998; 16(1):106–107.
99. Caruso I, Sarzi Puttinji P, Cazzola M, Azzolini V. Double blind study of 5-hydroxytryptophan versus placebo in the treatment of primary fibromyalgia syndrome. J Int Med Res 1990; 18:201–209.
100. Bessette L, Carette S, Fossel AH, Lew RA. A placebo controlled crossover trial of subcutaneous salmon calcitonin in the treatment of patients with fibromyalgia. Scand J Rheumatol 1998; 27:112–116.
101. Bennett RM, Clark SC, Walczyk J. A randomized, double blind, placebo controlled study of growth hormone in the treatment of fibromyalgia. Am J Med 1998; 104:227–231.
102. Bou-Holaigah I, Calkins H, Flynn JA, et al. Provocation of hypotension and pain during upright tilt table testing in adults with fibromyalgia. Clin Exp Rheumatol 1997; 15:239–246.
103. Martinez-Lavin M, Vidal M, Barbosa RE, Pineda C, Casanova JM, Nava A. Norepinephrine-evoked pain in fibromyalgia. A randomized pilot study. BMC Musculoskelet Disord 2002; 3:2.

104. Wood PB. Fibromyalgia syndrome: a central role for the hippocampus: a theoretical construct. J Musculoskeletal Pain 2004; 12(1):19–26.
105. Dziedzicka-Wasylewska M, Ferrari F, Johnson RD, et al. Mechanisms of action of pramipexole: effects on receptors. Rev Contemp Pharmacother 2001; 12(1–2):1–31.
106. Holman AJ, Myers RR. A randomized, double-blind, placebo-controlled trial of pramipexole, a dopamine agonist, in patients with fibromyalgia receiving concomitant medications. Arthritis Rheum 2005; 52(8):2495–2505.
107. Holman AJ. Treatment of fibromyalgia with the dopamine agonist ropinirole: a 14-week double-blind, pilot, randomized controlled trial with 14-week blinded extension. Arthritis Rheum 2004; 50(9)(suppl):A1870.
108. Paulson GW, Gill W. Botulinum toxin is unsatisfactory therapy for fibromyalgia. Mov Disord 1996; 11(4):459.
109. Goebel A, Netal S, Shedel R, Sprotte G. Human pooled immunoglobulin in the treatment of chronic pain syndromes. Pain Med 2002; 3(2):119–127.
110. Kempenaers C, Simenon G, Vander Elst M, et al. Effect of an antidiencephalon immune serum on pain and sleep in primary fibromyalgia. Neuropsychobiology 1994; 30(2–3):66–72.
111. Janzen V, Scudds RA. Sphenopalatine blocks in the treatment of pain in fibromyalgia and myofascial pain. Laryngoscope 1997; 107:1420–1422.
112. Bengtsson A, Bengtsson M. Regional sympathetic blockade in primary fibromyalgia. Pain 1988; 33:161–167.
113. Yunus MB, Aldag JC. Restless legs syndrome and leg cramps in fibromyalgia syndrome: a controlled study. BMJ 1996; 312:1339.
114. Kaplan PW, Allen R, Bucholz DW, Walters JK. A double blind, placebo-controlled study of the treatment of periodic limb movements in sleep using carbidopa/levodopa and propoxyphene. Sleep 1993; 16:713–716.
115. Becker PM, Jamieson AO, Brown WD. Dopaminergic agents in restless legs syndrome and periodic limb movements of sleep: response and complications of extended treatment in 49 cases. Sleep 1993; 16:713–716.
116. Earley CJ, Yaffee JB, Allen RP. Randomized, double blind, placebo-controlled trial of pergolide in restless legs syndrome. Neurology 1998; 51:1599–1602.
117. Montplaisir J, Nicolas A, Denesle R, Gomez-Mancilla. Restless legs syndrome improved by pramipexole: a double blind randomized trial. Neurology 1999; 52(5):938–943.
118. Spath M, Welzel D, Farber L. Treatment of chronic fatigue syndrome with 5-HT3 receptor antagonists-preliminary results. Scand J Rheumatol 2000; 113:72–77.
119. Guymer EK, Clauw DJ. Treatment of fatigue in fibromyalgia. Rheum Dis Clin North Am 2002; 28(2):367–378.
120. Martinez-Lavin M, Hermosillo AG. Autonomic nervous system dysfunction may explain the multisystem features of fibromyalgia. Semin Arthritis Rheum 2000; 29: 197–199.
121. Martinez-Lavin M, Hermosillo AG, Mendoza C, et al. Orthostatic sympathetic derangement in subjects with fibromyalgia. J Rheumatol 1997; 24:714–718.
122. Karas B, Grubb BP, Boehm K, et al. The postural orthostatic tachycardia syndrome: a potentially treatable cause of chronic fatigue, exercise intolerance and cognitive impairment in adolescents. Pacing Clin Electrophysiol 2000; 23:344–351.
123. Raj SR, Brouillard D, Simpson CS, et al. Dysautonomia among patients with fibromyalgia: a non-invasive assessment. J Rheumatol 2000; 27:2660–2665.
124. Wilke WS, Fouad-Tarazi, Cash JM, Calabrese LH. The connection between chronic fatigue syndrome and neurally mediated hypotension. Cleve Clin J Med 1998; 65: 261–266.
125. Barkhuizen A. Rational and targeted pharmacologic treatment of fibromyalgia. Rheum Dis Clin North Am 2000; 28(2):261–290.
126. Bennett RM, Clark SR, Campbell SM, et al. Symptoms of Raynaud's syndrome in patients with fibromyalgia. A study utilizing the Nielsen test, digital photoplethysmography and measurement of platelet alpha 2-adrenergic receptors. Arthritis Rheum 1991; 34:264–269.
127. Sletvold H, Stiles TC, Landro NI. Information processing in primary fibromyalgia, major depression and healthy controls. J Rheumatol 1995; 22:137–142.

128. Landro NI, Stiles TC, Sletvold H. Memory functioning in patients with primary fibro-myalgia an major depression and healthy controls. J Psychosom Res 1997; 42:297–306.
129. Wahner-Roedler DL, Elkin PL, Vincent A, et al. Use of complementary and alternative medical therapies by patients referred to a fibromyalgia treatment program at a tertiary care center. Mayo Clin Proc 2005; 80(6):826.
130. Forseth K, Gran JT. Management of fibromyalgia: what are the best treatment choices? Drugs 2002; 6(4):577–592.
131. Hadhazy VA, Ezzo J, Creamer P, Berman BM. Mind-body therapies for the treatment of fibromyalgia. A systematic Review. J Rheumatol 2000; 27(12):2911–2918.
132. Berman BM, Swyers JP. Complementary medicine treatments for fibromyalgia syndrome. Baillieres Best Pract Res Clin Rheumatol 1999; 13(3):487–492.
133. White KP, Harth M. An analytical review of 24 controlled clinical trials for fibromyalgia syndrome (FMS). Pain 1996; 64(2):211–219.
134. Rossy LA, Buckelew SP, Dorr N, et al. A meta-analysis of fibromyalgia treatment interventions. Ann Behav Med 1999; 21:180–191.
135. Sim J, Adams N. Systematic review of randomized controlled trials of nonpharmaco-logical interventions for fibromyalgia. Clin J Pain 2002; 18(5):324–336.
136. Rosen NB. Physical medicine and rehabilitation approaches to the management of myofascial pain and fibromyalgia syndromes. Baillieres Clin Rheumatol 1994; 8(4):881–916.
137. Field T, Diego M, Cullen C, et al. Fibromyalgia pain and Substance P decrease and sleep improves after massage therapy. J Clin Rheumatol 2002; 8(2):72–76.
138. Caballero-Uribe CV, Abuchaibe I, Abuchaibe S, Navarro E. Treatment of tender points in patients with fibromyalgia syndrome (FMS) with therapeutic infrared laser ray. Arthritis Rheum 1997; 40(9)(suppl):S44.
139. Kaada B. Treatment of fibromyalgia by low-frequency transcutaneous nerve stimula-tion. Tidsskrift For Den Norske Laegeforening 1989; 109(29):2992–2995.
140. Yurkuran M, Celiktas M. A randomized, controlled therapy of Balneotherapy in the treatment of patients with primary fibromyalgia syndrome. Physikalische Medizin Rehabilitationsmedizin Kurortmedizin 1996; 6(2):109–112.
141. Guieu R, Blin O, Pouget J, Serratrice G. Nociceptive threshold and physical activity. Can J Neurol Sci 1992; 19:69–71.
142. Koltyn KF, Garvin AW, Gardiner RL, Nelson TF. Perception of pain following aerobic exercise. Med Sci Sports Exerc 1996; 28:1418–1421.
143. Schwarz L, Kindermann W. Changes in beta-endorphin levels in response to aerobic and anaerobic exercise. Sports Med 1992; 13:25-36.
144. Koltyn KF. Analgesia following exercise: a review. Sports Med 2000; 29:85–98.
145. Geel SE. The fibromyalgia syndrome: musculoskeletal pathophysiology. Semin Arthritis Rheum 1994; 23:347–353.
146. Watkins LR, Maier SF, Goehler LE. Immune activation: the role of pro-inflammatory cytokines in inflammation, illness responses and pathological pain states. Pain 1995; 63:289–302.
147. Bennett RM. The contribution of muscle to the generation of fibromyalgia symptoma-tology. J Musculoskel Pain 1996; 4:35–59.
148. McCain GA, Bell DA, Mai FM, et al. A controlled study of the effects of a supervised cardiovascular fitness training program on the manifestations of primary fibromyalgia. Arthritis Rheum 1988; 31:1135–1141.
149. Norregaard J, Lyddegaard JJ, Mehlsen J, et al. Exercise training in treatment of fibromy-algia. J Musculoskel Pain 1997; 5:71–79.
150. Nichols DS, Glenn TM. Effects of aerobic exercise on pain perception, affect and level of disability in individuals with fibromyalgia. Phys Ther 1994; 74:327–332.
151. Martin L, Nutting A, Macintosh BR, et al. An exercise program in the treatment of fibromyalgia. J Rheumatol 1996; 23:1050–1053.
152. Wigers SH, Stiles TC, Vogel PA. Effects of aerobic exercise versus stress management treat-ment in fibromyalgia. A 4.5 year prospective study. Scand J Rheumatol 1996; 25:77–86.
153. Jones KD, Burckhardt CS, Clark SR. A randomized controlled trial of muscle strength-ening versus flexibility training in fibromyalgia. J Rheumatol 2002; 29:1041–1048.

154. Richards SC, Scott DL. Prescribed exercise in people with fibromyalgia: parallel group randomized controlled trial. BMJ 2002; 325(7357):185.
155. Millea PJ, Holloway RL. Treating fibromyalgia. Am Fam Physician 2000; 62:1575–1582.
156. Gowans SE, Dehueck A, Voss S, Silaj A, Abbey SE. Six-month and one-year follow-up of 23 weeks of aerobic exercise for individuals with fibromyalgia. Arthritis Rheum 2004; 51(6):890–898.
157. Mannerkorpi K. Exercise in fibromyalgia. Curr Opin Rheumatol 2005; 17(2):190–194.
158. Da Costa D, Abrahamowicz M, Lowensteyn I, et al. A randomized clinical trial of an individualized home-based exercise programme for women with fibromyalgia. Rheumatology 2005; 44(11): 1422–1427. (Epub ahead of print: abstr. www.ncbi.nlm.nih.gov/entrez).
159. Maquet D, Croisier JL, Demoulin C, et al. Value of aerobic rehabilitation in the management of fibromyalgia. Rev Med Liege 2006; 61(2):109–116.
160. Glass JM, Lyden AK, Petzke F, et al. The effect of brief exercise cessation on pain, fatigue, and mood symptom development in healthy fit individuals. J Psychosom Res 2004; 57(4):391–398.
161. Busch A, Schachter CL, Peloso PM, Bombardier C. Exercise for treating fibromyalgia syndrome. Cochrane Database Syst Rev 2002, 3:CD003786.
162. Gowans SE, deHueck A, Voss S, Richardson M. A randomized, controlled trial of exercise and education for individuals with fibromyalgia. Arthritis Care Res 1999; 12(2):120–128.
163. Ramsay C, Moreland J, Ho M, et al. An observer blinded comparison of supervised and unsupervised aerobic exercise regimen in fibromyalgia. Rheumatology 2000; 39(5):501–505.
164. Berman BM, Ezzo J, Hadhazy V, Swyers JP. Is acupuncture effective in the treatment of fibromyalgia? J Fam Pract 1999; 48:213–218.
165. Sprott H, Franke S, Kluge H, Hein GF. Pain treatment in fibromyalgia by acupuncture [letter]. Rheumatol Int 1998; 18(1):35–36.
166. Targhino RA, Imamura M, Kaziyama HH, et al. Pain treatment with acupuncture for patient with fibromyalgia. Curr Pain Headache Rep 2002; 6(5):379–383.
167. Assefi NP, Sherman KJ, Jacobsen C, et al. A randomized clinical trial of acupuncture compared with sham acupuncture in fibromyalgia. Ann Intern Med 2005; 143(1): 10–19.
168. Martin DP, Sletten CD, Williams BA, Berger IH. Improvement in fibromyalgia symptoms with acupuncture: results of a randomized controlled trial. Mayo Clin Proc 2006; 81(6):749–757.
169. Deluze C, Bosia LO, Zirbs A, et al. Electroacupuncture n fibromyalgia: results of a controlled trial. BMJ 1992; 305(6864):1249–1252.
170. NIH consensus conference. Acupuncture. JAMA 1998; 280: 1518-1524.
171. Blunt KL, Rajwani MH, Guerriero RC. The effectiveness of chiropractic management of fibromyalgia patients: a pilot study. J Manipulative Physiol Ther 1997; 20(6):389–399.
172. Hains G, Hains F. A combined ischemic compression and spinal manipulation in the treatment of fibromyalgia: a preliminary estimate of dose and efficacy. J Manipulative Physiol Ther 2000; 23(4):225–230.
173. Ferraccioli G, Ghirelli L, Scita F, et al. EMG-biofeedback training in fibromyalgia syndrome. J Rheumatol 1987; 14(4):820–825.
174. Sarnoch H, Adler F, Scholz OB. Relevance of muscular sensitivity, muscular activity and cognitive variables for pain reduction associated with EMG biofeedback in fibromyalgia. Percept Mot Skills 1997; 84(3 Pt 1):1043–1050.
175. Molina E, Cecchettin M, Fontana S. Failure of EMB BF after sham BF training in fibromyalgia. Fed Proc 1987; 46:13–57.
176. Buckelew SP, Conway R, Parker J, et al. Biofeedback/relaxation training and exercise interventions for fibromyalgia: a prospective trail. Arthritis Rheum 1998; 11:196–209.
177. Haanen HC, Hoenderdos HT, van Romunde LK, et al. Controlled trial of hypnotherapy in the treatment of refractory fibromyalgia. J Rheumatol 1991; 18(1):72–75.
178. Nielson WR, Walker C, McCain GA. Cognitive behavioral treatment of fibromyalgia syndrome: preliminary findings. J Rheumatol 1992; 19:98-103.

179. Vlaeyen JW, Teeken-Gruben NJ, Goossens ME, et al. Cognitive educational treatment of fibromyalgia: a randomized trial. I. Clinical effects. J Rheumatol 1996; 23:1237–1245.

180. Goldenberg DL, Kaplan KH, Nadeau M. A controlled study of a stress-reduction, cognitive-behavioral treatment program in fibromyalgia. J Musculoskel Pain 1994; 2(2):53–66.

181. White KP, Nielson WR. Cognitive behavioral treatment of fibromyalgia syndrome: a followup assessment. J Rheumatol 1995; 22:717–721.

182. Singh BB, Berman BM, Hadhazy VA, Creamer. A pilot study of cognitive behavioral therapy in fibromyalgia. Altern Ther Health Med 1998; 4:67–70.

183. Turk DC, Okifuji A, Sinclair JD, Starz TW. Interdisciplinary treatment for fibromyalgia syndrome: clinical and statistical significance. Arthritis Care Res 1998; 11:186–195.

184. Mengshoel AM, Forseth KO, Haugen M. Multidisciplinary approach to fibromyalgia. A pilot study. Clin Rheumatol 1995; 14:165–170.

185. Lemstra M, Olszynski WP. The effectiveness of multidisciplinary rehabilitation in the treatment of fibromyalgia: a randomized controlled trial. Clin J Pain 2005; 21(2):166–174.

186. Luedtke CA, Thompson JM, Postier JA, et al. A description of a brief multidisciplinary treatment program for fibromyalgia. Pain Manag Nurs 2005; 6(2):76–80.

187. Shupak NM, McKay JC, Nielsen WR, et al. Exposure to a specific pulsed low-frequency magnetic field: A double-blind placebo-controlled study of effects on pain ratings in rheumatoid arthritis and fibromyalgia patients. Pain Res Manag 2006; 11(2):85–90.

188. Usui C, Doi N, Nishioka M, et al. Electroconvulsive therapy improves severe pain associated with fibromyalgia. Pain 2006; 121(3):276–280.

10

Soft-Tissue Pain Syndromes: Brain, Mind, and Body Connections

As with most things, clinically there are "lumpers and splitters"; that is, some authorities place myofascial pain syndrome (MPS) and fibromyalgia syndrome (FMS) as two aspects of the same pathophysiological entity, while others feel that they are separate entities with some areas of correspondence. The pathophysiology of these two soft-tissue pain problems has been discussed in some detail. It would appear that there are significant differences in the pathoetiology of these disorders. Another significant difference is the ability to clinically effect successful treatment of the MPS, an element that is, to date, less definitive in the treatment of FMS.

The purpose of this chapter is to look beyond these specific entities and consider how the brain, mind, and body play significant roles in the pathoetiology of soft-tissue pain, particularly FMS.

CENTRAL SENSITIVITY SYNDROMES

The terminology central sensitivity syndromes (CSS) has been used most particularly by Yunus (1–3). It reflects that FMS is only one of a group, or spectrum, of similar syndromes. This spectrum is thought to include FMS, chronic fatigue syndrome, irritable bowel syndrome (IBS), female urethral syndrome, MPS, temporomandibular pain and dysfunction syndrome, restless legs syndrome, periodic limb movement disorder, multiple chemical sensitivities, tension-type headaches, migraine, and primary dysmenorrhea (3). Yunus and Inanici (3) note that these syndromes are most likely associated with each other, although the specific physiological associations are not all known. However, they are felt to share overlapping features and common pathoetiological mechanisms of neuroendocrine dysfunction and central sensitivity. Furthermore, they note that FMS has been shown to be associated with a number of other CSS including IBS, tension-type headaches, chronic fatigue syndrome, primary dysmenorrhea, restless legs syndrome, and female urethral syndrome (1).

Yunus notes that the various CSS entities share clinical characteristics including gender (female preponderance), age distribution, and symptomatology (pain, fatigue, sleep disorder, paresthesia, and global hyperesthesias) (1,3). Furthermore, he notes that there is no discernable structural pathology that can be found by typical laboratory and radiological testing. The CSS cannot be classified as psychiatric syndromes, in spite of the fact that psychological factors may play a role in "a minority subgroup of patients with CSS (3)."

Medically, there are two classical models used to explain illness—pathology, with associated structural damage, infection or inflammation, or psychiatry. Yunus states that there is a "third paradigm" consisting of illness characterized by neurohormonal changes and central sensitivity, which are different from psychiatric illnesses (1,2). In Chapter 8, the specific functional neuroendocrine abnormalities were discussed, along with specific neurochemical dysfunctions and abnormalities in brain function associated with FMS. Similar specific pathophysiological changes have not been demonstrated, to date, for the majority of other CSS entities, including MPS and tension-type headache (see Chapter 12) or migraine, nor, to date, restless legs syndrome. In fact, looking at tension-type headache, a totally different set of neurochemical changes are noted (see Chapter 12).

It would also appear that the boundaries between the classical medical paradigms and the "third paradigm" are not definitive. Pain in chronic diseases can certainly be increased, or affected, by psychological factors, as can questions of disability and overall morbidity. Environmental and psychological stressors can increase the perception of pain. Frequent exposures to stressors may contribute to the development or augmentation of abnormal pain sensitivity in some genetically predisposed individuals.

As noted several times in this text, chronic pain is a biological, psychological, and sociological entity, all aspects of which must be dealt with to best achieve appropriate amelioration.

THE NEUROMATRIX

As discussed in Chapter 1, Melzack has advanced his gate-control theory to include a more global pain construct. The neuromatrix consists of pathways linked to the thalamus, cortex, and limbic system, which generate patterns of neural activity. These patterns underlie awareness of the body and produce pain perception and pain behavior. Any factor that would increase or decrease the functional aspects of pain transmission or pain modulation in the neuromatrix would be able to influence pain sensitivity (4). Conceptually, FMS may be secondary to alterations in the neuromatrix that cannot be restored to normal function, possibly due to plasticity or the older concept of "fixed" or "reverberating" circuits.

DYSFUNCTIONAL PAIN MODULATION

The concept of dysfunctional pain modulation encompasses two aspects: the development of central sensitization secondary to neurochemical and neuroanatomical changes initiated and induced by pain, and dysfunctional inhibition, the inability of the normal inhibitory descending antinociceptive pathways to effectively inhibit nociception (5).

It has been hypothesized that chronic musculoskeletal pain is associated with central dysmodulation (6). This led to the question of classification of pain based on its specific pathophysiological mechanisms and not on etiology. Disorders characterized by dysfunctional pain modulation were thought best to be described as "disorders of dysfunctional pain (7)."

Not all patients with long-standing nociception develop dysfunctional pain symptoms. Genetic predisposition, pain experienced in the neonatal period, intensity and persistence of initial pain, as well as emotional factors may be important in the development of dysfunction pain states (8,9).

Myofascial Pain Syndrome

Symptoms of MPS that radiate distally are typically diffuse and frequently found to have nonanatomical borders. This is unlike neuropathic pain secondary to nerve root compression or nerve entrapment. Peripheral sensory abnormalities associated with MPS are typically variable or transient, unlike those seen in neuropathic pain.

There may be some similarities between the problem of chronic muscle pain and neuropathic pain: both may have common causal central mechanisms. Experimental evidence has demonstrated that primary muscle nociception can induce dorsal horn abnormalities that may be associated with hyperalgesia and the development of persistent pain in enlarged regions (10,11).

Other clinical research may indicate that dysfunctional central pain modulation may explain chronic musculoskeletal pain disorders. Evidence has been noted, indicating a lowered pain threshold and allodynia in patients with chronic cervico-brachial pain syndromes thought to be indicative of central excitability (12). Central sensitization with regions of secondary hyperalgesia have been felt to be associated with myofascial trigger points (13). A study has also shown that patients with MPS have quantitatively altered nociception that induces central hyperexcitability (14). Finally, other reports are indicative of dysfunctional pain in MPS (6,13,15).

Fibromyalgia
Peripheral muscular changes do not appear to be the cause of widespread pain in FMS (5). In a subgroup of 30% to 40% of patients who develop FMS, there is a prior history of regional MPS (5).

Lidbeck states that there is an increasing body of evidence indicating that the poorly understood chronic musculoskeletal pain disorders such as FMS have, as their pathoetiology, dysmodulation of the central pain processing/modulating systems (5).

As was discussed in detail in Chapter 8, there is evidence indicating the allodynia and hyperalgesia found in FMS is secondary, possibly, to dysfunctional inhibition (16,17). The fact that infusions of ketamine, an N-methyl-D-aspartate (NMDA) receptor antagonist, reduced pain in the experimental treatment of FMS patients (18) indicates that central sensitization may play an important role in the pathophysiology of FMS pain. FMS patients also appear to have qualitatively changed nociception, which enhances support for central hyperexcitability in these patients (19).

Multiple factors indicate that FMS is associated with a generalized central dysfunction of pain modulation including widespread allodynia and hyperalgesia involving both the superficial tissues and deeper structures. Also, as detailed in Chapter 8, there are many reasons to consider multiple neuroendocrine dysfunction as well as abnormal central stress responses.

LIMBICALLY AUGMENTED PAIN SYNDROME

The Rome brothers described a hypothesis that would tie the biopsychosocial aspects of the problem of chronic pain together in a way that would encompass all aspects of chronic soft-tissue pain and other forms of chronic pain in at least a subset of such patients (20).

The question of the relationship between depression and chronic pain has long been debated. It is known that nociceptive sensory information, after reaching the thalamus, goes to the limbic system where any emotional significance to such input is assessed; this will result in the type and degree of CNS, endocrine, immune system, and neuropeptide response (21). Research has shown, from brain-imaging studies, limbic system abnormalities in previously traumatized individuals (22).

Hippocampal dysfunction in humans may induce impairment in the evaluation and categorization of experience into memory. Such traumatic memories may be encoded by the amygdala, leaving these individuals unable to place them within a meaningful context. Decreased hippocampal functioning may thus induce hyper-responsiveness to stimuli, causing incoming stimuli to be interpreted in terms of "fight or flight" responses, with pain patients unable to do more than experience more pain in a situation in which they have no apparent control (21).

Research has described the bidirectional nature of the facilitatory and inhibitory processes that are responsible for hyperalgesia, allodynia, pathologic involvement of the sympathetic branch of the autonomic nervous system in a number of various pain states, and the chronicity of pain after the cessation or significant reduction of the initiating activity in nociceptive afferents (23).

Linkages between the various sensory, emotional/affective, and cognitive aspects of chronic pain have been explained via the gate control mechanisms in the spinal cord dorsal horn (23); factors mediating cognitive and behavioral activities (24), and psychophysiological mechanisms such as chronic muscle tension/spasm (25), and common neurobiological substrates (26) may also be linked. The Rome brothers (20) hypothesized a kindling model, which achieves such a linkage via neuroplastic changes that are accumulated during a life of various experiences that may, under some circumstances, lead to a state of corticolimbic sensitization.

"Kindling", in this context, is a generic term referring to specific stimulus-induced neuroplastic mechanisms that will modify neuronal membrane functions, intracellular chemical messenger systems, synaptic activity, and the microscopic neuroanatomy of the CNS (20). Neuroplastic processes would transduce intero-ceptive and exterceptive stimuli into cellular memory (20).

Animal research using kindling revealed that an organism's prior experience with a stimulus, and the environmental context in which the stimulus is delivered help to determine the augmentation of a response (27,28).

It was suggested that kindling would be an appropriate model for nociception-induced neuroplastic changes that can develop in the limbic system and other CNS systems, leading to corticolimbic sensitization, which can engender a clinical picture of persistent pain, affective dysregulation, and disturbances in behavior (20). The concept of the limbically augmented pain syndrome (LAPS) is considered to be a clinical manifestation of corticolimbic sensitization secondary to kindling mechanisms in the supraspinal structures that effect both nociceptive processing and affective regulation (20). Clinical observations as well as neurobiological evidence suggests that both nociceptive/chronic pain disorders and affective/emotional disorders have significant similarities in clinical phenomenology, pharmacological treatments, and neuroanatomic loci as well as in their chemical/molecular substrates (20).

The LAPS construct leads to clinical features that include chronic alterations in pain perception, which are often atypical, resistance to analgesic treatments, disturbances of mood, sleep, energy, libido, memory/concentration, behavior, and stress intolerance (20).

CONCLUSIONS

Of major importance to this discussion is the close similarity in the clinical aspects of LAPS and patients with FMS, but not those with simple MPS. The fact that many FMS patients do have a history of trauma, emotional or physical, would appear to give some credence to the LAPS hypothesis. That the clinical similarities are so close to those seen in this group of patients is of great interest, as the LAPS gives a neuro-biological construct that takes into account not only the various clinical hypotheses that account for the physiological/nociceptive aspects of FMS and other chronic painful disorders, but also the questions of past history, pre-existing and concurrent psychiatric morbidity, and the close association of the biological, psychological, and sociological (including environmental) aspects of chronic pain.

Central sensitization or sensitivity secondary to nociceptive/neuroplastic changes (secondary to nociceptive changes in the dorsal horn) as a primary pain mechanism is not an isolated etiology in the production of the various aspects of chronic pain. Recalling that the nociceptive and antinociceptive pathways have a very close anatomical relationship in the CNS with the limbic system, whether one looks at the concept of neuromodules in Melzack's neuromatrix hypothesis or the possibly more encompassing LAPS, a neurobiological construct, which can give etiological information for all aspects of the biological–psychological–sociological aspects of chronic pain is an important clinical model.

On a purely clinical basis, this represents a subpopulation of chronic pain patients who are frequently seen in the tertiary care chronic pain facilities and who represent the most difficult patient population to successfully treat. The extremely close integration of the noted symptomatology associated with neuroplastic changes would make it difficult for pharmacological treatment to work, as by itself it changes little. Physical treatment, such as physical or occupational therapy, inter-ventional procedures, or even psychotherapy performed in isolation from a comprehensive interdisciplinary treatment paradigm may not be helpful in this patient population.

Many questions persist; although the use of ketamine to diminish pain in FMS patients, presumably via its activity as an NMDA receptor antagonist, may give some pain relief (18), what does this do to the other complex manifestations of the chronic pain syndrome over time? We have discussed the neuroplastic changes associated with chronic pain, starting in the spinal cord dorsal horn. If the LAPS construct or hypothesis is correct, and neuroplastic changes occur in the supraspinal regions inducing corticolimbic sensitization, what, if anything, can be done to either reverse these processes or ameliorate their impact?

Clinically, it would appear that a multifaceted, concurrent interdisciplinary treatment paradigm utilizing cognitive–behavioral therapy as one part of the paradigm is most helpful, at least with our present state of knowledge. Cognitive restructuring while dealing with the physiological aspects of the pain (i.e., central sensitization, for example) would appear to be helpful in possibly retraining the affected supraspinal CNS substrates, at least in terms of treatment success in these very difficult clinical pain problems.

The brain, the mind, and the body are all parts of the complicated chronic pain problem. Therefore, all aspects of these entities, individually and collectively, must be dealt with in the hope of successfully helping patients with these complex clinical problems.

REFERENCES

1. Yunus MB. Central sensitivity syndromes: a unified concept for fibromyalgia and other similar maladies. J Indian Rheum Assoc 2000; 8:27–33.
2. Yunus MB, Inanici F. Clinical characteristics and biopathophysiological mechanisms of fibromyalgia syndrome. In: Baldry P, ed. Myofascial Pain and Fibromyalgia Syndromes: A clinical Guide to Diagnosis and Management. London, UK: Churchill Livingstone, 2001:351–377.

3. Yunus MB, Inanici F. Fibromyalgia syndrome: clinical features, diagnosis, and biopatho-physiologic mechanisms. In: Rachlin ES, Rachlin IS, eds. Myofascial Pain and Fibromyalgia: Trigger Point Management. 2nd ed. St. Louis, Mo: Mosby, 2002:3–32.

4. Melzack R. Gate control theory: on the evolution of pain concepts. Pain Forum 1996; 5:125–128.

5. Lidbeck J. Central hyperexcitability in chronic musculoskeletal pain: a conceptual breakthrough with multiple clinical implications. Pain Res Manag 2002; 7(2):81–92.

6. Henriksson KG. Muscle activity and chronic muscle pain. J Musculoskel Pain 1999; 7:101–109.

7. Sjolund B. Chronic pain in society—a case for chronic pain as a dysfunctional state? Qual Life Res 1994; 3(suppl 1):S5–S9.

8. Wiesenfeld-Hallin Z, Hao J.-X, Xu X.-J, Aldskogius H, Seiger A. Genetic factors influence the development of mechanical hypersensitivity, motor deficits and morphological damage after transient cord ischemia in the rat. Pain 1993; 55:235–241.

9. Fitzgerald M. Developmental neurobiology of pain. In: Wall PD, Melzack R, eds. Textbook of Pain, 4th ed. Edinburgh, UK: Churchill Livingstone, 1999:235–251.

10. Wall PD, Woolf CJ. Muscle but not cutaneous C-afferent input produces prolonged increases in the excitability of the flexion reflex in the rat. J Physiol 1984; 356:289–295.

11. Dubner R. Hyperalgesia in response to injury to cutaneous and deep tissues. In: Fricton JR, Dubner R, eds. Orofacial Pain and Temporomandibular Disorders. New York, NY: Raven Press, 1995:61–71.

12. Sheater-Reid RB, Cohen MI. Psychophysical evidence for a neuropathic component of chronic neck pain. Pain 1998; 75:341–347.

13. Kramis RC, Roberts WJ, Gillette RG. Non-nociceptive aspects of persistent musculoskel-etal pain. J Orthop Sports Phys Ther 1996; 24:255–267.

14. Bendtsen L, Jensen R, Olesen J. Quantitatively altered nociception in chronic myofascial pain. Pain 1996; 65:259–264.

15. Littlejohn GO. Clinical update on other pain syndromes. J Musculoskel Pain 1996; 4:163–179.

16. Lautenbacher S, Rollman GB. Possible deficiencies of pain modulation in fibromyalgia. Clin J Pain 1997; 13:189–196.

17. Yunus MB. Towards a model of pathophysiology of fibromyalgia: aberrant central pain mechanisms with peripheral modulation. J Rheumatol 1992; 19:846–850.

18. Graven-Nielsen T, Aspergren Kendall S, Henriksson KG, et al. Ketamine reduces muscle pain, temporal summation, and referred pain in fibromyalgia patients. Pain 2000; 85:483–491.

19. Bendtsen E, Norregaard J, Jensen R, Olesen J. Evidence of qualitatively altered nociception in patients with fibromyalgia. Arthritis Rheum 1997; 40:98–102.

20. Rome HP, Rome JD. Limbically augmented pain syndrome (LAPS): kindling, corticolim-bic sensitization, and the convergence of affective and sensory symptoms in chronic pain disorders. Pain Med 2000; 1:7–23.

21. Aronoff GM, Feldman JB. Preventing iatrogenic disability from chronic pain. Curr Rev Pain 1999; 3:67–77.

22. van der Kolk B. The body keeps the score: memory and the evolving psychobiology of posttraumatic stress. Harvard Rev Psychiatry 1994; 1:253–265.

23. Coderre TJ, Katz J, Vaccarino AL, Melzack R. Contribution of central neuroplasticity to pathological pain: review of clinical and experimental evidence. Pain 1993; 52:259–285.

24. Rudy TE, Kerns RD, Turk DC. Chronic pain and depression: toward a cognitive-behavioral mediation model. Pain 1988; 35:129–140.

25. Flor H, Turk DC: Psychophysiology of chronic pain: do chronic pain patients exhibit symptom-specific psychophysiological responses? Psychol Bull 1989; 105:215–259.

26. Chapman CR. The affective dimension of pain: a model. Adv Pain Res Ther 1995; 22:283–301.

27. Racine RJ, Ivy GO, Milgram NW. Kindling: clinical relevance and anatomical substrate. In: Bolwig TG, Trimble MR, eds. The Clinical Relevance of Kindling. Chichester, UK, John Wiley & Sons, 1989; 15–34.

28. Gilbert ME. The phenomenology of limbic kindling. Toxicol Ind Health 1994; 10:343–358.

11

Neuropathic Pain[†]

INTRODUCTION

Reports of more than a century of medical observation and research have demonstrated that neuropathic pain is much more than a concept or a single disorder. It is instead an evolving collection of established clinical and experimental conditions, all of which share the perpetuation of pain symptoms or pain-related behavior created by injury to neural tissue other than that involved with simple nociception (1,2).

While neuropathic pain has been operationally defined as an abnormal pain state that arises from a damaged peripheral nervous system (PNS) or central nervous system (CNS) (3), there is evidence to suggest that several disease states within this category have active residual involvement of nociceptors at the site of the original injury, creating a mixed nociceptive-neuropathic pattern. As well, several painful disorders categorized as neuropathic are created or maintained by aberrant neural communication involving autonomic nervous system pathways that are not considered to be purely peripheral or central. These include complex regional pain syndromes types I and II (reflex sympathetic dystrophy and causalgia, respectively) and sympathetically maintained pain (SMP) (4,5).

NEUROPATHIC PAIN SYNDROMES

In primary care as well as many types of specialty practice, the term neuropathic pain has been most often thought of as simply meaning painful peripheral neuropathy, as commonly occurs in severe diabetes mellitus (DM). This association may have developed based on the high incidence of diabetes, the bilateral, distal distribution of other symptoms (sensory loss), and signs (reduced temperature, circulatory compromise) commonly seen in this illness. In general clinical practice, the pains of well-known neurologic disorders, such as those created by herpes zoster and inflammatory involvement of the trigeminal nerves, are more likely to be thought of as focal neuralgias, rather than neuropathic pain. Similarly, the pain created by local compression of nerve roots is considered to represent just one aspect of a radiculopathy rather than being part of a neuropathic pain syndrome. Even when contralateral pain is created by unilateral thalamic or other deep hemispheric infarctions, the symptoms are first thought to represent a specific (central poststroke) syndrome, rather than being part of a more general (neuropathic) pain category.

[†]This chapter was co-written by David R. Longmire, Department of Internal Medicine, University of Alabama School of Medicine, Huntsville, Alabama, U.S.A. Dr. Longmire is in private practice specializing in pain management, clinical neurophysiology, and adult and child neurology.

In addition to those syndromes mentioned in the preceding paragraph, there are several common, clearly identified conditions which are known to be associated with severe, persistent neuropathic pain (5,5a,6,6a).

NEUROPATHIC PAIN DISORDERS BY ETIOLOGY

In theory, almost any of the pathologic processes known to create damage or dysfunction to neural tissue can be considered as potential causes for neuropathic pain. Viral/ bacterial, aseptic inflammation, pressure due to neoplasm or other structural lesions, degenerative, ischemia, autoimmune, toxic, traumatic, and endocrine/metabolic mechanisms have all been implicated in the production of pain (Table 1) (7–9).

PATHOPHYSIOLOGIC PROCESSES SUBSERVING NEUROPATHIC PAIN

As one might expect, there is substantial evidence that abnormal nerve activity is an important mechanism underlying the spontaneous pain typical of neuropathic pain states (10,11,12). It is hypothesized that sites of ectopic foci develop on injured or regenerating nerves in the periphery, at the level of the nociceptor, neuromas, or segments of injured nerves; at the dorsal root ganglion; and in the dorsal horn of the spinal cord. Indeed, after nerve transection, increased sensitivity occurs, followed in a few days by spontaneous activity. These abnormal ectopic foci may be thought of as spontaneous pain generators, resulting in paroxysmal and spontaneous pain (see Chapter 3 for more detail).

TABLE 1   Common Causes of Neuropathic Pain

Polyneuropathy
   Diabetes (insulin-dependent and noninsulin-dependent)
   Alcoholism
   HIV
   Hypothyroidism
   Renal failure
   Chemotherapy (vincristine, cisplatinum, paclitaxel, metronidazole)
   Anti-HIV drugs
   B12 and folate deficiencies
   Small-fiber neuropathy
Mononeuropathy
   Entrapment syndromes
   Traumatic injury
   Diabetes
   Vasculitis
Plexopathy
   Diabetes
   Avulsion
   Tumor
Root syndromes and radiculopathy
   Compressive lesions
Cervical and lumbar radiculopathy
   Neuropathic low-back pain
   Inflammatory
   Diabetes
Postherpetic neuralgia (PHN)
Trigeminal neuralgia
Phantom limb pain
RSD/causalgia/CRPS

Source: Adapted from Ref. 5a.

Precise pathophysiology is unclear, but pharmacologic evidence suggests that ectopic activity is due to an increased number of sodium channels, or more likely an abnormal subtype of sodium channel, resulting in unstable sodium channel activity. Pharmacologic evidence supporting this hypothesis is the effectiveness of local anesthetics and some anticonvulsants (sodium channel-blocking drugs) in neuropathic pain. These drugs presumably produce frequency and voltage-dependent blockade of sodium channels on damaged neurons (11). The abnormal sodium channel involved in neuropathic pain states may be a tetrodotoxin-insensitive subtype, found only in neural tissue (14). Accumulation of atypical as well as tetrodotoxin-sensitive sodium channels (responsible for normal nerve conduction) may explain often inadequate therapeutic benefit of current sodium channel-blocking drugs.

Work in animal models demonstrates that voltage-dependent calcium channels may also be important in modulating neuropathic transmission. Unfortunately, the currently available calcium channel blockers are cardioselective, and are not particularly effective in neuropathic pain. There appear to be at least six calcium channel subtypes, and studies with novel N-type calcium channel blockers are promising in animals (13). Preliminary studies with conotoxin (SNX-111) are positive, although the drug must be administered intrathecally.

Gabapentin, a novel anticonvulsant, appears to bind to the a2d subunit of a voltage-dependent calcium channel. Work by Chaplan and his colleagues (13) demonstrated that messenger RNA and protein for the a2d subunit are increased more than 10-fold in dorsal root ganglia following nerve injury, but are not changed after other forms of tissue injury. Blockade of a retrograde signal from the injury site (which may involve nerve growth factor) prevents upregulation of the a2d subunit. Chaplan pointed out that the a2d subunit does not seem to play a role in normal channel kinetics but may affect calcium channel assembly and insertion into the neuronal membrane. Thus, the subunit may act as a drug-binding site and secondarily modify channel kinetics.

NEUROPATHIC PAIN DISORDERS
Diabetic Neuropathy

The most recent International Association for the Study of Pain (IASP) definition of neuropathic pain, as noted earlier, is "pain initiated or caused by a primary lesion or dysfunction in the nervous system (15)."

It is felt that there are three general phases of pain (16,17): phase 1—transient activation of the nociceptive system occurs secondary to appropriate stimuli and CNS processing of this stimulus-induced information occurs appropriately; phase 2—each injury evokes mechanisms representing nociceptive system plasticity, and which induces reversible modulation of the nociceptive system; phase 3—modification of the nociceptive system induces chronic abnormal pain sensations.

These mechanisms may be activated in a different order, which would help to explain the clinical differences between nociceptive and neuropathic pain.

In nociceptive pain, tissue damage occurs, activation of phase 1 is noted, after peripherally occurring pain, which is conducted to the CNS—pain modulation in phase 2 occurs, including peripheral and central sensitization—these changes may last hours to days—and then modification of pain sensation (in phase 3) can occur, particularly in disorders involving chronic inflammatory processes, causing prolonged changes to responsiveness, leading to chronic pain (17). In neuropathic pain, damage to the nervous system induces the changes to phase 3 first, secondary to loss of function, inducing modification of pain sensation, which is followed by activation of phase 1 (activation of the nociceptive system) by ectopic activity secondary to changes in the nociceptive system and then modulation in phase 2 occurs, which is effected by central sensitization, disinhibition, and descending facilitation (17).

Diabetic neuropathy (DN) is a broad term for several different clinical syndromes, with different pathophysiologic mechanisms.

Diabetes is probably the most common cause of neuropathy, and DN is probably the most common neurologic problem associated with diabetes. The incidence of DN increases with the duration of diabetes and the degree and duration of hyperglycemia. Further epidemiologic data indicate that between 30% and 40% of type 2 diabetics have a distal peripheral neuropathy (18,19). The Diabetes Control and Complications Trial (DCCT) study found that the annual incidence of neuropathy was 2% per year, but with intensive treatment of type 1 diabetics, it dropped to 0.56%. They found that other risk factors included the duration of diabetes, age, cigarette smoking, hypertension, height, and hyperlipidemia (20).

In general, the prevalence of DN varies from 5% to 100%, secondary to questions regarding the diagnosis.

The definition of DN, according to the San Antonio Consensus Statement on DN, is a demonstrable disorder, subclinical or clinical, occurring in the presence of DM without other causes for peripheral neuropathy. Furthermore, the diabetic peripheral neuropathy includes somatic and/or autonomic manifestations (21).

In Chapter 3, we discussed some of the mechanisms of peripheral neuropathic pain, including: peripheral neuronal sensitization, spontaneous ectopic electrical discharges, collateral sprouting, and ephaptic communication. Centrally, there are also problems including disinhibition, central sensitization, and reorganization of synaptic connectivity in the spinal cord dorsal horn.

The pathophysiology of painful diabetic neuropathy (PDN) is also multifactorial, with somatic and autonomic neuropathies.

Somatic neuropathies include both mononeuropathies and polyneuropathies, while the autonomic neuropathies affect the cardiovascular system, along with the gastrointestinal and genitourinary systems, among others.

Still another classification includes symmetrical neuropathies and focal and multifocal neuropathies.

The most common form of DN is the distal sensory or sensorimotor polyneuropathy, which involves both small and large nerve fibers (22).

Small fiber sensory neuropathies can include a number of characteristics, and include hypoxia as well as distal axonopathy with dying back of the nerve as primary pathoetiology. The small fiber sensory neuropathy includes: hyperalgesia, paresthesia, burning pain, lancinating pain, loss of pain and temperature sensation, loss of visceral pain, and eventual foot ulceration leading to an increased incidence of amputation.

In the presence of a large fiber sensory neuropathy, one can find loss of vibration and proprioception and areflexia on neurologic examination and abnormal nerve conduction studies.

The distal symmetrical sensorimotor polyneuropathy begins insidiously and can involve both large and small fibers. The distal lower extremities are the first to be affected. The sensory symptoms typically advance up above the knees and include the distal upper extremities and the anterior aspect of the trunk; the vertex of the head may also rarely be involved (23,24).

Symptoms may be positive (burning pain, paresthesia, lancinating pain, hyperesthesia, and allodynia) and/or negative (numbness).

There are also a number of symmetrical neuropathies associated with diabetes. Hyperglycemic neuropathy is associated with paresthesias in the extremities and the trunk, and is most frequently seen in poorly controlled diabetic patients, or those who are newly diagnosed, and will improve with better glycemic control (22).

Acute painful neuropathy (diabetic neuropathic cachexia) is usually seen in older men with a history of significant weight loss associated with the sudden appearance of severe burning pain in the extremities, occasionally the trunk, autonomic dysfunction, sensory loss, and muscle weakness, which is less common (24–26).

Chronic inflammatory demyelinating polyneuropathy (CIDP) is associated with diabetes. Patient presentation includes symmetric weakness associated with demyelination (on nerve biopsy) and changes on electromyography. Pain distribution is less likely to be symmetric (26,27). Patients with CIDP associated with DM differs from idiopathic CIDP in that the diabetic patients are typically older, have a longer duration of symptoms, significant axonal loss, and poorer response to therapy (26,27).

Asymmetric, focal, and multifocal neuropathies are also found in diabetic patients. Diabetic amyotrophy (also known as asymmetrical proximal lower-limb neuropathy, diabetic polyradiculopathy, and diabetic lumbosacral radiculoplexus neuropathy) is most frequently seen in type 2 diabetics in their fifth or sixth decades. At first, it is associated with unilateral symptoms, becoming bilateral. An asymmetrical proximal motor neuropathy is seen in association with pain in the back, hip, and knees. Muscle wasting and weakness are seen in the hip flexors, adductors, and quadriceps. There is a loss of the quadriceps reflex. The patellar reflex is also decreased ipsilaterally. Pain is acute or subacute. The disorder appears to be immunologic in nature (28,29).

Diabetic cranial neuropathies most typically affect the oculomotor nerves (third, fourth, and sixth), facial nerve (seventh), and fifth cranial nerves. The optic nerve can also be affected. Clinically, patients may develop mild or severe periorbital pain and/or headache followed by diplopia. It is associated with muscle paresis with sparing of the pupillary reflex, decreased blink reflex and, more rarely, nonarteritic acute anterior ischemic optic neuropathy without the presence of pre-existing diabetic retinopathy (30,33).

Truncal mononeuropathy (also known as thoracoabdominal neuropathy, thoracolumbar neuropathy, thoracolumbar radiculopathy, and thoracic radiculopathy) is most frequently seen in middle-aged patients, typically those with essentially mild diabetes. Both positive and negative sensory signs can be seen, including pain in the back, abdomen, or chest in the distribution of thoracic and/or upper lumbar nerve roots, and associated areas of sensory loss or dysesthesia in dermatomal distributions. The pain can be severe burning, stabbing, belt-like, deep and aching, and is more intense at night. The pain begins unilaterally and then becomes bilateral. In some patients, hyperalgesia and allodynia may occur. Weakness of the abdominal wall can be seen, associated with abdominal muscle paresis. Diabetic distal symmetric polyneuropathy is also frequently present (26,34,35).

Mononeuritis multiplex is an asymmetrical sensory and motor peripheral neuropathy associated with damage to at least two nerves. It can later become symmetric. The disorder, which is associated with systemic disorders such as diabetes, rheumatoid arthritis, and vasculitis, can get worse over time. The associated nerve damage appears to be secondary to axon destruction (36).

Diabetic autonomic neuropathy is frequently overlooked. It can affect any organ of the body, which is enervated by autonomic nerves. Parasympathetic dysfunction has been found in 65% of type 2 diabetics at 10 years post diagnosis of diabetes; combined sympathetic and parasympathetic neuropathic is found in 15.2% of patients (37). There are numerous symptoms found in autonomic neuropathy in various systems: cardiovascular: postural hypotension, resting tachycardia, painless myocardial infarction; prolonged QT interval, sudden death; gastrointestinal: esophageal motor incoordination, gastric hypomotility, pyloro-spasm, uncoordinated intestinal motility or diabetic diarrhea, constipation, fecal incontinence, gallbladder hypocontraction; genitourinary: impaired bladder sensation, atonic bladder, postmicturation dribbling detrusor hyporeflexia or hyperreflexia,' male impotence, problems with ejaculation, dyspareunia, and reduced vaginal lubrication in women; thermoregulatory: sudomotor and vaso-motor changes; pupillary: miosis, disturbances with dilatation and the Argyll Robertson pupil. There is a question as to the presence of impaired breathing and sleep apnea. Gustatory sweating is the most common symptom followed by postural hypotension, diarrhea, sexual dysfunction, anhidrosis of the feet, bladder abnormalities, and gastroparesis (24,37–41).

Clinical evaluation of the cardiovascular signs of diabetic autonomic neuropathy, particularly in patients with a five-year history of diabetes or longer, should be performed, and include at least postural blood pressure changes as well as heart rate variability with respiration (42).

Type 1 diabetic patients with cardiac autonomic neuropathy can have a greater risk of sudden death possibly associated with prolongations of the QTc interval (43–49). Type 1 diabetic patients with autonomic neuropathy have decreased myocardial perfusion capacity when given a vasodilator, which may be part of the cause for increased mortality in these patients, possibly secondary to defective myocardial sympathetic vasodilatation; the lack of the ability to maintain blood pressure during vasodilatation, or both (50). It has even been suggested that cardiac autonomic neuropathy may contribute to a "dead in bed syndrome" associated with decreased vagal tone and predominant sympathetic tonus increasing the possibility of cardiac arrhythmia during significant bouts of hypoglycemia (51,52). This would also be associated with a higher risk of arrhythmia and sudden death after acute myocardial infarction (53,54).

As the risk of cardiovascular events in patients with diabetes is estimated to be two to four times higher than in normals, a thorough clinical evaluation should be routinely done (55,56). It should also be noted that the diabetic cardiac autonomic neuropathy develops independently from the painful, somatic DN (57).

Compression neuropathies (entrapment neuropathies) are uncommon. The median nerve is most commonly affected. The ulnar or lateral femoral cutaneous nerve may also be affected (24,58).

MECHANISMS OF DIABETIC PERIPHERAL NEUROPATHY

The theoretical constructs include metabolic, vascular, altered neurotrophic support, autoimmune, and free radicals associated with oxidative stress.

Hyperglycemia and the polyol pathway: Hyperglycemia is the primary reason for the development of DN as has been demonstrated by the DCCT (20). This group also showed that with excellent control of hyperglycemia there is a significant reduction of autonomic dysfunction (53%), neuropathy (64%), and motor conduction velocity changes (44%) in type 1 diabetics (24,59).

Insulin is not responsible for glucose uptake in the peripheral nerves. For this reason, high glucose levels in the blood cause high nerve glucose concentrations. The polyol pathway, via reactions catalyzed by aldose reductase, converts glucose to sorbitol. Nerve fructose levels are also increased. Excess fructose and sorbitol induce a decrement in the expression of the sodium/myoinositol cotransporter, which causes decreased myoinositol levels. This, in turn, creates decreased levels of Na/K ATPase activity. Aldose reductase, when activated, depletes its cofactor nicotinamide adenine dinucleotide phosphate (NADPH), which causes decreased levels of nitric oxide and glutathione, which work to stop oxidative injury. The lack of nitric oxide stops vascular relaxation, which helps in the induction of chronic ischemia (60–65).

Microvascular ischemic changes in the nerves of diabetes can include endothelial cell hyperplasia, thickening of the capillary basement membrane and neuronal ischemia and infarction (60,66). Endoneurial vascular resistance to hyperglycemic blood may induce endoneurial ischemia (26).

Neurotrophic factors are needed for the maintenance of nerve function and structural maintenance. NGF has been found to be decreased, and, along with insulin-like growth factor-1, shown to correlate with the severity of DN in animals (24). Insulin has neurotrophic effects and in a diabetic state, its deficiency may be associated with the development of neuropathy (60).

Autoimmune neuropathy is felt to emerge from immunogenic changes of the cells in the endothelial capillaries (26).

Dysfunction of the sodium channels has been found in animal models of painful neuropathy (67). Increased activity of voltage-gated calcium channels has also been demonstrated in DN, which can lead to tissue injury (68).

Oxygen-free radicals may induce nerve damage directly or by inhibiting nitric oxide production, and thus causing a reduced nerve blood flow. Free radical generation is increased in diabetics by the processes of nonenzymatic glycation and polyol pathway. At the same time, the ability to neutralize free radicals is decreased because NADPH, which deals with cell oxidation/reduction status, is diminished as it is consumed by increased activity of aldose reductase (24,69).

Activation of protein kinase C (PKC) occurs secondary to hyperglycemia, which leads to increased diacylglycerol synthesis and PKC activation. PKC may also be activated by oxidative stress. It increases vascular permeability, blood flow changes, and impairment of nitric oxide synthesis (70–72).

Another possible mechanism is derangement of the essential fatty acid pathways from linolenic acid to prostaglandins and thromboxane, which can induce cellular dysfunction in a number of areas including membrane fluid abnormalities, a decrease in prostaglandin E2, and changes in the membrane of red blood cells (73,74).

Finally, circulating NGF is decreased in diabetic patients with neuropathy (75). Treatment with NGF has shown improvements in peripheral nerve growth and function (76).

Regardless of the pathophysiologic mechanism, or combination of mechanisms that coalesce to induce the production of DN, chronic hyperglycemia appears to have a significant if not pivotal role in its pathoetiology.

SMALL-FIBER NEUROPATHY

Small-fiber neuropathy (SFN) is a common peripheral nerve disease, typically idiopathic in etiology, which commonly presents in middle-aged and older people with burning pain in their feet and/or symptoms of autonomic dysfunction (77,78,79).

The disorder selectively involves small diameter myelinated and unmyelinated nerve fibers. Frequently, autoimmune disorders/mechanisms are suspected but rarely found. SFN can be caused by disorders of metabolism (diabetes), chronic infections (such as human immunodeficiency virus), genetic abnormalities, amyloidosis, drug toxicity, inherited sensory, and autonomic neuropathies. It may be focal or multifocal (15,16).

Diagnosis is most commonly made on the basis of the clinical picture, normal nerve conduction studies (standard electrophysiologic tests for nerve injury do not detect small-fiber function), and abnormally specialized tests of small nerve fibers, including biopsy assessment of epidermal nerve fiber density, temperature sensation tests for sensory fibers [quantitative sensory testing (QST) for heat and cold], sudomotor testing, and cardiovagal testing for autonomic fibers (78,79).

The associated pain is typically secondary to injury to small, unmyelinated C-fiber nerve axons. The pathogenesis of neuropathic pain commonly involves the loss of peripheral axons and inappropriate peripheral and central adaptation of neuronal signaling secondary to this loss (80).

Clinically, patients with SFN may present with either positive sensory symptoms (burning, tingling, prickling, lancinating, or aching pain) or negative symptoms (numbness, tightness, coldness). They may develop allodynia. A feeling of cramping is not uncommon. The symptoms are usually distal. They can be patchy or diffuse. The symptoms are typically worse at night (78).

Of interest is that even subclinical SFN may present with late-onset restless-legs syndrome (RLS) (81). While RLS is primarily classified as a sleep disorder, it may be associated with subclinical small fiber neuropathy, as well as, possibly, dysfunction of the postsynaptic dopamine receptors related to iron metabolism of the CNS as well as opiate receptors (82). Another study noted RLS frequently associated with acquired neuropathies, especially dysimmune neuropathies—particularly small-fiber sensory neuropathies (83).

Pain can also occur with large nerve-fiber dysfunction. Autonomic symptoms may include increases or decreases in sweating, facial flushing, skin discoloration, dry eyes, and mouth as well as possible changes in skin temperature, and erectile dysfunction (in up to 40% of males) (78,84,85).

On examination, clinical findings may include a decrease in temperature and pain sensitivity in a patient with normal strength, proprioception, and normal tendon reflexes. Vibration sensation is commonly normal, but some loss in the great toes can be consistent with mild large-fiber involvement. In many patients, especially those who cannot receive specialized testing, their clinical examination may be entirely normal or only minimal/mild findings are noted (78,86).

Testing for SFN may include nerve conduction studies, which assess large-fiber function, so they would be normal in the presence of only SFN. They are generally within normal limits. It should be noted that patients with SFN might also have some large-fiber loss/dysfunction (87).

Special testing for SFN includes:

1. *Sympathetic skin response.* This reflex change, which looks at small-fiber sudomotor function in the sweat-related skin electrical potentials, can be measured on electomyographic equipment (EMG). The sensitivity of this test for SFN is thought to be low (78).
2. *QST used for diagnosis of SFN.* Temperature testing (hot and cold) is preformed. This technique may be used for serial measurements (88,89,90).

3. *Quantitative sudomotor axon reflex test (QSART)*. Looks at postganglionic sympathetic sudomotor function. This test has a relatively high level of sensitivity in detecting SFN (85,86,89).

Other sudomotor function tests including the thermoregulatory sweat test and the Silastic skin imprint method and the EpiScan, a fast, painless, sensitive selective tissue conductance (STC) method for evaluating sudomotor dysfunction in SFN (89). Sudomotor testing was also found to be a very good tool in the evaluation/detection of SFN in another study by Low et al. (91).

The pathologic aspects of SFN have also been closely evaluated. An antibody against protein gene product 9.5, which is present in all axons, was developed in the early 1980s (92). This enabled immunohistochemical use to help determine, in skin punch biopsies, small-fiber density, which can be found to change as SFN develops. The reduction of intraepidermal nerve density is the most commonly reported abnormality in skin biopsy, with morphologic changes found in the epidermal nerves and underlying subepidermal nerve plexus (93). Another group indicated that intraepidermal nerve fiber density may be a useful endpoint measure for future neuropathy treatment trials—the main problem being the paucity of laboratories actually doing this work (94).

The most common cause of a SFN is typically not found, but when it is, DM is frequently the etiology. Idiopathic SFN is the largest diagnostic category (78,86). A subset of diabetic polyneuropathy patients appears to have symptomatic, primarily small-fiber involvement, with or without autonomic dysfunction (78).

Another group looked at the nerve axon reflex-related vasodilation (N-V response) as a method to evaluate C-nociceptive fiber function. They thought that the N-V response is a reliable tool to diagnose small-fiber dysfunction, which was found early in the natural history of DN (95) Sorensen et al. (96) found quantitative small nerve sensory testing a useful tool to detect the presence of neuropathy. They noted that small nerve fiber abnormalities do not predict the presence of pain in DN (96), and that more severe loss of intraepidermal nerve fibers can be associated with the presence of neuropathic pain in those patients with little or no sign of neuropathy (97).

Other research have found that impaired glucose tolerance (prediabetes) is associated with an "idiopathic" SFN (98,99).

Some other diagnoses related to SFN include:

- Chronic alcohol-dependent subjects, possibly via the direct toxic effect of alcohol on peripheral nerve fibers; painful alcoholic polyneuropathy effects the small myelinated and unmyelinated fibers more than large fibers, particularly early in the disease process. Hyperglycemia and impaired vitamin B (12) utilization may also be involved (100).
- Symptomatic HIV neuropathy, as a measure of small sensory fibers (decreased intraepidermal fiber density, abnormal cold, and heat pain thresholds) appears to be associated with transition to symptomatic HIV-associated distal sensory neuropathy up to 6 to 12 months later (101).
- Celiac disease, a T-cell mediated autoimmune disorder resulting from a lack of tolerance to gluten, is also associated with SFN as seen on skin biopsies. Idiopathic ataxia may also be seen (102,103).
- Sjogren syndrome patients with neuropathy exhibited either a decreased intraepidermal nerve fiber density or abnormal nerve morphology (104).

- Systemic lupus erythematosus, an inflammatory, autoimmune disease, is also found to be associated with a pure small-diameter nerve fiber neuropathy (105).
- Vasculitic neuropathy has infrequently been associated with skin denervation in spite of many manifestations of SFN, including reduced sensitivity to QST and neuropathic pain; epidermal nerve fiber densities were decreased, in addition to the more typical vasculitic effect on large diameter nerves (106,107).
- A case report of four patients with SFN responsive to steroid usage indicates that the patients had acute onset neuropathic pain, normal EMGs, and provocative/diagnostic QST and skin biopsies. The authors raised the question of this being a new entity (108).

Other hereditary disorders may be associated with SFN, including: hereditary sensory autonomic neuropathies I and II, burning feet syndrome, amyloidosis, Fabry's disease, and Tangier disease (78).

Treatment of SFN is not really different from that of large fiber neuropathies. If an identifiable cause is found, it should be treated. Most commonly, the goal of management of SFN is amelioration of pain, using the same drug classes used for more common neuropathic pain syndromes: anticonvulsants, tricyclic antidepressants, serotonin norepinephrine reuptake inhibitor (SNRIs), opiates, and topical agents.

HIV-ASSOCIATED NEUROPATHIC PAIN

Distal symmetrical polyneuropathy (DSP) associated with HIV infection is the most frequent neurologic complication of the disease (109). Spontaneous or evoked pain is the most common symptom of DSP (110). Aside from DSP, patients may develop Mononeuritis multiplex and progressive polyradiculopathy.

The actual pathophysiology of HIV neuropathy is not known. DSP, as noted above, is associated with injury or loss of primary afferent fibers inducing distal axonal degeneration, "dying back" of the neurons (111). This may be mediated by the HIV or by cytotoxic immune processes (110).

A direct mechanism is proposed in which the HIV viral envelope glycoprotein gp120 directly invades the peripheral nerve and the dorsal root ganglion, which induces neurotoxicity (112,113). The activity of chemokines and gp120 glycoprotein can act on the chemokines receptors of nociceptive neurons and induce both hyperesthesia and allodynia (114).

HIV may induce indirect damage by promoting macrophage infiltration in peripheral nerves and the dorsal root ganglia (115,116). The macrophages, once in the peripheral nerve, can cause local release of proinflammatory neurotoxic cytokines, such as tumor necrosis factor, interleukin-1, and interleukin-6, which can induce axonal degeneration (117–119).

Antiretroviral chemotherapy can also induce a toxic neuropathy (120).

NEUROPATHIC LOW-BACK PAIN

Low-back pain (LBP) is one of the most common disorders, effecting about two-thirds of the adult population at some time in their lives. It may or may not be associated with radiation to the sciatic and/or femoral nerves (121). The etiology of the pain may be secondary to a large number of possible problems, making the differential diagnosis large; however, it may be broken down to mechanical, compression, inflammatory, and neuropathic factors which may be directly effected by social and psychologic factors (121).

While the degeneration of the intervertebral disc is frequently considered to be the etiology of pain in patients with LBP, it may be more complicated. Degeneration/deterioration of a disc can influence the CNS by nociceptor stimulation in the annulus fibrosis, which can induce nociceptive pain which is considered to be discogenic pain. This stimulation may be secondary to mechanical or inflammatory factors. While pain with weight-bearing and specific movements is mechanical in nature, there is further growth of both nerve fibers and blood vessels into the deeper layers of the annulus fibrosis (122). Algetic substances including tumor necrosis factor and the interleukins (-1beta, -6, and -8) may also play a role in the development of LBP (122).

In the normal intervertebral discs, only the outer aspects of the annulus fibrosis receive sensory innervation. When discs degenerate, extensive nerve fiber growth is found in the middle third as well as the inner third of the diseased annulus (123,124). Some of this nerve growth is associated with the presence of substance P immunoreactivity (125). Algetic, inflammatory neuropeptides in the degenerated disc along with possible abnormal mechanical pressure in and upon a diseased, incompetent annulus can induce chemical and mechanical sensitization and stimulation of the nociceptive nerve fibers (123).

After the onset of discogenic abnormalities that can initiate pain, after the nociceptors in the disc have been stimulated, the somatosensory system can increase its sensitivity secondary to constant stimulation, causing a nonfunctional response: peripheral sensitization can occur. If the disc degeneration progresses to disc herniation, the nerve roots or dorsal root ganglion, adjacent nervous system structures, may be affected, leading to neuropathic pain of either mechanical or biochemical origin (122).

Disc degeneration can also influence other spinal structures including the facet joints, ligaments, and muscles, which individually or as a group can develop into pain generators. This can lead to disc degeneration leading to the development of chronic LBP without being the actual focus of the pain, with both nociceptive and neuropathic pain being modulated at higher centers (spinal and supraspinally) to develop central sensitization (122). The central sensitization can be associated with neural plasticity, which can play a significant role in the development and chronicity of pain (122).

It is also thought that in chronic sciatica, both nociceptive and neuropathic pain components can be distinguished. Neuropathic pain may be secondary to lesions of nociceptive sprouts in the degenerated disc (local neuropathic), mechanical compression of the nerve root (mechanical neuropathic root pain), or secondary to inflammatory mediators (inducing inflammatory neuropathic root pain) all originating from the degenerative disc even without the presence of mechanical compression. Because there can be several different pain mechanisms inducing sciatic pain, it can be called a "mixed pain syndrome (126)."

Kaki et al. (127) looked at the prevalence of neuropathic pain among a sample of 1169 LBP patients using the Leeds Assessment of Neuropathic Symptoms and Signs (LANSS) pain scale. They found that 54.7% of patients had LANSS pain scale scores suggesting a neuropathic type of pain, and 45.3% having neuropathic types of pain. Advanced age, female gender, increased height, white race, hypertension, diabetes, a history of smoking, previous back surgery, and previous medications were factors found to be associated with neuropathic LBP.

Bennett et al. (128) noted that in the past, pain was divided into two essentially mutually exclusive pain mechanisms: nociceptive and neuropathic. A new approach was looked at, essentially a model of chronic pain which was "more or less neuropathic." They looked at 200 patients (100 each of nociceptive and neuropathic) and used the LANSS pain scale and the Neuropathic Pain Scale. They felt that their data supported the theoretical construct that pain can be more or less neuropathic or predominantly neuropathic in origin.

Clinical Examination

On history, the patient may report both positive and negative sensory symptoms, including tingling, lancinating, burning pain (positive), or numbness (negative).

The clinician must look at the entire range of peripheral nerve sensation for possible dysfunction, including light touch, pinprick, temperature, and vibration. The use of sudomotor testing for possible associated sympathetic nervous system abnormalities may be useful (see below for more detail).

Treatment in Brief

For the chronic LBP patient, a whole-person, biobehavioral approach is best. Medications are important. This chapter details the useful anticonvulsant and antidepressant medications for the treatment of neuropathic pain.

Several studies have shown that the anticonvulsants topiramate (129) might reduce chronic sciatic in some patients, and bupropion SR (130) was not significantly better than placebo in the treatment of non-neuropathic chronic LBP. The authors of the latter study felt that ADMs that had both noradrenergic and serotonergic effects appeared to have greater efficacy in patients with chronic LBP.

Topical agents may also be useful in the chronic LBP patient, including lidocaine 5% and capsaicin 0.075%. The use of topical ketamine and gabapentin and/or doxepin may also be given a trial if necessary (see below for more detail).

CENTRAL POST-STROKE PAIN

Central post-stroke pain (CPSP) was originally thought to be "thalamic" pain, as described by Dejerine and Roussy (131), although it was described even earlier in 1883 (132). Dejerine and Roussy (131) characterized their eponymous thalamic pain syndrome by including: hemiplegia; hemiataxia and hemiasterognosis; difficulties with both superficial and deep sensation; persistent, paroxysmal, typically intolerable pain; and choreoathetoid movements.

The reported incidence of CPSP varies widely from 2% (133) to 8% (134) of stroke patients and to 25% (135) in patients with lateral medullary infarctions (Wallenberg's syndrome).

The onset of the pain may be immediate or be delayed for months to years. (136–138). The pain may encompass a large part of the contralateral body, but it may also involve only a small area. The pain attributes include dysesthesias, spontaneous or evoked, and burning (136).

Sensory abnormalities are also associated with CPSP. These may include altered sensory processing—warm and cold stimulation applied to the skin may be perceived as paresthesias or dysesthesias rather than cold or warm (134,136). Allodynia is found (139,140) in 55% to 70% of patients. Hyperalgesia and dysesthesia are also frequently seen (141).

Location of the lesions inducing the CPSP is definitively referable to the spinothalamo-cortical tract/pathway, typically associated with abnormal evoked sensations in the peripherally affected area (134,142,143). While at least three thalamic regions which directly or indirectly receive spinothalamic projections appear to be involved in the development of CPSP—the ventroposterior thalamus including posteriorly and inferiorly located nuclei bordering on that region, the reticular nucleus and the medial intralaminar region—it is the ventroposterior thalamic region that is proposed to be most significantly involved in central pain (144–146). It should also be noted that cerebrovascular lesions located above the diencephalon, that is, in the parietal lobe, may also induce CPSP (139,142,147).

Sympathetic dysfunction has also been felt to play a role in central pain secondary to signs of abnormal sympathetic activity: edema, hypohydrosis, trophic skin changes, changes in skin color, and decreased skin temperature (148,140). It is also noted that some or many of these changes may be secondary to "movement allodynia" (138), which makes the patient keep the affected limb motionless.

Reports of CPSP associated with abnormal "epileptiform" activities in thalamic cells may be involved with central pain (149–151). This would also indicate that some aspects of the problem might be secondary to cortical involvement, as epileptiform discharges typically are associated with that region.

Treatment of the CPSP is difficult and may include antidepressants, anticonvulsants, antiarrihythmics, analgesics, and nonmedication treatment including transcutaneous electrical nerve stimulation (TENS), dorsal column stimulation, and deep brain stimulation (DBS).

One undesirable effect of repetitive DBS is the reduction of the seizure threshold, known as kindling (151a–151d). One of our patients experienced pain that was only partially reduced with the original stimulus parameters of DBS. In an attempt to improve pain control, that individual used the external controller to increase the amount of stimulation above the amount by the attending neurosurgeon. After several days of this maneuver, the patient suffered a first-ever focal onset, secondarily generalized seizure. To the authors' knowledge this patient may represent the first case of self-induced kindling of seizures in a human patient using DBS for pain control. Other treatments include sympathetic blockade, as well as surgical interventions including cordotomy, dorsal root entry zone lesions, thalamotomy, or cortical and subcortical ablations (152–168).

COMPLEX REGIONAL PAIN SYNDROMES AS NEUROPATHIC PAIN

Following peripheral nerve injury, concomitant alternations may be evident in dorsal root ganglia, including transmitter changes and increased density of sympathetic nerve terminals (169). Tyrosine hydroxylase positive cell terminals that produce norepinephrine migrate from vessels supplying the dorsal root ganglion to nerve ganglion cells following sciatic nerve injury. The dorsal root ganglia then express a-adrenergic receptors. This may be a putative link between peripheral tissue injury, nerve injury, and SMP states, such as reflex sympathetic dystrophy and causalgia (complex regional pain syndromes types 1 and 2, respectively). In the periphery, sprouting nerve terminals may exhibit sensitivity to prostaglandins, cytokines, and catecholamines. These kinds of changes further increase the complexity of the neuropathic pain picture and blur the distinctions between nociceptive and neuropathic pain.

It should be noted that not all stimulus-independent pain is mediated by spontaneous activity in primary sensory neurons. Loss of normal inhibitory mechanisms, whether segmental, supraspinal, or both, may also cause neuropathic pain

(170). After deafferentation injury, particularly following loss of C fibers, arborization of Ab fibers into the substantia gelatinosa of the dorsal horn may result in central sensitization and allodynia (171). Available evidence supports the contention that tactile allodynia is mediated by large myelinated Ab afferents with input that is modulated at supraspinal sites in the dorsal columns (172).

This may explain why TENS and spinal cord stimulation, which produce a low-threshold, tingling sensation characteristic of large fiber afferent activation, may be effective in chronic pain states, particularly neuropathic pain. Tactile allodynia should be differentiated from thermal allodynia, which appears to be mediated by nonmyelinated C fibers and amplified by pathologic spinal dynorphin.

POST-HERPETIC NEURALGIA

Post-herpetic neuralgia (PHN) is a model of neuropathic pain. Its mechanisms differ from those of DN as well as other models of distal symmetric neuropathy.

This disorder is secondary to a latent infection and reactivation after infection with varicella-zoster virus (VZV), which typically inhabits sensory ganglion neurons. Pain is a common clinical concomitant of VZV virus reactivation (173).

The prevalence is currently debatable. It is noted that approximately 10% of patients with VZV/herpes zoster infection will develop PHN. The incidence rises with age, with more than 50% of cases in patients older than 60. Fifty percent of these patients are reported to have pain that is refractory to treatment (174). Another study showed that the pain can precede the eruption of the vesicular rash. It noted that 10% to 15% of patients with herpes zoster develop chronic PHN (pain lasting three months or more after the rash resolves) (175).

While the incidence of PHN does increase with age (176), a longitudinal study of patients with PHN found that only 48% were symptomatic after one year (177).

Another author noted that the incidence of PHN to be 400/100,000 per year, with the incidence rising to 12/1000 people over 80 years of age (178). Finally, the lifetime risk of the development of PHN may approach 20% of the population (179).

The natural variations of resolution of PHN (180) makes the disorder very difficult to evaluate in a clinical trial, as the natural history of resolution of the diathesis may confound the ability to generalize treatment results of controlled trials in PHN (175).

PHN is most commonly found in the thoracic dermatomes, followed by the ophthalmic division of the trigeminal nerve (181,182).

The pathophysiology of PHN is noted to be in reality a spectrum with three subtypes: a group with "irritable nociceptors," who experience minimal deafferentation and touch-evoked allodynia secondary to peripheral nociceptor input, pain which is intensified by capsaicin and relieved by injection of local anesthetics (182); a deafferentation group with significant sensory loss and no allodynia—anesthesia dolorosa—with possible deafferentation-induced hyperactivity of the CNS nociceptive neurons, and/or disinhibition of CNS neurons secondary to loss of pain inhibitory A-β primary afferents or a disruption in descending inhibition (182,183); or patients with deafferentation with profound thermal sensory deficit and allodynia, wherein large diameter afferents produce allodynia via new, direct connections to the CNS nociceptors beginning in the dorsal horn of the spinal cord, with central neuronal reorganization (183). Because of the central changes here, it is felt that these patients will respond better to drugs working against central sensitization rather than drugs with peripheral mechanisms of action (184).

As treatment is different for this disorder, and should be done in a mechanistic fashion, we will briefly look at it here. In the acute stages, an antiviral agent should be used within 72 hours, as it can help prevent PHN (185). The concurrent use of amitriptyline may also be helpful (185).

The treatment of PHN should include tricyclic antidepressants (amitriptyline, nortriptyline, desipramine; gabapentin, pregabalin (drugs working on the a2d subunit of the calcium ion channels); opioids and topical lidocaine may also be useful (186–196).

Capsaicin cream has low benefit, while epidural steroid and epidural morphine injections have no benefit (197–201). The effectiveness of carbamazepine is unproven (175), as is the use of ketamine (184,202) using nonclinical, evidence-based medicine principles.

GLIAL ACTIVATION IN NEUROPATHIC PAIN

In almost a counterpoint to the above noted mechanisms of neuropathic pain, it has been reported that astrocytes and microglia in the CNS/spinal cord can be activated and induce the creation and maintenance of pain facilitation secondary to inflammation and damage to peripheral nerves, other peripheral tissues, spinal nerves, and the spinal cord. Glial cells appear to be of immune cell origin (203,204).

Glial activation can occur via a number of processes: bacteria and viruses that bind to specific receptors expressed by both microglia and astrocytes; substance P, excitatory amino acids (EAAs), fractalkine [a unique chemokine expressed by neurons; its only receptor is expressed by microglia (205)] and ATP released by A-δ and/or C fibers presynaptically or by brain to spinal cord pain enhancement pathways; as well as nitric oxide, prostaglandins, and fractalkine released from "pain transmission neurons" (206–209). After the microglia and astrocytes are activated, they induce hyperexcitability from nociceptive neurons and increased release of substance P and EAAs from the presynaptic terminals (206,207). These changes are helped by glial release of nitric oxide, EAAs, prostaglandins, proinflammatory cytokines such as interleukin-1 and -6, tumor necrosis factor, and NGF (206,207).

These changes create the presence of continuous "pathologic pain" (210).

Research indicates that intrathecal gene therapy driving the production of interleukin-10, an anti-inflammatory cytokine, can stop neuropathic/pathologic pain (211).

Finally, data suggest that in response to morphine, glia release neuroexcitatory substances, causing opposition to morphine's analgesic effects (212).

DIAGNOSTIC EVALUATION OF NEUROPATHIC PAIN

There exist two lines of thought relative to the clinical diagnosis of pain syndromes of this type: one suggests that, since the symptom characteristics of neuropathic pain are not pathognomonic for the condition, their lack of specificity make the diagnosis difficult to reach (213). Another provides evidence to support certain symptom characteristics as strong indicators of neuropathic pain (213a,215). Regardless of which attitude is correct, the pain practitioner hoping to differentiate neuropathic from non-neuropathic disorders must begin, as always, with the clinical history.

MEDICAL PAIN HISTORY

The style of medical history, which has been modified for the specific documentation of pain, has been described in detail elsewhere (8,216).

Within that system the clinician acquires patient information regarding at least eight aspects of the pain problem: a mnemonic often used to ensure that completeness of data collection regarding each characteristic is PQRST, in which P=Provocative, Palliative factors; Q=Quality, R=Region (of onset), Radiation and Referred Pain; S=Severity, and T=Timing. Of these characteristics, those that are most commonly considered in the diagnosis of neuropathic pain are quality (burning, shooting, tingling, sharp, or shock-like), timing (continuous or intermittent/paroxysmal), and provocative (stimulus-evoked or stimulus-independent) (2). While verbal reports of the regional (spatial) distribution may be helpful in determining the relationship of pain to specific neurologic syndromes, the use of a standardized Pain Drawing Instrument is preferred for documentation. One tragic error made by clinicians in the past is the dismissal of pain as being organic simply because it did not resemble an anatomic or dermatomal distribution. In fact, many neuropathic pains, which are maintained or mediated through autonomic pathways, may follow a pattern of sympathetic sclerotomes or blocks of pain referred from deep muscular or visceral afferent reflexes. In recording pain severity or intensity, it is important to document the patient's subjective report using standardized scales such as a verbal Numeric Rating Scale (NRS-11) or nonverbal Visual Analog Scale. Even more important is to avoid the cardinal sin of confusing results of a verbal and visual scale by reporting: "the patient stated that his/her Visual Analog Score was 6 out of 10." For patients with multifocal neuropathic pain or mixed neuropathic/myofascial pain a verbal scale is preferred, since it can be used easily to record intensity *for each region*, not just the peak or average pain (216a). Finally, it has been suggested that this mnemonic should be changed to add the letter O, for *other*, (associated) symptoms, such as loss of sensation or nonpainful paresthesias or dysesthesia occurring in the same general area as the pain.

PHYSICAL EXAMINATION OF PATIENTS WITH NEUROPATHIC PAIN

In general, all major parts of the physical examination are important for adequate determination of the presence of local disease, which may cause pain. (8,216). Any patient in whom the symptom characteristics suggest neurologic origin may also demonstrate regional abnormalities of motor or reflex functions. However, the portions of the examination, which are most relevant to the evaluation of neuropathic pain, are those which are related to sensory dysfunction, such as hypoesthesia, hyperesthesia, hyperalgesia, and allodynia (1,5,215,216).

There are three important aspects in performing the sensory examination in patients with neuropathic pain: (*i*) the information that is obtained is still subjective, (*ii*) stimulation with different modalities may create a mixed or uninterpretable response pattern, and (*iii*) that there may also be hypoesthesia or even areas of total anesthesia in the middle of areas that the patient describes as being so painful.

Techniques that should be utilized during the examination should include: vibration perception threshold using a 128 Hz tuning fork (looks at large fibers); light touch sensation using Nylon Semmes Weintein mono-filaments or Von Frey hairs (for testing large myelinated A-α and A-β fibers); thermal sensation thresholds—mediated by the unmyelinated C fibers (warmth) and cold by the Aδ fibers. Autonomic function should be tested, looking at sudomotor function, blood pressure responses. It may also, in some cases, be advisable to perform skin punch biopsies with immunohistochemical staining looking for nerve fiber density, as well as decreased levels of substance P and CGRP particularly in DN (217–219).

The severity of a pain condition can be related to the size of a painful area, but the intensity is independent, no matter how large or small the territory.

INTEGRATION OF HISTORY/PHYSICAL DATA FOR NEUROPATHIC PAIN EVALUATION

It is evident from the preceding paragraphs that the duration and complexity of the clinical evaluation of human neuropathic pain are very dependent upon the patient's ability to tolerate long and potentially uncomfortable procedures. For screening purposes however, different methods have been developed to provide a combination of individual components of the history and physical examination. The more simple and direct methods are exemplified by Galer and Jensen (220), and Krause and Backonja (214). Development of a Neuropathic Pain Questionnaire demonstrates burning pain, shooting pain, numbness, electric pain, tingling pain, squeezing pain, freezing pain, and significant sensitivity to touch. Analysis of the elements reveals that the three most valuable features were the symptoms of numbness, tingling pain, and the mixed response of symptoms/signs expressed as increased pain due to touch on physical examination.

LABORATORY, RADIOLOGIC, AND ELECTRODIAGNOSTIC ASSESSMENT

Once the history, physical findings, and neuropathic pain questionnaire have yielded sufficient evidence to support the potential presence of NP, specific biochemical, structural, and neurophysiologic tests may be applied to confirm or eliminate certain disorders from the differential diagnosis.

Laboratory evaluation is necessary to determine the presence of hematologic, chemical, or pathologic processes with a high potential for causing or contributing to the pain (7,9). Such tests are also used to monitor (*i*) systemic response to treatment since there are often effects on renal and hepatic function and (*ii*) serum levels of primary analgesics and certain adjuvant medications such as anticonvulsants. DNA and other specific biochemical tests for neuropathic pain disorders, which have a familial tendency or pattern of inheritance can be helpful for genetic counseling, but are not often ordered in primary care pain practice. Similarly, direct and electron microscopic assessment of nerve tissue obtained at biopsy is only used selectively for the definitive pathologic diagnosis of certain illnesses such as neuropathy.

Radiologic evaluation (221) provides valuable information about the presence or absence of structural lesions compressing or invading tissues of the brain, brainstem, spine, spinal cord, root, plexus, or nerve. Certain specialized tests are known to be helpful in the diagnostic assessment of specific conditions, for example, triple phase contrast bone scan as a tertiary way of testing for CRPS Type I/RSD.

Electroneurodiagnostic tests are helpful in localizing structural lesions or regional dysfunction in many disorders of the nervous system, not just those related to neuropathic pain. However, common procedures such as electroencephalography and electromyography/nerve conduction studies to the medical assessment of painful conditions of brain and spinal cord, root and nerve respectively are known to be helpful in confirming and localizing many neurologic illnesses presenting with pain (222). For painful disorders such as CRPS types I and II, and SMP, a wide range of electrophysiologic tests of sympathetic sudomotor function can be found (223) including STC assessment of the skin over painful and nonpainful regions (224,225).

INITIAL SYMPTOM MANAGEMENT

There is some disagreement as to which treatment approaches (pharmacologic or interventional) represent the best and worst chances for symptom control. Nevertheless, the mainstay of treatment of neuropathic pain is pharmacologic. Effective regimens often require multiple medications.

Attempts at monotherapy with standard analgesics including opioids tend to be less effective, since neuropathic pain can be resistant to medications of that type (158,226,227).

Neuropathic pain may be treated with some success using adjuvant analgesics, that is, medications not traditionally considered to be pain relievers (228). Adjuvant analgesics, such as tricyclic antidepressants and anticonvulsants, do not have strong antinociceptive analgesic properties in experimental or clinical studies, but have been shown to be helpful in neuropathic pain states (229,230). In addition, the possible effectiveness of opioids for neuropathic pain should not be overlooked, although doses may be considerably higher than typical antinociceptive doses.

The clinician should also keep in mind that successful management of chronic pain often requires treating neuropathic pain as well as pain associated with tissue injury, because both conditions may coexist and interact to maintain the painful condition. Chronic pain syndromes are often a product of integrated nociceptive and neuropathic mechanisms, and as such require consideration of both types for any pain lasting greater than three to six months.

MECHANISTIC BASIS OF NEUROPATHIC PAIN MANAGEMENT

Management of neuropathic pain is a complicated endeavor and often is frustrating to patient and physician alike. This stems from our relatively poor understanding of mechanisms and the limited efficacy of currently available analgesics. Therapeutic approaches vary greatly among physicians, which reflects the paucity of randomized clinical trials, particularly those comparing different drug regimens. Given our current level of understanding of neuropathic pain mechanisms and the limitations of available drugs, nonpharmacologic methods may be as effective as pharmacologic approaches. Recalcitrant chronic pain syndromes warrant an interdisciplinary approach, which may include attempts to treat the underlying disease (e.g., causes of the peripheral neuropathy) as well as formulation of a rational approach to medications, interventions such as nerve blocks, and psychologic and physical therapies.

ADJUVANT ANALGESICS: ANTICONVULSANTS AND TRICYCLIC ANTIDEPRESSANTS

It is often helpful to consider the various medications useful for neuropathic pain in terms of their traditional pharmacologic indications (e.g., anticonvulsants and antidepressants). However, it is necessary to keep in mind that all these drugs have incompletely understood mechanisms of action, and the drug categories are more conventional than mechanistic.

PHARMACOLOGY OF NEUROPATHIC PAIN

From a practical standpoint, medications remain the pillar of pain management strategies, despite their limitations. From a conceptual standpoint, adjuvant analgesic drugs may be categorized into two broad classes, membrane stabilizing agents and medications that enhance inhibitory mechanisms in the dorsal horn. This classification system may provide a simple framework with which to approach therapy; however, it should be kept in mind that most of these drugs have multiple mechanisms of action, and their effects often may overlap. Given the limitations of our current drugs, pain management often becomes an exercise in polypharmacy, where the clinician uses multiple medications to target different symptoms. This strategy may optimize the chances for success, but complicates management issues when side effects develop.

MECHANISMS OF ACTION

Membrane stabilizing agents include local anesthetics such as lidocaine and some anticonvulsant drugs, including carbamazepine, phenytoin, and valproic acid (12). Their molecular mechanism of action involves blockade of frequency and voltage-dependent sodium channels on damaged or regenerating neuronal membranes (10,11). It appears that minimal doses of suppressive drugs may inhibit ectopic discharges without interfering with normal neuronal function. It is also possible that the sodium channel targets are atypical and not involved in normal neuronal conduction. Although the evidence is less substantial, corticosteroids also appear to have effects on membrane conductance (231,232). In addition, tricyclic antidepressants, such as amitriptyline, have effects on sodium channels (233), an action that is distinct from their effects on the reuptake of serotonin and norepinephrine. The latter are traditionally thought to be responsible for their effects on depression and pain.

Conventional wisdom maintains that the adjuvant analgesics, particularly the tricyclic antidepressants, and clonazepam and baclofen, modulate inhibitory mechanisms in the spinal cord and brain. Inhibitory pathways descend from the periaqueductal gray, reticular formation, and nucleus raphe magnus in the dorsolateral funiculus to the dorsal horn. These pathways mediate antinociception by adrenergic, serotonergic, gamma-amino butyric acid (GABAergic), and opioid mechanisms (234). Although the putative mechanisms are complex and poorly understood, serotonergic effects are mediated in part by action on GABAergic interneurons (235). For example, facilitory effects of large myelinated afferent fibers may be suppressed by tonic GABAergic activity, removal of which results in allodynia (236).

As noted earlier, tricyclic antidepressants alter monoamine transmitter activity at neuronal synapses by blocking presynaptic reuptake of norepinephrine and serotonin, thereby modulating descending inhibitory spinal pathways. However, additional mechanisms include effects on membranes, interaction with NMDA activity (237), and sodium channel blockade (233).

TREATMENT OF COMORBID DEPRESSION AND ANXIETY

It is crucial that psychosocial and emotional factors be explored, because there is a high comorbidity of depression and anxiety disorders in patients with chronic pain. Moreover, given the similarities between the pharmacology of mood and depression and pain transmission (e.g., serotonin and norepinephrine), patients with concomitant systemic illness and stress may be at risk for depression and development of an abnormal chronic pain state. Pharmacologic management of depression may improve neuropathic pain by addressing overlapping, but distinct mechanisms.

ABLATIVE PROCEDURES

After multiple medication trials in which there has been minimal therapeutic benefit and perhaps significant drug-related side effects, patients may believe that they have little recourse but to undergo invasive, ablative procedures in attempts to relieve their pain. Specific treatment modalities aimed at the underlying pathophysiology are usually not possible in most neuropathies, particularly with chronic sensory polyneuropathies. In general, ablative procedures are not warranted, because of the high probability of long-term worsening of pain. Except for patients with advanced cancer-related pain, nerve ablation is likely to provide only temporary benefit, leaving the patient with sensory and perhaps motor deficits. Exceptions to this phenomenon appear to be ablation of sympathetic fibers, visceral plexi, and medial branch nerve blocks, which denervate painful facet joints in the spine. In cases of nerve entrapment, where ongoing nerve compression is likely to be responsible for pain, neurolysis or transposition of the nerve may provide benefit, as long as pain is not due to irreversible underlying nerve damage. In all cases of neuropathic pain, even when neuropathy is evident, it is appropriate from time to time to re-evaluate the presumed etiology of the neurologic problem.

When a medication trial proves to be ineffective, a multidimensional or interdisciplinary approach should be considered. Again, this includes an attempt to treat the underlying disease, as well as specific pharmacologic, psychologic, and physical therapy interventions. The outcome measure for successful treatment should include increased activity as well as decreased subjective pain ratings and improved patient satisfaction. The treatment goal in chronic neuropathic pain is different from that in acute pain. In the usual acute pain setting, the goal is nearly complete relief of pain, to allow recovery of normal function during the healing process. With chronic neuropathic pain, limitations of current analgesics usually make complete pain relief a very unrealistic goal. Therefore, attention to increasing function and comfort and treating associated problems, such as depression, become paramount. Reducing dependence on opioid medications may or may not be an important goal. The objectives to consider with chronic opioid therapy include determining whether nonopioid approaches have been tried, whether the pain syndrome is opioid responsive, and whether the patient demonstrates appropriate improvement in function, without undo side effects or evidence of abuse of medications.

Nonpharmacologic approaches to treating neuropathic pain include the use of a TENS unit, although relief may be poor when burning pain is a prominent complaint. This may be explained by the fact that burning pain is a C-fiber-mediated sensation, whereas TENS units probably modulate large fiber input into the dorsal horn.

Spinal cord stimulation may be efficacious for chronic pain, including neuropathic pain (238) and complex regional pain syndrome/reflex sympathetic dystrophy

(239). Mechanisms involved are poorly understood, which reflects current understanding of neuropathic pain states in general. However, central effects may include alteration in dorsal horn processing and transmission in the tract of Lissauer (240) and suppression of sympathetic outflow from the intermediolateral gray column of the spinal cord. The latter effect may explain improved peripheral blood flow in patients with chronic peripheral vascular insufficiency. The Craig PENS technique, a novel application of electroacupuncture [percutaneous neural stimulation (PNS)] has been shown effective in herpes zoster, diabetic peripheral neuropathy, and sciatica (241–243).

Available evidence indicates that nonpharmacologic approaches such as TENS and Craig PENS can provide an initial rational therapeutic strategy, and may obviate the need for potentially toxic medications, improve the effectiveness of current analgesic regimens, or reduce the amount of medications required. Spinal cord stimulation still tends to be a treatment of last resort, although judicious use earlier in the course of treatment is probably warranted in carefully selected patients. Considering the current high cost of medication, alternative approaches, if efficacious, may prove to be cost-effective.

A peculiar property of the nervous system is its plasticity. Damage to nerves often results in alteration or amplification of the signal encoded by the nerve. For example, peripheral nerve ablation, performed with good therapeutic intentions, may result in a pain syndrome that is worse than the one originally being treated. When dealing with the nervous system, "shooting the messenger" (the nerve) often intensifies and distorts the message. The new pain syndrome may be more severe, and associated with allodynia, hyperalgesia, and spontaneous and paroxysmal pain, all in the presence of mild to moderate cutaneous numbness. This complex of signs and symptoms is paradoxical to the patient and confusing to the clinician, but quite typical of neuropathic pain.

MECHANISTIC APPROACH TO THE SELECTION OF TREATMENT

When standard therapies are found to be only partially effective in controlling symptoms it is often helpful to select other medications or interventions based on the compatibility of the mechanisms of the illness and the treatment being considered (243a,242).

For example, it has become popular to contrast neuropathic pain with typical postinjury, nociceptive pain. Nociceptive pain, typically thought to indicate a properly functioning nervous system, is considered physiologic because it results from activation of nociceptors, specialized nerve endings that respond to high threshold noxious stimuli and generally serve a protective function.

In contrast, neuropathic pain may be thought of as pathophysiologic, because it arises from a damaged PNS or CNS and provides no obvious protective benefit (2,12).

On the other hand, pain associated with peripheral neuropathy may be maintained by sustained peripheral nociceptive input (245). Strong nociceptive input often produces central sensitization, an abnormal pain amplification process in the CNS. Therefore, the definitional borders of neuropathic pain are becoming more diffuse, not more distinct, as we gain a better understanding of the remarkable plasticity of the nervous system and its close association with the various tissues that it innervates.

Neuropathic pain may also be classified as stimulus-evoked or stimulus-independent pain. Stimulus-evoked pain can result from stimulation of nervi nervorum present in connective tissue surrounding otherwise intact nerves. Painful stimuli that activate nociceptors around nerves include inflammation and tissue injury from tumor or trauma (170).

Stimulus-independent neuropathic pain may result from damage to afferent sensory fibers in the PNS or CNS. In this case, ongoing inflammation is usually absent. Days to months after peripheral nerve injury, persistent abnormal primary afferent activity from the periphery may arise from hypersensitive nerve terminals or nerves (246).

STIMULUS-EVOKED NEUROPATHIC PAIN AND OPIOID ANALGESICS

Various studies suggest that stimulus-evoked neuropathic pain is more sensitive to opioids than stimulus-independent pain (227). Opioid responsiveness may be maintained in some forms of stimulus-evoked pain, because opioid receptors in the substantia gelatinosa are preserved. On the other hand, segmental loss of presynaptic central opioid receptors occurs following injury or loss of C fibers, typically seen after deafferentation injury. However, the magnitude of receptor loss is minimal and largely segmental, and only partly explains the diminished opioid-responsiveness characteristic of neuropathic pain (172).

Supraspinal facilitative mechanisms may also be involved in maintenance of neuropathic pain and opioid resistance. Evidence suggests that sustained afferent drive induces facilitation of spinal cord pain transmission involving a descending pathway from the rostroventral medial medulla (RVM) (172). Tonic facilitation may involve supraspinal cholesystokinin (CCK), traditionally thought of as a visceral hormone that regulates emptying of the gallbladder. CCK antagonists injected into the RVM in animals reverse tactile and thermal allodynia produced by spinal nerve ligation (247). Mechanistically, these antiopioid and pronociceptive actions may occur at spinal and supraspinal sites. Spinal CCK may antagonize opioid effects at the level of the primary afferent terminal in the spinal cord. Both CCK and opioids colocalize on primary nociceptive afferent neurons in the dorsal horn. In addition, CCK may act on supraspinal opioid-dependent pathways in the RVM to reduce opioid responsiveness, and thus impair descending inhibition, an important mechanism involved in opioid pain relief. Ultimately, CCK antagonists may prove useful for treating neuropathic pain states.

The phenomenon of reduced opioid responsiveness in neuropathic pain has prompted extensive studies in animals, particularly the effects of intrathecal opioids on pain associated with thermal and tactile stimulation. The similarities between opioid tolerance and neuropathic pain are also an area of active study (248). It is well known that N-methyl-D-aspartate (NMDA) antagonists appear to minimize the development of opioid tolerance. Spinal dynorphin may be a common link between NMDA, central sensitization, and reduced opioid responsiveness. Following spinal nerve ligation, dynorphin levels in the spinal cord increase, suggesting that dynorphin may act as a pronociception mediator (172). Although, under certain circumstances, dynorphin appears to have analgesic properties, it is becoming increasingly clear that dynorphin also has nonopioid, antianalgesic properties. Antiserum to dynorphin blocks thermal hyperalgesia after nerve injury in rats. Moreover, antiserum to dynorphin or MK801, an NMDA antagonist, restores normal spinal morphine analgesia following spinal nerve ligation. Furthermore, both agents restore morphine synergy between the brain and spinal cord (172), which is required for the full clinical analgesic effects of morphine. Therefore, current evidence suggests that the pain-promoting effect of dynorphin is mediated by the NMDA receptor. Although the full clinical ramifications of dynorphin are far from understood, it is clear that sustained nociceptive drive from the periphery maintains elevated levels of spinal dynorphin, which in turn, may have toxic effects on the spinal cord. Thus, reducing sustained peripheral nociceptive input into the spinal (i.e., pain relief) may be an important way to reduce the incidence of neuropathic pain (249).

Currently, NMDA antagonists, such as ketamine, have only limited indications because of significant side effects. Ultimately, however, medications such as NMDA antagonists may become available that can reduce the effects of pathologic spinal dynorphin.

ANTICONVULSANTS

Anticonvulsants are useful for trigeminal neuralgia, postherpetic neuralgia, DN, and central pain (228,230). Although anticonvulsants have traditionally been thought of as most useful for lancinating pain, they may also relieve burning dysesthesias. Chemically, anticonvulsants are a diverse group of drugs, are typically highly protein bound, and undergo extensive hepatic metabolism. Carbamazepine has a long history of use for neuropathic pain, particularly trigeminal neuralgia. Trigeminal neuralgia is an FDA-approved indication for the drug. Carbamazepine is chemically related to the tricyclic antidepressant imipramine, has a slow and erratic absorption, and may produce numerous side effects, including sedation, nausea, vomiting, and hepatic enzyme induction. In 10% of patients, transient leukopenia and thrombocytopenia may occur, and in 2% of patients hematologic changes can be persistent, requiring stopping the drug (250–252). Aplastic anemia is the most severe complication associated with carbamazepine, which may occur in 1:200,000 patients. Although requirements for hematologic monitoring remain debatable, a complete blood cell count, hepatic enzymes, blood urea nitrogen (BUN), and creatinine are recommended at baseline, and these are checked again at two, four, and six weeks, and every six months thereafter. Carbamazepine levels should be drawn every six months and after changing the dose to monitor for toxic levels and verify that the drug is within the therapeutic range (4–12 mg/cc). Patients with low pretreatment white blood cell counts are at increased risk of developing leukopenia (WBC < 3000/mm^3). Because toxicity is entirely unpredictable, it is important to instruct patients to recognize clinical signs and symptoms of hematologic toxicity, such as infections, fatigue, ecchymosis, and abnormal bleeding, and to notify the physician if they develop. To improve compliance, carbamazepine should be started at a low dose (e.g., 50 mg twice daily) and increased over several weeks to a therapeutic level (200–300 mg four times a day).

Phenytoin also has well-known sodium-channel-blocking effects and is useful for neuropathic pain (252a). However, it is less effective than carbamazepine for trigeminal neuralgia (253). We have also noted that neuropathic pain caused by structural lesions causing nerve or root compression can paradoxically increase when phenytoin is administered. Phenytoin has a slow and variable oral absorption, some of which is dependent upon GI motility and transit time. Toxicity includes CNS effects and cardiac conduction abnormalities. Side effects are common and include hirsuitism, gastrointestinal and hematologic effects, and gingival hyperplasia (254). Allergies to phenytoin are common, and may involve skin, liver, and bone marrow. Phenytoin doses in the range of 100 mg twice or three times a day may be helpful for neuropathic pain; therapeutic blood levels are in the range of 10 to 20 mg/ml. There are numerous potential drug interactions, including induction of cytochrome P450 enzymes, which may accelerate the metabolism of other drugs. Because of side effects and toxicity, phenytoin is not a first-line drug for neuropathic pain.

Valproic acid appears to interact with sodium channels but may also alter GABA metabolism. The principle nonantiepileptic FDA approved use of valproic acid is for the prophylaxis of migraine headache (255). Potential toxicity includes hepatic injury and thrombocytopenia, particularly in children on multiple antiepileptic medications, although valproic acid is generally considered safe for adults.

Divalproex sodium is better tolerated than valproic acid. The recommended starting dose is 250 mg twice daily, although some patients may benefit from doses up to 1000 mg/day. As a prophylactic drug, valproic acid can reduce the frequency of migraine attacks by about 50% (255). Although there is little published information on the efficacy of valproic acid for neuropathic pain syndromes, based on its mechanism of action it may be useful alone or in combination with other adjuvant drugs.

Clonazepam may be useful for radiculopathic pain and neuropathic pain of a lancinating character. Clonazepam enhances dorsal horn inhibition by a GABAergic mechanism. The drug has a long half-life (18–50 hr), which reduces the risk of inducing an abstinence syndrome on abrupt withdrawal. The major side effects of clonazepam include sedation and cognitive dysfunction, especially in the elderly. Although the risk of organ toxicity is minimal, some clinicians recommend periodic complete blood count (CBC) and liver function tests for monitoring. Starting doses of 0.5 to 1.0 mg at bedtime are appropriate to reduce the incidence of daytime sedation.

Topiramate was found to be identical to placebo in three placebo-controlled trials for PDN, while a fourth, independent placebo-controlled trial used different methods to assess topiramate efficacy and tolerability. It was found that in this study topiramate monotherapy reduced pain and body weight more effectively than placebo (256).

Gabapentin is a popular anticonvulsant for neuropathic pain. Gabapentin was released for use in the United States in 1994, for the treatment of adults with partial epilepsy. Almost immediately after its release, physicians began to use gabapentin for various neuropathic pain disorders, such as diabetic peripheral neuropathy and PHN. The structural similarity of gabapentin to GABA suggested that the drug might be useful for neuropathic pain. Although tricyclic antidepressants have been proven clinically effective for neuropathic pain for years, they often fail to provide adequate pain relief or cause unacceptable side effects. Therefore, when gabapentin became available, its benign side effect profile quickly made it very popular among physicians. Although initial enthusiasm for the drug was based largely on word of mouth, anecdotal published reports, and discussions at clinical meetings, animal studies have substantiated the efficacy of gabapentin in various types of neuropathic pain. Over time, a growing consensus concerning the usefulness of gabapentin has emerged.

It is clear that gabapentin is not a direct GABA agonist, although indirect effects on GABA metabolism or action may occur. A leading hypothesis suggests that gabapentin interacts with a novel receptor on a voltage-activated calcium channel (13,257). Research has shown that it interacts with the alpha2delta subunit on the voltage-gated calcium channel (192). Inhibition of voltage-gated sodium channel activity (such as occurs with classical anticonvulsants, for example, phenytoin and carbamazepine) and amino acid transport, which alters neurotransmitter synthesis, may also occur. Although gabapentin is not an NMDA antagonist, there is evidence that gabapentin interacts with the glycine site on the NMDA receptor (258).

Ligation of rat spinal nerves L5 and L6 (the Chung model) produces characteristic pain behaviors, including allodynia, which are typical of neuropathic pain. Chapman et al. (259) demonstrated that gabapentin reduces pain in the Chung model. Gabapentin appears to act primarily in the CNS, in contrast to amitriptyline, which seems to act centrally and peripherally (260). Gabapentin also is effective in reducing pain behavior in phase 2 of the formalin test, a model of central sensitization and neuropathic pain (261). Gabapentin reduces spinally mediated hyperalgesia seen after sustained nociceptive afferent input caused by peripheral tissue injury. Gabapentin also enhances spinal morphine analgesia in the rat tail-flick test, a laboratory model of nociceptive pain (262).

Gabapentin is effective in reducing painful dysesthesias and improving quality of life scores in patients with painful diabetic peripheral neuropathy (263). Of patients randomized to receive gabapentin, 56% achieved a daily dosage of 3600 mg divided into three doses per day. The average magnitude of the analgesic response was modest, with a 24% reduction in intensity at the completion of the study compared with controls. Side effects were common. Dizziness and somnolence occurred in about 25% of patients, and confusion occurred in 8% of patients.

Morello et al. (264) compared gabapentin with amitriptyline for DN and found both equally effective. However, the number needed to treat (NNT) for the tricyclic antidepressants is 2.5 and 4.2 for gabapentin (265–267). Although gabapentin probably has fewer contraindications than tricyclic antidepressants, it is considerably more expensive.

PHN is another difficult neuropathic syndrome. PHN affects approximately 10% to 15% of patients who develop herpes zoster, and is a particularly painful syndrome associated with lancinating pain and burning dysesthesias. The incidence of PHN is age-related, with up to 50% of patients older than 60 years of age developing persistent pain after a bout of herpes zoster. Pain relief usually requires pharmacologic therapy. Unfortunately, most medications are not very effective. For example, only about one half of patients obtain adequate relief with antidepressants.

Rowbotham et al. (268) evaluated the efficacy of gabapentin for the treatment of PHN. Of patients taking gabapentin, 65% achieved a daily dosage of 3600 mg. Although the average magnitude of pain reduction with gabapentin was modest, with approximately a 30% reduction in pain compared with controls, statistically pain reduction was highly significant. In addition, gabapentin improved sleep parameters and quality of life scores. Adverse effects that occurred more commonly in the gabapentin group included somnolence (27%), dizziness (24%), ataxia, peripheral edema, and infection (7–10%). Based on the data of Rowbotham and his colleagues, it is reasonable to consider gabapentin as first-line therapy for PHN. Gabapentin probably is at least as effective as antidepressants, with fewer contraindications. Gabapentin may be used as monotherapy or add-on treatment.

Although gabapentin can theoretically be started at 300 mg three times a day with most patients, it has been the clinical experience of one of the authors (DRL) that giving lower initial doses (100 mg) and gently escalating the drug to a schedule of four times a day (three times a day with meals and again at bedtime) has improved compliance. Use of the bedtime dose may assist with sleep and reduces nocturnal pain. In addition, this reduces the risk of patients stopping the drug because of side effects, before a therapeutic dose (i.e., 25 mg/kg/day) is achieved. In our experience, the most gentle schedule involves starting with a bedtime dose of 100 mg for two days. The daily dose is then increased to 100 mg twice a day with breakfast and supper or breakfast and at bedtime, for two days. Thereafter, the dose can be increased to three times a day with meals and at bedtime. Further titration every three to seven days can be continued until pain relief, side effects, or a maximum daily dose in the range of 2400 to 3600 mg/day is reached. An instruction sheet for the patients is helpful in clarifying the dosage schedule.

Gabapentin is generally well tolerated, even in the geriatric population, and has a safer side effect profile than tricyclic antidepressants. In the PHN study, the majority of patients were titrated to 3600 mg/day, and the median patient age was 73 years. The kidneys excrete gabapentin, and the dosage must be reduced for patients with renal insufficiency (269).

Pregabalin is also a GABA analog, with similar structure and function to gabapentin. A new class of anticonvulsants was named, the "Gabapentinoids" of which these two drugs are the first known for inclusion. Pregabalin (Lyrica) is indicated for the treatment of neuropathic pain associated with both DN and PHN (270).

Pregabalin has negligible hepatic metabolism; it is not protein bound and has a plasma half-life of about six hours. Most of the oral dose (95%) is found unchanged in the urine. Peak plasma levels are found in about one hour post oral doses; oral bioavailability is about 90%.

Pregabalin binds to the alpha2delta subunit protein of the voltage-gated calcium channels, like gabapentin, and therefore reduces release of excitatory neurotransmitters (271).

Several randomized clinical trials show pregabalin to be superior to placebo in the treatment of neuropathic pain (PHN and DPN) at doses of 300 to 600 mg/day. Sleep was improved. Common adverse events included dizziness, peripheral edema, weight gain, and somnolence (271).

Randomized controlled studies of pregabalin in painful diabetic peripheral neuropathy were also done and showed the drug to be superior to placebo in doses of 300 to 600 mg/day. Improvements in sleep were also seen (272–275).

Pregabalin was also evaluated for use in Canada for the treatment of peripheral neuropathic pain. The past treatment was reviewed. It was noted that the number of subjects with >50% reduction in pain was increased when pregabalin was compared to placebo. Withdrawal due to adverse events was more frequent with pregabalin than placebo. The authors concluded that while pregabalin appeared effective in the treatment of peripheral neuropathic pain, no evidence was found that it offered advantages over the treatments currently being used in Canada (Table 2) (276).

ANTIDEPRESSANTS

Tricyclic antidepressants have been used for years for the management of neuropathic pain syndromes, including DN, PHN, and migraine headache (229,277,278). However, pain relief is often modest and accompanied by side effects. Controlled studies indicate that approximately one-third of patients will obtain more than 50% pain relief, one-third will have minor adverse reactions, and 4% will discontinue the antidepressant because of major side effects (229). Fortunately, some patients obtain excellent pain relief.

Because comparisons between tricyclic antidepressants have not shown great differences in efficacy (229,277), the choice of which antidepressant to use often depends on the side effect profile of a given drug. For example, when a patient is

TABLE 2 Adjuvant Analgesics for Neuropathic Pain

Drug class	Mechanism of drug action
Anticonvulsants	Multiple possible MOA
Carbamazepine	Sodium channel blockade
Carbatrol	Sodium channel blockade
Trileptal	Sodium channel blockade
Topiramate	Sodium channel blockade
Lamotrigine	Sodium channel blockade
Levotiracetam	Unknown
Phenytoin	Sodium channel blockade
Valproic acid	Sodium channel blockade
Gabapentin	Calcium channel binding
Pregabalin	Calcium channel binding
Clonazepam	GABAergic mechanism
Antidepressants	
Amitriptyline	As a group, norepinephrine and serotonin
Nortriptyline	reuptake effects, possible NMDA effects, and
Imipramine	sodium channel blockade
Desipramine	
Fluoxetine	Serotonin selective effects
Paroxetine	Serotonin selective effects
Venlafaxine	Adrenergic and opioid receptor binding effects
Antiarrhythmics	As a group, sodium channel-blocking effects
Lidocaine	
Mexiletine	
EMLA cream	
Miscellaneous	
Tramadol	Acts at mu opioid receptors and as a serotonin and norepinephrine reuptake inhibitor
Corticosteroids	Anti-inflammatory and membrane-stabilizing effects
Baclofen	GABA-B agonist
Capsaicin	Vanilloid agonist and C-fiber neurotoxin

Abbreviation: MOA, mechanisms of action.

having difficulty in sleeping because of pain, a more sedating drug, such as amitriptyline, may be indicated. On the other hand, desipramine, which is less sedating, may be better tolerated in elderly patients.

The tricyclic antidepressants are generally highly protein bound with large volumes of distribution and long elimination half-lives. They undergo extensive hepatic first-pass metabolism and typically have active metabolites. Although effective doses may be lower than typically used for depression, this is often not the case. Patients must be warned of potential side effects including sedation, cognitive changes, and orthostatic hypotension from a-adrenergic blockade. Anticholinergic side effects are common and include constipation, urinary retention, and exacerbation of glaucoma. Antihistaminic effects may cause sedation. Because of their long half-lives, these drugs may be given as a single bedtime dose. To minimize side effects, small doses (e.g., 10–25 mg) are used initially and increased over several weeks to a therapeutic dose, generally in the range of 50 to 150 mg/day. An electrocardiogram (ECG) is recommended if there is a history of cardiac disease. ECG changes such as QRS widening, PR and QT prolongation, and T wave flattening can be induced by these agents. Tricyclic antidepressants may have quinidine-like actions, consistent with their sodium channel-blocking effects, particularly in patients with underlying ischemic cardiac disease or arrhythmias (279). Because abrupt discontinuation of antidepressants may precipitate withdrawal symptoms, such as insomnia, restlessness, and vivid dreams, a gradual taper over 5 to 10 days is recommended. Occasional blood levels are recommended, as well as CBC and hepatic studies to monitor for organ toxicity.

Amitriptyline is a tertiary amine that inhibits norepinephrine and serotonin reuptake equally (280). Amitriptyline is probably the most commonly used tricyclic agent for neuropathic pain. Amitriptyline also is the most sedating of the tricyclic antidepressants and has the most potent anticholinergic effects. A starting dose of 25 mg at bedtime is recommended. Amitriptyline is metabolized into nortriptyline, a secondary amine with twice as much inhibition of norepinephrine reuptake, compared with serotonin. Nortriptyline is less sedating than amitriptyline with less anticholinergic side effects. A starting dose of 10 mg at bedtime is generally well tolerated.

Imipramine is a tertiary amine with equal inhibition of norepinephrine and serotonin uptake. This drug is moderately sedating and has average anticholinergic effects. The suggested starting dose is 25 mg at bedtime. Because of unpredictable metabolism, occasional blood levels are suggested. Imipramine is metabolized to a secondary amine, desipramine, which is a much more selective inhibitor of norepinephrine uptake. Desipramine is less sedating and has fewer anticholinergic effects than imipramine or amitriptyline, is at least as effective for pain control, and is better tolerated by elderly patients.

Compared with tricyclic agents, serotonin-selective reuptake inhibitors (SSRIs) for neuropathic pain have been relatively disappointing. In addition, they are more expensive than the older generic agents. Nonetheless, at relatively high doses (e.g., 60 mg) paroxetine is effective for DN (281). Fluoxetine may also be useful in the treatment of rheumatic pain conditions, many of which have neuropathic components (282). SSRIs are better tolerated than tricyclic antidepressants and should be considered as first-line drugs in patients with concomitant depression. In this group, they may serve double duty.

Venlafaxine is a novel phentylethylamine antidepressant that is chemically distinct from the older tricyclic antidepressants and the serotonin selective uptake inhibitors. Although venlafaxine blocks serotonin and norepinephrine reuptake, its analgesic actions may be mediated by both an opioid mechanism and adrenergic effects (283). The drug may be at least as well tolerated as tricyclic agents and more effective for pain than standard doses of serotonin-selective drugs. Indeed, an initial report suggests that venlafaxine is effective for neuropathic pain (284). Venlafaxine should be started at one half of a 37.5 mg tablet twice daily and titrated weekly to a maximum of 75 mg, taken twice a day. Nausea appears to be the most common side effect. An extended release formulation of the drug was effective in relieving the pain associated with DN. The NNT values for the higher dose of venlafaxine ER is comparable with those of the TCAs and gabapentin (285).

Duloxetine is a serotonergic and noradrenergic reuptake inhibitor with low affinity for other neurotransmitter systems. The most common adverse events are referable to the gastrointestinal and nervous systems. Duloxetine is primarily eliminated via the urine after significant hepatic metabolism via multiple oxidative pathways, methylation, and conjugation. The half-life is 12.1 hours. Duloxetine does cause inhibition of CYP2D6. It should not be used in combination with nonselective monoamine oxidase inhibitors or CYP 1A2 inhibitors (286). It is effective for major depressive disorders as well as for the treatment of diabetic peripheral neuropathic pain (287–289).

Several double-blind, randomized multicenter trails comparing duloxetine to placebo for the treatment of diabetic peripheral neuropathy have been done. In one, patients received duloxetine 60 mg daily, twice a day or placebo. Duloxetine was superior to placebo in both dosages; discontinuations secondary to adverse events were more frequent in the duloxetine 60 mg/bid group (290).

In the second, a 12-week double-blind placebo-controlled study in types 1 and 2 diabetics with PDN, both 60 and 120 mg/day dosages demonstrated statistically significant improvement in pain compared to placebo (291).

Duloxetine has also been found to be an effective and safe treatment for many symptoms associated with fibromyalgia in subjects with or without a major depressive disorder, particularly for women, who had the best outcomes, with significant improvement over most outcome measures (288,292,293).

Antidepressant drugs (ADMs) have been used for many years in the treatment of neuropathic pain. Reasons include the traditional monoaminergic hypothesis. It is also known that antidepressants can interfere with the opioid system, inhibit ion channel activity, and interact with the NMDA receptors. The tricyclic antidepressants (TCAs) have the lowest NNT, the number of patients that need to be treated to achieve a 50% decrement in pain in one patient. The NNT for TCAs is 2.4 versus 6.7 for the selective serotonin reuptake inhibitors. It appears that the ADMs with noradrenergic reuptake inhibition in addition to serotonergic reuptake inhibition, such as venlafaxine, bupropion, and duloxetine demonstrate a better analgesic effect. The TCAs remain the first choice treatment for neuropathic pain (294,295). However, no head-to-head comparisons between ADMs and other analgesics have been done (294).

TRAMADOL

Tramadol appears to be the most widely used analgesic for chronic noncancer pain of all types in the relatively opiophobic European Union.

Tramadol is a centrally acting analgesic that is related structurally to codeine and morphine. It consists of two enantiomers, both of which are important in the drugs analgesic mechanisms. The (+)-tramadol and the metabolite (+)-O-desmethyl-tramadol (also called M1) are mu opioid receptor agonists. (+)-tramadol also inhibits serotonin reuptake, while the (−)-tramadol enantiomers inhibits norepinephrine reuptake, enhancing inhibitory effects on spinal cord pain transmission (296).

Tramadol is rapidly absorbed after oral administration. It is rapidly distributed in the plasma, with about 20% plasma protein binding. It is metabolized by O- and N-demethylation and by conjugation forming glucuronides and sulfates. Tramadol and its metabolites are excreted mainly by the kidneys, with a mean elimination half-life of about six hours (265,296).

The O-demethylation of the drug to M1 is catalyzed by cytochrome P450 (CYP) 2D6 (265).

The analgesic potency of tramadol is only 10% of that of morphine status-post parenteral administration. Tramadol produces less constipation and problems with dependence than equianalgesic dosages of opioids (265). There are no respiratory or cardiovascular problems associated with the drug (297).

M1 has a greater affinity to the mu receptor and is felt to be mainly responsible for tramadol opiate activity (296).

It is felt that the dual activity (opioid and nonopioid) explains its effectiveness in pain that may not be responsive to opiates alone: neuropathic pain (298).

Tramadol is felt to be one of the first-choice drugs for the treatment of neuropathic pain; it has been to be effective in several placebo-controlled studies (298–304).

In a Cochrane evidence-based review, tramadol was found to be "an effective treatment for neuropathic pain" (305). The reviewers found five "eligible" RCTs, three comparing tramadol with placebo, one comparing tramadol with clomipramine, and one comparing tramadol with morphine. All three trials comparing tramadol to placebo were positive, with tramadol being superior to placebo. There was not enough evidence to develop a conclusion regarding tramadol versus morphine or clomipramine (305). It was determined that the NNT was 3.5 (the number needed to treat, to find one patient with a greater than 50% diminution of pain) (305,306).

For moderate to severe pain, start at 25 mg PO qam, then increase by 25 mg/day every three days to 25 mg qid, then increase by 50 mg/day every three days to 50 mg qid. Maximum dosage should not exceed 50 to 100 mg every four to six hours as needed. Typically, no more than 300 to 400 mg a day should be used.

ANTIARRHYTHMICS

Antiarrhythmics block ectopic neuronal activity at central and peripheral sites (307). Lidocaine, mexiletine, and phenytoin—type I antiarrhythmics—stabilize neural membranes by sodium channel blockade. Lidocaine suppresses spontaneous impulse generation on injured nerve segments, dorsal root ganglia, and dorsal horn wide dynamic range neurons (308,309). Lidocaine infusions have been used to predict the response of a given neuropathic pain disorder to antiarrhythmic therapy (310). Lidocaine may be effective at subanesthetic doses, and following nerve blocks analgesia may outlast conduction block for days or weeks (310–312). It has been reported that patients with PNS injury experience better pain relief than those with central pain syndromes (313). If a trial infusion of lidocaine is effective, a trial of oral mexiletine is worth considering.

Prior to starting mexiletine, a baseline ECG is recommended to determine if the patient has underlying ischemic heart disease. Dosages may be increased from 150 to 250 mg three times a day over several days. Taking the medication with food may minimize gastric side effects, which are common and a major reason for discontinuing the drug. Other side effects of mexiletine are nervous system effects such as tremor and diplopia. Once on a stable dose, a serum level should be obtained (the therapeutic range is between 0.5 and 2.0 mg/mL).

TOPICAL PREPARATIONS OF LOCAL ANESTHETICS

Topical preparations of local anesthetics may be effective for neuropathic pain when there is localized allodynia or hypersensitivity. Topical blockade of small- and large-fiber nerve endings should reduce mechanical and thermal allodynia. A topical lidocaine patch (Lidoderm 5% lidocaine) has become available, which can be applied to painful areas in shingles (herpes zoster) and in more chronic forms of neuropathic pain such as DN or the ischemic neuropathies created by prolonged peripheral vascular insufficiency. Up to three patches may be applied at one time to the painful area. The patches can be worn for up to 12 hours a day. However, the treating physician must ensure that the patient understands that chronic forms of neuropathic pain may require a longer therapeutic trial, for example, 30 days, before optimal symptomatic control can be determined. In patients with DN (313a) have found that the addition of topical lidocaine patches to exogenous GABAergic oral agents may provide further improvement of symptom control.

A topical cream, eutectic mixture of local anesthetic (EMLA cream), a mixture of lidocaine and prilocaine, may also be useful for cutaneous pain. The cream may be applied three or four times a day to the painful area.

CORTICOSTEROIDS

Corticosteroids are clearly useful for neuropathic pain, particularly in stimulus-evoked pain such as lumbar radiculopathy. The anti-inflammatory effects of corticosteroids are well known, which may partly explain their efficacy for pain. When administered epidurally for treatment of discogenic radiculopathy, corticosteroids inhibit phospholipase A2 activity, and suppress the perineural inflammatory response caused by leakage of disk material around the painful nerve root (314). However, corticosteroids also act as membrane stabilizers by suppressing ectopic neural discharges (231,232). Therefore, some of the pain-relieving action of corticosteroids may be due to a lidocaine-like effect.

Depot forms of corticosteroids injected around injured nerves provide pain relief and reduce pain associated with entrapment syndromes. Corticosteroids are also effective if given orally or systemically. In cancer pain syndromes, steroids such as dexamethasone may be first-line therapy for neuropathic pain. The potential side effects of corticosteroids are well known and may be seen whether given orally, systemically, or epidurally.

BACLOFEN

Baclofen is useful for trigeminal neuralgia and other types of neuropathic pain (315), particularly as an add-on drug. Baclofen is a GABA-B agonist and is presumed to hyperpolarize inhibitory neurons in the spinal cord (236), thereby reducing pain. This GABA effect appears to be similar to benzodiazepines, such as clonazepam. Side effects of baclofen can be significant and include sedation, confusion, nausea, vomiting, and weakness, especially in the elderly. A typical starting dose is 5 mg three times a day. Thereafter, the drug can be increased slowly to 20 mg four times a day. Abrupt cessation may precipitate withdrawal with hallucinations, anxiety, and tachycardia. The drug is excreted by the kidney and the dosage must be reduced in renal insufficiency.

CAPSAICIN

Capsaicin is a C-fiber-specific neurotoxin and is one of the components of hot peppers that produces a burning sensation on contact with mucous membranes. Topical preparations are available over the counter and are widely used for chronic pain syndromes. Capsaicin is a vanilloid receptor agonist and activates ion channels on C fibers that are thermotransducers of noxious heat (>43°C) (316). With repeated application in sufficient quantities, capsaicin can inactivate primary afferent nociceptors. For patients with pain due to sensitized nociceptors, capsaicin may be effective, if they can tolerate the pain induced by the medication. The drug causes intense burning, which may abate with repeated applications and gradual inactivation of the nociceptors. However, in patients with tactile allodynia, which is probably mediated by large fibers, capsaicin may not be as effective. Capsaicin extracts are available commercially as topical preparations, containing 0.025% and 0.075% and should be applied to the painful area three to five times a day. The preparation may be better tolerated if it is used after application of a topical local anesthetic cream.

PKC INHIBITORS

Activation of PKC has been implicated in noted changes in pain perception. When activated by phorbol esters, PKC enhances thermal hyperalgesia in diabetic mice. Activated PKC also leads to enhancement of EAAs in dorsal horn neurons as well as trigeminal neurons. It is therefore possible that PKC may induce neuronal sensitization that produces hyperalgesia in DN. Ruboxistaurin, a PKC inhibitor, may be a valid treatment for diabetic neuropathic pain (317–319).

TRANSCRANIAL MAGNETIC STIMULATION

A recent study found that repetitive transcranial magnetic stimulation (rTMS) was effective for neuropathic pain, particularly for central poststroke pain and trigeminal neuralgia. The effective rTMS for the treatment of neuropathic pain consisted of a train of 200 pulses/min at 20 Hz for 10 minutes over the identified motor cortex contralateral to the affected side of the body (320). Motor cortex stimulation has also been noted to induce an increase in cerebral blood flow in the ipsilateral thalamus, orbitofrontal, and cingulate gyri as well as in the upper brain stem (320).

SUMMARY AND RECOMMENDATIONS

Neuropathic pain is a common cause of chronic pain and tends to be resistant to usual doses of traditional analgesic medications. Three classic examples of neuropathic pain include trigeminal neuralgia, PHN, and DN. Neuropathic pain is often described as lancinating or burning in nature. Both types of pain may be present at the same time, often accompanied by allodynia.

Neuropathic pain may be manageable with one or more adjuvant analgesic drugs, often prescribed as part of a comprehensive treatment plan. From a theoretical point of view, it may be helpful to categorize adjuvant analgesics into two broad classes of drugs, agents that act as membrane-stabilizing agents and drugs that enhance dorsal horn inhibition. Membrane-stabilizing drugs may act by blocking sodium and calcium channels on damaged neural membranes. Medications that enhance dorsal horn inhibition appear to act by augmenting spinal biogenic amine and GABAergic mechanisms. From a clinical standpoint, given the paucity of our understanding of neuropathic pain mechanisms and how the medications actually work, it is probably more useful to classify adjuvant drugs according to their traditional therapeutic indications (e.g., antidepressants and anticonvulsants). This point of view is strengthened by the fact that most drugs appear to have multiple mechanisms and sites of action, making further subclassification arbitrary and probably inaccurate.

Anticonvulsants, particularly carbamazepine (and more recently gabapentin and pregabalin), are useful for neuropathic pain. Although conventional wisdom suggests that anticonvulsants may be most effective for lancinating pain, anticonvulsants are also useful for burning dysesthesias. The mechanism of action of gabapentin and pregabalin is poorly understood, but the drug has been demonstrated to bind to the alpha2delta subunits of the voltage-dependent calcium channel receptors (192). Gabapentin reduces the pain due to diabetic peripheral neuropathy and PHN; the overall safety record with gabapentin is good, making it an attractive alternative to carbamazepine and tricyclic antidepressants, particularly for elderly patients.

Clonazepam is another option and also poses minimal risk from the standpoint of organ toxicity. Clonazepam may be useful for radicular pain and pain associated with tumors, such as plexopathy. In addition, clonazepam may be used to supplement other adjuvant drugs. When given at bedtime, the mild sedating effect of clonazepam can be helpful for patients who have difficulty sleeping because of pain.

Antidepressants have been used effectively for years in the management of multiple pain syndromes, including DN, PHN, rheumatoid arthritis, osteoarthritis, migraine headache, LBP, and fibromyalgia. However, pain relief is often modest and accompanied by side effects. Studies indicate that only one-third of patients obtain more than 50% pain reduction. However, some patients obtain dramatic pain relief.

The choice of which antidepressant to use for neuropathic pain often depends on the particular side effect profile of a given drug, because comparisons of individual tricyclic antidepressants have not shown great differences in efficacy. When a patient is having difficulty in sleeping because of pain, a more sedating drug, such as amitriptyline is appropriate. On the other hand, desipramine, which is considerably less sedating and has fewer anticholinergic effects, may be much better tolerated in elderly patients. Serotonin-selective reuptake inhibitors for neuropathic pain have been disappointing, although paroxetine at relatively high doses is useful for DN. Fluoxetine may be useful in the treatment of rheumatic pain conditions, many of which have neuropathic components. As with the tricyclic agents, the SSRIs are probably interchangeable. However, SSRIs are better tolerated than tricyclics and may be extremely effective in treating patients with chronic pain and concomitant depression.

It remains unclear whether anticonvulsants or antidepressants should be first-line therapy for neuropathic pain. Similar results have been obtained with both, and current evidence concerning drug efficacy does not support the use of one drug over another. In many cases, selection of a particular drug may depend more on expected side effects (e.g., sedation) or the clinician's experience with the drug, than theoretical considerations about mechanisms of drug action. It must be remembered that treatment of neuropathic pain remains largely empirical. In addition, for maximum analgesic benefit, more than one drug may be necessary. Until more effective medications become available, polypharmacy will remain the rule instead of the exception. This is probably understandable, given the multiple mechanisms involved in the pathophysiology of neuropathic pain.

In general, for neuropathic pain either gabapentin or amitriptyline (or a similar tricyclic antidepressant) should be first-line therapy. When considering issues such as time to effective analgesic action and toxicity, gabapentin is more attractive. Gabapentin often is our first choice, followed by a tricyclic antidepressant, such as nortriptyline. Both drugs must be started slowly and titrated to effect, perhaps to rather high levels, for full benefit. However, tricyclics have many potential side effects that must be considered, particularly anticholinergic and cardiac interactions and organ toxicity. Clearly, gabapentin is a safer drug, but may cause sedation or dysphoria in some patients. Occasionally patients complain of weight gain and nonpitting edema. Until recently another disadvantages of gabapentin included its cost (approximately 10 times the cost of a generic tricyclic antidepressant at usual starting doses) and the need to take the drug three or four times a day. Keep in mind that the dosage of gabapentin must be reduced appropriately for patients with renal insufficiency. Newer marketed medications such as duloxetine and pregabalin may also, as time and treatment experience grows, become primary treatments.

An evidence-based treatment algorithm for neuropathic pain treatment was performed and identified 105 RCTs using MEDLINE and EMBASE. The tricyclic antidepressants and the anticonvulsants gabapentin and pregabalin were found to be the most frequently studied. In the treatment of neuropathic pain, the lowest number needed to treat (NNT) was for the TCAs, followed by the opiates, and then the anticonvulsants gabapentin and pregabalin. It was felt that the NNT along with the NNH (number needed to harm) were the best way to assess relative efficacy between trails, but they have significant limitations (321).

When an appropriate medication trial has been ineffective, and all other appropriate medications have been tried and failed or delivered minimal effectiveness, an interdisciplinary pain medicine approach should be considered (see Chapter 17). Reducing dependence on opioid medications may or may not be a primary goal, depending on whether the pain syndrome is opioid responsive, the patient is demonstrating appropriate improvements in function, and there are not undue side effects or evidence of drug abuse.

Current evidence indicates that nonpharmacological approaches may be reasonable, obviate or reduce the need for potentially toxic medications, and improve the effectiveness of analgesic regimens. Spinal cord stimulation may reduce pain in selected patients. Less invasive techniques, including TENS units and percutaneous nerve stimulation, are also beneficial.

DISCUSSION

The goals of providing medical care for patients with neuropathic pain are often directed by changes in the quality, intensity, timing, and regional distribution of the patients' symptoms, rather than objective signs or test results of the underlying etiology.

When considering those limitations it is helpful to target specific symptoms, for example, burning pain with tricyclic antidepressants and sharp, shooting pain with anticonvulsants. However, from a practical standpoint, pharmacologic choices are often based on physician experience and comfort with the safety and efficacy profiles of a given drug. Moreover, the high cost of new drugs (213) for which no generic yet exists may make older tricyclic antidepressants, such as amitriptyline, the only cost-effective alternative for some patients. Until more effective drugs become available, the pharmacologic approach remains largely one of trial and error. In the meantime, nonpharmacologic strategies may assume a larger role in clinical practice. The authors agree that effective management of neuropathic pain requires patience and persistence on the part of the clinician and the patient. The ability of some patients to accept incomplete pain relief during many therapeutic trials, simply with the hope that an optimal treatment may be determined, provides an example of courage that should be emulated by all health care givers. When a patient's internal strengths flag due to protracted suffering, physicians should be prepared to treat, or arrange consultative treatment for, the anxiety and depression that often accompany prolonged pain illness.

REFERENCES

1. Fields HL. Painful Dysfunction of the Nervous, In: Fields HL, Chap 6, Pain. New York: McGraw-Hill Book Company, 1987:133–167.
2. Bennett GJ. Neuropathic pain. In: Wall PD, Melzack R, eds, Textbook of pain, 3rd ed. Edinburgh: Churchill Livingstone 1994:201–224.
3. Merskey HH, Bogduk N.Classification of Chronic Pain: Descriptions of Chronic Pain Syndromes and Definitions of Pain Terms. 2nd ed. Seattle: Washington IASP Press, 1994:212–213.
4. Jay GW. The Autonomic Nervous System. In: Raj PP, ed., Chap 47 Pain Medicine: A Comprehensive Review. St. Louis: Mosby-Year Book, 1996:461–464.
5. Dworkin RH, Backonja M, Rowbotham MC, et al. Advances in neuropathic pain: diagnosis, mechanisms, and treatment recommendations. Arch Neurol 2003; 60:1524–1534.
5a. Galer BS. Neuropathic pain of peripheral origin: Advances in pharmacologic treatment. Neurology 1995; 45(suppl 9):S17–S25.
6. Schreiber S, Backer MM, Pick CG. The antinociceptive effect of venlafaxine in mice is mediated through opioid and adrenergic mechanisms. Neurosci Lett 1999; 273:85–88.
6a. Scadding JW. Neuropathic Pain. In Asbury, AK, McKhann, GM, McDonald, WI, eds., Diseases of the Nervous system: Clinical Neurobiology, 2nd ed. Philadelphia: Harcourt Brace Jovanovich, WB Saunders Company, 1992:858–872.
7. Kennedy LD, Longmire DR. Medical/Laboratory Evaluation of Pain Patients. Pain Digest 1 1992; 4:306–312.
8. Longmire DR. Evaluation of the Pain Patient. In: Raj PP, ed., Chap 3, Pain Medicine, a Comprehensive Review, 1996:26–34.
9. Kennedy LD. Laboratory Investigations. In: Raj PP, ed., Chap 5. Pain Medicine, a Comprehensive Review 1996:47–54.
10. Devor M. The pathophysiology of damaged peripheral nerves. In Wall PD, Melzack R, eds, Textbook of pain, 3rd ed. Edinburgh: Churchill Livingstone, 1994:79–100.
11. Devor M. Neurobiological basis for selectivity of sodium channel blockers in neuropathic pain. Pain Forum 1995; 4:83–86.
12. Tasker R. Pain resulting from central nervous system pathologycentral pain. In: Bonica, JJ, ed. The Management of Pain. Philadelphia: Lea and Febiger, 1990:264–280.
13. Chaplan SR. Neuropathic pain: Role of voltage-dependent calcium channels. Regional Anesthesia and Pain Medicine 2000; 25:283–285.
14. Novakovic SD, Tzoumaka E, McGivern JG, et al. Distribution of the tetrodotoxin-resistant sodium channel PN3 in rat sensory neurons in normal and neuropathic conditions. J Neurosci 1998; 18:2174–2187.
15. Mersky H, Bogduk N. Classification of Chronic Pain. 2nd ed. Seattle, WA: IASP Press, 1994.
16. Woolf CJ, Salter MW. Neuronal Plasticity: increasing the gain in pain. Science 2000; 127:1159–1171.
17. Klein T, Magerl W, Rolke R, Treede RD. Human surrogate models of neuropathic pain. Pain 2005; 115:227–233.
18. Thomas PK, Tomlinson DR. Diabetic and hypoglycemic neuropathy. In: Dyck PJ, Thomas PK, eds. Peripheral Neuropathy. Philadelphia: WB Saunders, 1993:1219–1250.
19. Ziegler D, Gries FA, Spuler M, Lessmann F. The epidemiology of diabetic neuropathy. DiaCAN Multicenter Study Group. Diabet Med 1993; 10(suppl 2):S82–S86.
20. The DCCT Research Group. The effect of intensive treatment of diabetes on the development and progression of long-term complications in insulin-dependent diabetes mellitus. N Eng J Med 1993; 329:977–986.
21. Report and recommendations of the San Antonio conference on diabetic neuropathy. Consensus statement. Diabetes 1988; 37(7):1000–1004.
22. Thomas PK. Classification, differential diagnosis, and staging of diabetic peripheral neuropathy. Diabetes 1997; 46(suppl 2):S54–S57.

23. Boulton AJM, Ward JD. Diabetic neuropathies and pain. Clin Endocrinol Metab 1986; 16:917–931.
24. Bhadada SK, Sahay RK, Jyotsna VP, Agrawal JK. Diabetic neuropathy: current concepts. J Indian Acad Clin Med 2001; 2(4):305–316.
25. Archer AG, Watkins PJ, Thomas PK, Sharma AK, Payan J. The natural history of acute painful neuropathy in diabetes mellitus. J Neurol Neurosurg Psychiatry 1983; 46:491–499.
26. Soliman E. Gellido. Diabetic Neuropathy 2004. eMedicine.com.
27. Krendel DA, Zacharias A, Younger DS. Autoimmune diabetic neuropathy. Neurol Clin 1997; 15(4):959–971.
28. Dyck PJ, Norell JE, Dyck PJ. Non-diabetic lumbosacral radiculoplexus neuropathy: natural history, outcome and comparison with the diabetic variety. Brain 2001; 124 (Pt 6):1197–1207.
29. Dyck PJ, Windebank AJ. Diabetic and nondiabetic lumbosacral radiculoplexus neuropathies: new insights into pathophysiology and treatment. Muscle Nerve 2002; 25(4): 477–491.
30. Kazem SS, Behzad D. Role of blink reflex in diagnosis of subclinical cranial neuropathy in diabetic mellitus type II. Electromyogr Clin Neurophysiol 2005; 45(5):299–303.
31. Janaky M, Fulop Z, Palffy A, Benedek K, Benekek G. Non-arteritic ischaemic optic neuropathy NAION in patients under 50 years of age. Acta Ophthalmol Scand 2005; 83(4):499–503.
32. Kao HJ, Chang YY, Lan MY, Kao YF, Wu HS, Liu JS. Diabetic inferior division palsy of the oculomotor nerve. Acta Neurol Taiwan 2005; 14(2):79–83.
33. Ramunni A, Giancipoli G, Guerriero S. LDL-apheresis accelerates the recovery of non-arteritic acute anterior ischemic optic neuropathy. Ther Apher Dial 2005; 9(1):53–58.
34. Ellenberg M. Diabetic truncal mononeuropathy—a new clinical syndrome. Diabetes Care 1978; 1(1):10–13.
35. Massey EW. Diabetic truncal mononeuropathy: electromyographic evaluation. Acta Diabetol Lat 1980; 17(3–4):269–272.
36. Brooks PV. Mononeuritis Multiplex. 2002. eMedicine.com.
37. Toyry JP, Niskaner LK, Mantysaari MJ, et al. Occurrence predictors and clinical significance of autonomic neuropathy in NIDDM: ten years follow up from diagnosis. Diabetes 1996; 45:308–315.
38. Vinik AI, Erbas T. Recognizing and treating diabetic autonomic neuropathy. Clev Clinic J Med 2001; 68(11):928–944.
39. Vinik AI, Freeman R, Tomris E. Diabetic autonomic neuropathy. Semin Neurol 2003; 23 (4):365–372.
40. Ziegler D, Gries FA, Spuler M, Lessmann F, Diabetic Cardiovascular Autonomic Neuropathy Multicenter Study Group. The epidemiology of diabetic neuropathy. J Diabetes and Its Compl 1992; 6:49–57.
41. Sampson MJ, Wilson S, Karagiannis P, Edmonds M, Watkins PJ. Progression of diabetic autonomic neuropathy over a decade in insulin-dependent diabetics. Quart J Med 1990; 75:635–646.
42. Kocer A, Zekeriya A, Maden E, Tasci A. Orthostatic hypotension and heart rate variability as indicators of cardiac autonomic neuropathy in diabetes mellitus. Eur J Gen Med 2005; 2(1):5–9.
43. Lee SP, Yeoh L, Harris ND, et al. Influence of autonomic neuropathy on QTc interval lengthening during hypoglycemia in type 1 diabetes. Diabetes 2004; 53:1535–1542.
44. Sivieri R, Veglio M, Chinaglia A, et al. Prevalence of QT prolongation in a type 1 diabetic population and its association with autonomic neuropathy: the neuropathy study group of the Italian society for the study of diabetes. Diabet Med 1993; 10:920–924.
45. Ewing DJ, Neilson JM. QT interval length and diabetic autonomic neuropathy. Diabet Med 1990; 1L:23–26.
46. Weston PJ, James MA, Panerai R, et al. Abnormal baroreceptor-cardiac reflex sensitivity is not detected by conventional tests of autonomic function in patients with insulin-dependent diabetes mellitus. Clin SciLond 1996; 91:59–64.
47. Ziegler D. Diabetic cardiovascular autonomic neuropathy: prognosis, diagnosis and treatment. Diabetes Metab Rev 1994; 10:339–383.

48. Malpas SC, Maling TJ. Heart-rate variability and cardiac autonomic function in diabetes. Diabetes 1990; 39:1177–1181.
49. Coumel P, Johnson N, Extramiana F, et al. Electrocardiography changes and rhythm problems in the diabetic. [Abstract]. Arch Mal Coeru Vaiss 2000; 93 Spec No 4:59–66.
50. Taskiran M, Fritz-Hansen T, Rasmussen B, et al. Decreased myocardial perfusion reserve in diabetic autonomic neuropathy. Diabetes 2002; 51:3306–3310.
51. Ewing DJ, Boland O, Neilson JM, et al. Autonomic neuropathy, QT interval lengthening, and unexpected deaths in male diabetic patients. Diabetologia 1991; 34(3):182–185.
52. Weston PJ, Gill GV. Is undetected autonomic dysfunction responsible for sudden death in type 1 diabetes mellitus? The "dead in bed" syndrome revisited. Diabet Med 1999; 16:626–631.
53. Farrell TG, Odemuyiwa O, Bashir Y, et al. Prognostic value of baroreflex sensitivity testing after acute myocardial infarction. Br Heaerth J 1992; 67:129–137.
54. La Rovere MT, Bigger JT, Marcus FI, et al. Baroreflex sensitivity and heart-rate variability in predciton of total cardiac mortality after myocardial infarction. Lancet 1998; 351: 478–484.
55. Aring AM, Jones DE, Falko JM. Evaluation and prevention of diabetic neurpathy. Am Fam Physician 2005; 71:2131–2138, 2129–2130.
56. Consensus development conference on the diagnosis of coronary heart disease in people with diabetes: 10–11 February 1998, Miami, Florida. American Diabetes Association. Diabetes Care 1998; 21:1551–1559.
57. Lagi A, Cipriani M, Paggetti C, et al. Power spectrum analysis of heart rate variations in the early detection of diabetic autonomic neuropathy. Clin Auton Res 1994; 4(5):245–248.
58. Vinik A, Mehrabyan A, Colen L, Boulton A. Focal entrapment neuropathies in diabetes. Diabetes Care 2004; 27(7):1783–1788.
59. DCCT Research Group. The effect of intensive diabetes therapy on the development and progression of neuropathy. Ann Intern Med 1995; 122:651–688.
60. Kelkar P. Diabetic Neuropathy. Semin Neurol 2005; 25(2):168–173.
61. Oates PJ. Polyol pathway and diabetic peripheral neuropathy. Int Rev Neurobiol 2002; 50:325–392.
62. Yamagishi S, Imaizumi T. Diabetic vascular complications: pathophysiology, biochemical basis and potential therapeutic strategy. Curr Pharm Des 2005; 11(18):2279–2299.
63. Ahmad FK, He Z, King GL. Molecular targets of diabetic cardiovascular complications. Curr Drug Targets 2005; 6(4):487–494.
64. Defraigne JO. A central pathological mechanism explaining diabetic complications? Rev Med Liege 2005; 60(5–6):472–478.
65. Chung SS, Chung SK. Aldose reductase in diabetic microvascular complications. Curr Drug Targets 2005; 6(4):475–486.
66. Cameron NE, Eaton SE, Cotter MA, Tesfaye S. Vascular factors and metabolic interactions in the pathogenesis of diabetic neuropathy. Diabetologia 2001; 44:1973–1988.
67. Craner JM, Klein JP, Renganathan M, et al. Changes of sodium channel expression in experimental painful diabetic neuropathy. Ann Neurol 2002; 52:786–792.
68. Hall KE, Liu J, Sima AA, Wiley JW. Impaired G-protein function contributes to increased calcium currents in ra5ts with diabetic neuropathy. J Neurophysiol 2001; 86:760–770.
69. Gingliano D, Ceriello A, Pawlisso G. Oxidative stress and diabetic vascular complications. Diabetes Care 1996; 19:257–267.
70. Inoguchi T, Sonta T, Tsubouchi H, et al. Protein Kinase C–Dependent Increase in Reactive Oxygen SpeciesROS Production in Vascular Tissues of Diabetes: Role of Vascular NAD (PH Oxidase. J Am Soc Nephrol 2003; 14:S227–S232.
71. Idris I, Gray S, Donnely R. Protein Kinase C activation: isozyme-specific effects on metabolism and cardiovascular complications in diabetes. Diabetologia 2001; 44(6): 657–658.
72. Qu X, Seale JP, Donnely R. Tissue and isoform-selective activation of protein kinase C in insulin-resistant obese Zucker rats—effects of feeding. J Endocrinology 1999; 162(2): 207–214.
73. Cameron NE, Cotter MA, Horrobin DH, Tritschler HJ. Effects of alpha-lipoic acid on neurovascular function in diabetic rats: interaction with essential fatty acids. Diabetologia 1998; 41:390–399.

74. Jamal GA. The use of gamma linolenic acid in the prevention and treatment of diabetic neuropathy. Diabet Med 1994; 11:145–149.
75. Faradji V, Sotelo J. Low serum levels of nerve growth factor in diabetic neuropathy. Acta Neurol Scand 1990; 81:402–413.
76. Apfel SC, Kessler JA, Adornato BT, et al. Recombinant human nerve growth factor in the treatment of diabetic polyneuropathy. NGF Study Group. Neurology 1998; 51(3): 695–702.
77. Lacomis D. Small-fiber neuropathy. Muscle Nerve 2002; 26:173–188.
78. Hoitsma E, Reulen JP, de Baets M, et al. Small fiber neuropathy: a common and important clinical disorder. J Neurol Sci 2004; 15; 227(1):119–130.
79. Singleton JR. Evaluation and treatment of painful peripheral polyneuropathy. Semin Neurol 2005; 25(2):185–195.
80. Polydefkis M, Allen RP, Hauer P, et al. Subclinical sensory neuropathy in late-onset restless-legs syndrome. Neurology 2000; 55:1115–1121.
81. Koves P, Szakacs Z. Pathophysiology of restless leg syndrome and periodic leg movement disorder in view of the latest research findings. Ideggyogy Sz 2005; 58(5–6): 148–163. [Abstract]
82. Gemignani F, Brindani F, Negrotti A, et al. Restless legs syndrome and polyneuropathy. Mov Disord 2006; [Epub ahead of print].
83. Stewart JD, Low PA, Fealey RD. Distal small-fiber neuropathy: results of tests of sweating and autonomic cardiovascular reflexes. Muscle Nerve 1992; 15:661–665.
84. Novak V, Friemer ML, Kissel JT, et al. Autonomic impairment in painful neuropathy. Neurology 2001; 56:861–868.
85. Periquet MI, Novak V, Collins MP, et al. Painful sensory neuropathy: prospective evaluation using skin biopsy. Neurology 1999; 53:1641–1647.
86. Oh SJ, Melo AC, Lee DK, et al. Large-fiber neuropathy in distal sensory neuropathy with normal routine nerve conduction. Neurology 2001; 56:1570–1572.
87. Jamal GA, Hansen S, Weir AI, et al. The neurophysiologic investigation of small fiber neuropathies. Muscle Nerve 1987; 10:537–545.
88. Longmire DR. An electrophysiological approach to the evaluation of regional sympathetic dysfunction: a proposed classification. Pain Physician 2006; 9:69–82.
89. Low VA, Sandroni P, Fealey RD, Low PA. Detection of small-fiber neuropathy by sudomotor testing. Muscle Nerve 2006; 34(1):57–61.
90. Smith G, Robinson S. Idiopathic neuropathy, prediabetes and the metabolic syndrome. J Neurol Sci 2006; 242(1–2):9–14.
91. Thompson RJ, Doran JF, Jackson P, et al. PGP 9.5—a new marker for vertebrate neurons and neuroendocrine cells. Brain Res 1983; 278:224–228.
92. Wendelschafer-Crabb G, Kennedy WR, Walk D. Morphological features of nerves in skin biopsies. J Neurol Sci 2006; 242(1–2):15–21.
93. Smith AG, Howard JR, Kroll R, et al. The reliability of skin biopsy with measurement of intraepidermal nerve fiber density. J Neurol Sci 2005; 228(1):65–69.
94. Caselli A, Spallone V, Marfia GA, et al. Validation of the nerve axon reflex for the assessment of small nerve fiber dysfunction. J Neurol Neurosurg Psychiatry 2006; 77(8): 927–932.
95. Sorensen L, Molyneaux L, Yue DK. The level of small nerve fiber dysfunction does not predict pain in diabetic neuropathy: a study using quantitative sensory testing. Clin J Pain 2006; 22(3):261–265.
96. Sorensen L, Molyneaux L, Yue DK. The relationship among pain, sensory loss, and small nerve fibers in diabetes. Diabetes Care 2006; 29(4):883–887.
97. Cheliout-Heraut F, Zrek N, Khemliche H, et al. Exploration of small fibers for testing diabetic neuropathies. Joint Bone Spine 2005; 72(5):412–415.
98. Hoffman-Snyder C, Smith BE, Ross MA, et al. Value of the oral glucose tolerance test in the evaluation of chronic idiopathic axonal polyneuropathy. Arch Neurol 2006; Jun 12 [Epub ahead of print].
99. Zambelis T, Karandreas N, Tzavellas E, et al. Large and small fiber neuropathy in chronic alcohol-dependent subjects. J Peripher Nerv Syst 2005; 10(4):375–381.
100. Herrmann DN, McDermott MP, Sowden JE, et al. Is skin biopsy a predictor of transition to symptomatic HIV neuropathy? A longitudinal study. Neurology 2006; 66(6):857–861.

101. Brannagan TH 3rd, Hays AP, Chin SS, et al. Small-fiber neuropathy/neuronopathy associated with celiac disease: skin biopsy findings. Arch Neurol 2005; 62(10):1574–1578.
102. Chin RI, Latov N. Peripheral neuropathy and celiac disease. Curr Treat Options Neurol 2005; 7(1):43–48.
103. Chai J, Herrmann DN, Stanton M, et al. Painful small-fiber neuropathy in Sjogren syndrome. Neurology 2005; 65(6):925–927.
104. Goransson LG, Tjensvoll Ab, Herigstad A, et al. Small diameter nerve fiber neuropathy in systemic lupus erythematosus. Arch Neurol 2006; 63(3):401–404.
105. Lee JE, Shun CT, Hsieh SC, Hsieh ST. Skin denervation in vasculitic neuropathy. Arch Neurol 2005; 62(10):1570–1573.
106. Kararizou E, Davaki P, Karandreas N, et al. Nonsystemic vasculitic neuropathy: a clinicopathological study of 22 cases. J Rheumatol 2005; 32(5):853–858.
107. Dabby R, Gilad R, Dadeh M, et al. Acute steroid responsive small-fiber sensory neuropathy: a new entity? J Peripher Nerv Syst 2006; 11(1):47–52.
108. Scutellari PN, RIzzati R, Antinolfi G, et al. The value of computed tomography in the diagnosis of low back pain. A review of 2,012 cases. Minerva Med 2005; 96(1):41–59.
109. Estanislao L, Carter K, McAthur J, et al. A randomized controlled trial of 5% lidocaine gel for HIV-associated distal symmetric polyneuropathy. J Acquir Immune Defic Sundr 2004; 37(5):1584–1586.
110. Verma S, Estanislao L, Simpson D. HIV-associated neuropathic pain: epidemiology, pathophysiology and management. CNS Drugs 2005; 19(4):325–334.
111. Pardo CA, McArthur JC, Griffin JW. HIV neuropathy: insights in the pathology of HIV peripheral nerve disease. J Peripher Nerv Syst 2001; 6:21–27.
112. Herzberg U, Sagen J. Peripheral nerve exposure to HIV viral envelope protein gp120 induces neuropathic pain and spinal gliosis. J Neuroimmunol 2001; 116:29–39.
113. Apostolski S, McAlarney T, Quattrini A, et al. The gp120 glycoprotein of human immunodeficiency virus type 1 binds to sensory ganglion neurons. Ann Neurol 1993; 34 (6):855–863.
114. Oh SB, Tran PB, Gillard SE, et al. Chemokines and glycoprotein in 120 produce pain hypersensitivity by directly exciting primary nociceptive neurons. J Neurosci 2001; 21(14):5027–5035.
115. Imam I. The neurology of HIV infection—a review of the literature. Niger J Med 2005; 14(2):121–131.
116. Verma S, Micsa E, Estanislao L. Neuromuscular complications in HIV. Curr Neurol Neurosci Rep 2004; 4:62–67.
117. Verma S, Estanislao L, Mintz L, Simpson D. Controlling neuropathic pain in HIV. Curr HIV/AIDS Rep 2004; 1(3):136–141.
118. Power C, Gill MJ, Johnson RT. Progress in clinical neurosciences. The neuropathogenesis of HIV infection: host-virus interaction and the impact of therapy. Can J Neurol Sci 2002; 1:19–32.
119. Breen EC. Pro- and anti-inflammatory cytokines in human immunodeficiency virus infection and acquired immunodeficiency syndrome. Pharacol Ther 2002; 3:295–304.
120. Youle M. HIV-associated antiretroviral toxic neuropathy ATN: a review of recent advances in pathophysiology and treatment. Antivir Ther 2005; 10(suppl 2): M125–M129.
121. Brisby H. Pathology and possible mechanisms of nervous system response to disc degeneration. J Bone Joint Surg Am 2006; 88(suppl 2):68–71.
122. Baron R, Binder A. How neuropathic is sciatica? The mixed pain concept. Orthopade 2004; 33(5):568–575.
123. Freemont AJ, Peacock TE, Goupille P, et al. Nerve ingrowth into diseased intervertebral disc in chronic back pain. Lancet 1997; 350:178–181.
124. Coppes MH, Marani E, Thomeer R, Groen GJ. Innervation of "painful" lumbar discs. Spine 1997; 22:2342–2349.
125. Coopes MH, Marani E, Thomeer R, Groen GJ: Innervation of "painful" lumbar discs. Spine 1997; 22:2342–2349.
126. Kaki AM, El Yaski AZ, Youseif E. Identifying neuropathic pain among patients with chronic low-back pain: use of the Leeds Assessment of Neuropathic Symptoms and Signs pain scale. Reg Anesth Pain Med 2005; 30(5):422–428.

127. Bennett MI, SMither BH, Torrance N, Lee AJ. Can pain be more or less neuropathic? Comparison of symptom assessment tools with ratings of certainty by clinicians. Pain 2006; 122(3):289–294.
128. Khoromi S, Patsalides A, Parada S, et al. Topiramate in chronic lumbar radicular pain. J Pain 2005; 6(12):829–836.
129. Katz J, Pennella-Vaughan J, Hetzel RD, et al. A randomized, placebo-controlled trial of bupropion sustained release in chronic low back pain. J Pain 2005; 6(10):656–661.
130. Audette JF, Emenike E, Meleger AL. Neuropathic low back pain. Curr Pain Headache Rep 2005; 9:168–177.
131. Dejerine J, Roussy G. Le syndrome thalamique. Rev Neurol 1906; 14:521–532.
132. Greiff N. Zur localization der hemichorea. Archiv fur der Psychologie and Nervenkrankheiten 1883; 14:598.
133. Bowsher D. Sensory consequences of strokeLetter. Lancet 1993; 341:156.
134. Andersen G, Vestergaard K, Ingeman-Neilsen M, Jensen TS. The incidence of central post-stroke pain. Pain 1995; 61:187–193.
135. MacGowan DJ, Janal MN, Clark WC, et al. Central poststroke pain and Wallenberg's lateral medullary infarction: Frequency, character and determinants in 63 patients. Neurology 49:120–125.
136. Leijon G, Boivie J, Johansson I. Central Post-stroke pain-neurological symptoms and pain characteristics. Pain 1989; 36:13–25.
137. Holmgren H, Leijon G, Boivie J, et al. Central post-stroke pain-somatosensory evoked potentials in relation to location of the lesion and sensory signs. Pain 1990; 40: 43–52.
138. Bowsher D. The management of central post-stroke painReview. Postgrad Med J 1995; 71:598–604.
139. Woolf CJ, Mannion RJ. Neuropathic pain: aetiology, symptoms, mechanisms, and management. Lancet 1999; 353:1959–1964.
140. Bowsher D. Central pain: Clinical and Physiological characteristics. J Neurol Neurosurg Psychiatry 1996; 61:62–69.
141. Mersky HH, Lindblom U, Mumford JM, Nathan PW. Pain terms: a current note with definitions and notes on usage. Pain 1986; (suppl 3):216–221.
142. Boivie J. Central Pain. In: Wall PD, Melzack R, eds, Textbook of Pain, 3rd.ed. New York: Churchill Livingstone, 1994:871–902.
143. Jensen TS, Lenz FA. Central post-stroke pain: A challenge for the scientist and the clinicianEditorial. Pain 1995; 61:62–69.
144. Lenz FA. Ascending modulation of thalamic function and pain; experimental and clinical data. In: Sicuteri F, ed. Advances in pain research and therapy. New York: Raven, 1992: 177–196.
145. Jones EG. Thalamus and pain. APS Journal 1992; 1:58–61.
146. Boivie J. Hyperalgesia and allodynia in patients with CNS lesions. In: Willis WDJ ed. Hyperalgesia and Allodynia. New York: Raven, 1992: 363–373.
147. Sandy R. Spontaneous pain, hyperpathia and wasting of the hand due to parietal lobe haemorrhage. Euro Neurol 1985; 24:1–3.
148. Riddoch G. The clinical features of central pain. Lancet 1938; 234:1093–1098, 1150–1056, 1205–1209.
149. Gorecki J, Hirayama T, Dostrovsky JO. et al. Thalamic stimulation and recording in patients with deafferentation and central pain. Stereotact Funct Neurosurg 1989; 52:120–126.
150. Yaksh TL. Direct evidence that spinal serotonin and noradrenaline terminals mediate the spinal antinociceptive effects of morphine in the periaqueductal gray. Brain Res 1979; 160:180–185.
151. Hirato M, Watanabe K, Takahashi A, et al. Pathophysiology of centralthalamic pain: combined change of sensory thalamus with cerebral cortex around central sulcus. Stereotact Funct Neurosurg 1994; 62:300–303.
151a. Douglas, R.M. & Goddard, G. Long-term potentiation of the perforant path-granule cell synapse in the rat hippocampus. Brain Res 1975; 86:205–215.
151b. Goddard GV, Douglas RM. Does the engram of kindling model the engram of normal long term memory? Can J Neurol Sci 1975; 2(4):385–394.

151c. Racine RJ, Gartner JG, Burnham WM. Epileptiform activity and neural plasticity in limbic structures. Brain Res 1972; 27; 47(1):262–268.

151d. Racine R, Tuff L, Zaide J. Kindling, unit discharge patterns and neural plasticity. Can J Neurol Sci 1975; 2(4):395–405.

152. Leijon G, Boivie J. Central post-stroke pain-a controlled trial of amitriptyline and Carbamazepine. Pain 1989a; 36:27–36.

153. Davidoff G, Guarrachini M, Roth E, Sliwa J, Yarkony G. Trazodone hydrochloride in the treatment of dysesthetic pain in traumatic myelopathy: a randomized, double blind, placebo-controlled study. Pain 1987; 29:151–161.

154. Ekbom K. Tegretol, a new therapy of tabetic lightning pains. Acta Medica Scandinavica 1966; 179:251–252.

155. Tanelian DL, Victory RA. Sodium channel-blocking agents. Their use in neuropathic pain conditions. Pain Forum 1995; 4:75–80.

156. Kastrup J, Petersen P, Dejgard A, Angelo HR, Hilsted J. Intravenous lidocaine infusion– a new treatment of chronic painful diabetic neuropathy? Pain 1987; 28:69–75.

157. Awerbuch A. Treatment of thalamic pain syndrome with Mexilitene. Ann Neurol 1990; 28:233.

158. Portenoy RK, Foley KM, Inturrisi CE. The nature of opioid responsive-ness and its implications for neuropathic pain: new hypotheses derived from studies of opioid infusions. Pain 1990; 43:272–286.

159. Leijon G, Boivie J. Treatment of neurogenic pain with antidepressants. Nordisk Psykiatrisk Tidsskrift 1989b; 43(suppl 20):83–87.

160. Leijon G, Boivie J. Central post-stroke pain0 the effect of high and low frequency TENS. Pain 1989c; 38:187–191.

161. Siegfried J, Demierre B. Thalamic electrostimulation in the treatment of thalamic pain syndrome. Pain 1984; (suppl 2):116.

162. Taylor CP, Gee NS, Su TZ, et al. A summary of mechanistic hypotheses of gabapentin pharmacology. Epilepsy Res 1998; 29:233–249.

163. Shimoyama N, Shimoyama M, Davis AM, Inturrisi CE, Elliott KJ. Spinal gabapentin is antinociceptive in the rat formalin test. Neurosci Lett 1997; 222:65–67.

164. Tasker R, de Carvalho G, Dostrovsky JO. The history of central pain syndromes, with observations concerning pathophysiology and treatment. In: Casey KL, ed. Pain and central nervous disease: the central pain syndromes. 9th ed. New York: Raven, 1991:31–58.

165. Edgar RE, Best LG, Quail PA, Obert AD. Computer-assisted DREZ microcoagulation: posttramatic spinal deafferentation pain. J Spinal Dis 1993; 6:48–56.

166. Nashold BS, Bullitt E. Dorsal root entry zone lesions to control central pain in paraplegics. J Neurosurg 1981; 55:414–419.

167. Bowsher D, Nurmikko T. Central Post-stroke pain drug treatment options. Dis Manag 1996; 5:160–165.

168. Loh L, Nathan PW, Schott GD. Pain due to lesions of central nervous system removed by sympathetic block. BMJ 1981; 282:L1026–1028.

169. McLachlan EM, Janig W, Devor M, Michaelis M. Peripheral nerve injury triggers noradrenergic sprouting within dorsal root ganglia. Nature 1993; 363:543–546.

170. Woolf CJ, Shortland P, Coggeshall RE. Peripheral nerve injury triggers central sprouting of myelinated afferents. Nature 1992; 355:75–77.

171. Yamashiro K, Iwayama K, Kurihara M, et al. Neurones with epileptiform discharge in the central nervous system and chronic pain: Experimental and clinical investigations. Acta Neurochir SupplWien 1991; 52:130–132.

172. Ossipov MH, Lai J, Malan TP, Porreca F. Spinal and supraspinal mechanisms of neuropathic pain. Ann N Y Acad Sci 2000; 909:12–24.

173. Tenser RB, Dworkin RH. Herpes zoster and the prevention of postherpetic neuralgia. Editorial. Neurology 2005; 65:349–350.

174. Watson CP. Postherpetic neuralgia: the importance of preventing this intractable end-stage disorder. J Inf Dis 1998; 178:S91–S94.

175. Dubinsky RM, Kabbani H, El-Chami Z, et al. Practice parameter: treatment of postherpetic neuralgia. An evidence-based report of the quality standards subcommittee of the American Academy of Neurology. Neurology 2004; 63:959–965.

176. de Moragas JM, Kierland RR. The outcome of patients with herpes zoster. Arch Dermatol 1957; 75:193–196.

177. Watson CP, Evans RJ, Watt VR, Birkett N. Post-herpetic neuralgia: 208 cases. Pain 1988; 35:289–297.

178. Kurtzke JF. Neuroepidemiology. Ann Neurol 1984; 16:265–277.

179. Donahue JG, Choo PW, Manson JE, Platt R. The incidence of herpes zoster. Arch Intern Med 1995; 155:1605–1609.

180. Helgeson S, Petursson G, Gudmundsson S, Sigurdson JA. Prevalence of postherpetic neuralgia after a first episode of herpes zoster: prospective study with long term follow-up. BMJ 2000; 321:794–796.

181. Hope-Simpson RE. The nature of herpes zoster: a long-term study and a new hypothesis. Proc R Soc Med 1965; 58:9–20.

182. Beydoun SR. Postherpetic neuralgia- a model of neuropathic pain: overview of the pathogenesis and current therapeutic options. CME Article. www.pain.com.

183. Rowbotham MC, Petersen KL, Fields HL. Is post-herpetic neuralgia more than one disorder? Technical corner from IASP newsletter, Fall, 1999. www.iasp-pain.org/TC99Fall.html

184. Kost RG, Straus SE. Postherpetic neuralgia- pathogenesis, treatment and prevention. N Engl J Med 1996; 335:32–42.

185. Bowsher D. The effects of pre-emptive treatment of postherpetic neuralgia with amitriptyline: a randomized, double blind, placebo controlled trial. J Pain Symptom Manage 1997; 13:327–331.

186. Watson CP, Chipman M, Reed K, Evans RJ, Birkett N. Amitriptyline versus maprotiline in postherpetic neuralgia: a randomized, double-blind crossover trial. Pain 1992; 48:29–36.

187. Raja SN, Haythornthwaite JA, Pappagallo M, et al. Opioids versus antidepressants in postherpetic neuralgia: a randomized, placebo-controlled trial. Neurology 2002; 59:1015–1021.

188. Gnann JWJ, Whitely RJ. Clinical practice. Herpes zoster. N Engl J Med 2002; 347: 340–346.

189. Watson CP, Babul N. Efficacy of oxycodone in neuropathic pain: a randomized trial in postherpetic neuralgia. Neurology 1998; 50:1837–1841.

190. Rowbotham M, Harden N, Stacey B, et al. Gabapentin for the treatment of postherpetic neuralgia: a randomized controlled trial JAMA 1998; 280L:1837–1842.

191. Rice ACS, Maton S. Gabapentin in postherpetic neuralgia: a randomized, double blind, placebo controlled study. Pain 2001; 94:215–224.

192. Gee NS, Brown JP, Dissanayake VU, et al. The novel anticonvulsant drug, gabapentin-Neurontin binds to the alpha2delta subunit of a calcium channel. J Biol Chem 1996; 271:5768–5776.

193. Dworkin RH, Corbin AE, Young JP, et al. Pregabalin for the treatment of postherpetic neuralgia: a randomized, placebo-controlled trial. Neurology 2003; 60:1274–1283.

194. Pappagallo M, Campbell JN. Chronic opioid therapy as alternative treatment for post-herpetic neuralgia. Ann Neurol 1994; 35 (suppl):S54–S56.

195. Rowbotham MC, Fields HL. Topical lidocaine reduces pain in post-herpetic neuralgia. Pain 1989; 38:29–301.

196. Rowbotham MC, Davies PS, Verkempinck C, Galer BS. Lidocaine patch: double-blind, controlled study of a new treatment method for post-herpetic neuralgia. Pain 1996; 65:39–44.

197. Watson CP, Tyler KL, Bickers DR, et al. A randomized vehicle-controlled trial of topical capsaicin in the treatment of postherpetic neuralgia. Clin Ther 1993; 15:510–526.

198. Don PC. Topical capsaicin for treatment of neuralgia associated with herpes zoster injection. J Am Acad Dermatol 1988; 18(5Pt1):1135–1136.

199. Bernstein JE, Korman NJ, Bickers DR, et al. Topical capsaicin treatment of chronic post-herpetic neuralgia. J Am Acad Dermatol 1989; 21(2Pt1):265–270.

200. Kikuchi A, Kotani N, Sato T, et al. Comparative therapeutic evaluation of intrathecal versus epidural methylpresnisolone for long-term analgesia in patients with intractable postherpetic neuralgia. Reg Anesth Pain Med 1999; 24:287–293.

201. Kotani N, Kushikata T, Hashimoto H, et al. Intrathecal methylpresnisolone for intractable postherpetic neuralgia. N Engl J Med 2000; 343:1514–1519.

202. Klepstad P, Borchgrevink PC. Four years' treatment with ketamine and a trial of dextromethorphan in a patient with severe post-herpetic neuralgia. Acta Anaesthesiol Scand 1997; 41:422–426.
203. Carson MJ, Reilly CR, Sutcliffe JG, Lo D. Mature microglia resemble immature antigen-presenting cells. Glia 1998; 22:72–85.
204. Bartlett PF. Pluripotential hemopoetic stem cells in aduclt mouse brain. Proc Natl Acad Sci USA 1982; 79:2722–2725.
205. Verge GM, Milligan ED, Maier SF, et al. FractalkineCX3CL1 and fractalkine receptorCX3CR1 distribution in spinal cord and dorsal root ganglia under basal and neuropathic conditions. Eur J Neurosci 2004; 20(5):1150–1160.
206. Watkins LR, Milligan ED, Maier SF. Glial activation: a driving force for pathological pain. Trends Neurosci 2001; 24:450–455.
207. Watkins LR, Maier SF. Glia: A novel drug discovery target for clinical pain. Nat Rev Drug Disc 2003; 2:973–985.
208. Wieseler FJ, Maier SF, Watkins LR. Central proinflammatory cytokines and pain enhancement. Neurosignals 2005; 14(4):166–174.
209. Wieseler FJ, Maier SF, Watkins LR. Immune-to-brain communication dynamically modulates pain: physiological and pathological consequences. Brain Behav Immun 2005; 19(2):104–111.
210. Wieseler FJ, Maier SF, Watkins LR. Glial activation and pathological pain. Neurochem Int 2004; 45(2–3):389–395.
211. Milligan ED, Sloane EM, Langer SJ, et al. Controlling neuropathic pain by adeno-associated virus driven production of the anti-inflammatory cytokine, interleukin-10. Mol Pain 1 2005; 25: 9.
212. Watkins LR, Hutchinson MR, Johnson IN, Maier SF. Glia: novel counter-regulators or opioid analgesia. Trends Neurosci 2005; 28(12):661–669.
213. Boswell MV, Rosenberg SK, Chelimsky TC. In: Weiner R, ed. Neuropathic Pain: Mechanisms and Management. Chap 6: Pain Management, 1996.
213a. Dworkin RH, Galer BS, Rowbotham MC. Herpes zoster. N. Engl J Med 2000; 343(3):221–222.
214. Krause SJ, Backonja M-M. Development of a Neuropathic Pain Questionnaire. Clin J Pain 2003; 19:306–314.
215. Longmire DR. The Medical Pain History. Pain Digest 1 1991a; 1:29–34.
216. Longmire DR. The Physical Examination: Methods and application in the clinical evaluation of pain. Pain Digest 1 1991; 2:136–143.
216a. Jay GW, Krusz JC, Longmire DR, McLain DA: Current trends in the diagnosis and treatment of chronic neuromuscular pain syndromes. Am Academy of pain Management. ProCom International 2000.
217. Lindberger M, Schroder HD, Schultzberg M, et al. Nerve fiber studies in skin biopsies in peripheral neurpathies: immunohistochemical analysis of neuropeptides in diabetes mellitus. J Neurol Sci 1989; 93:289–296.
218. Wallengren J, Badendick K, Sundler F, et al. Innervation of the skin of the fore arm in diabetic patients: relation to nerve function. Acta Dermato-Venereoligica 1995; 75:37–42.
219. Levy DM, Terenghi G, Gu X-H, et al. Immunohistochemical measurements of nerves and neuropeptides in diabetic skin: relationship to tests of neurological function. Diabetologia 1992; 35:889–897.
220. Galer BS, Jensen MP. Development and preliminary validation of a pain measure specific to neuropathic pain: the neuropathic pain scale. Neurology 1997; 48:332–338.
221. Leak WD. Radiological assessment of the pain patient. Pain Digest 1 1992; 3:218–224.
222. Longmire DR. Electrodiagnostic studies in the assessment of painful disorders. Pain Digest 1993; 1:2–16
223. Longmire DR, Stanton-Hicks Md'A, Ranieri TA, Woodley WE, Leak WD. Laboratory methods used in the diagnosis of sudomotor dysfunction and Complex Regional Pain Syndromes: a critical review. Pain Digest 1996; 6:21–29.
224. Longmire DR, Parris WCV. Selective tissue conductance in the assessment of sympathetically mediated pain. In: Parris WCV, ed. Chap 10, Contemporary Issues in Chronic Pain. Boston: Kluwer Academic Press, 1991:147–160.
225. Longmire DR, Woodley, WE. Clinical neurophysiology of pain-related sympathetic sudomotor dysfunction. Pain Digest 1993; 3:202–209.

226. Arner S, Meyerson BA. Lack of analgesic effect of opioids on neuropathic and idiopathic forms of pain. Pain 1988; 33:11–23.
227. Dellemijn P. Are opioids effective in relieving neuropathic pain? Pain 1999; 80:453–462.
228. Hegarty A, Portenoy RK. Pharmacotherapy of neuropathic pain. Semin Neurol 1994; 14:213–224.
229. McQuay HJ, Tramer M, Nye BA, Carroll D, Wiffen PJ, Moore RA. A systematic review of antidepressants in neuropathic pain. Pain 1996; 68:217–227.
230. Swerdlow M. Anticonvulsants in the therapy of neuralgic pain. The Pain Clin 1986; 1:9–19.
231. Castillo J, Curley J, Hotz J, et al. Glucocorticoids prolong rat sciatic nerve blockade in vivo from bupivacaine microspheres. Anesthesiology 1996; 85:1157–1166.
232. Devor M, Govrin-Lippmann R, Raber P. Corticosteroids suppress ectopic neural discharge originating in experimental neuromas. Pain 1985; 22:127–137.
233. Pancrazio JJ, Kamatchi GL, Roscoe AK, Lynch C, III. Inhibition of neuronal Na+ channels by antidepressant drugs. J Pharmacol Exp Therap 1998; 284:208–214.
234. Yaksh TL, Malmberg AB. Central pharmacology of nociceptive transmission. In: Wall, PD, Melzack R, eds. Textbook of pain, 3rd ed. Edinburgh: Churchill Livingstone, 1994:165–200.
235. Alhaider AA, Lei SZ, Wilcox GL. Spinal 5-HT3 receptor-mediated antinociception: Possible release of GABA. J Neurosci 1991; 11:1881–1888.
236. Fink E, Oaklander AL. Small-fiber neuropathy: answering the burning questions. Sci Aging Knowledge Environ 2006; 6:7.
237. Eisenach JC, Gebhart GF. Intrathecal amitriptyline acts as an N-methyl-D-aspartate receptor antagonist in the presence of inflammatory hyperalgesia in rats. Anesthesiology 1995; 83:1046–1054.
238. North RB, Kidd DH, Zahurak M, James CS, Long DM. Spinal cord stimulation for chronic, intractable pain: experience over two decades. Neurosurg 1993; 32: 383–394.
239. Kemler MA, Barendse GAM, van Kleef M, et al. Spinal cord stimulation in patients with chronic reflex sympathetic dystrophy. N Engl J Med 2000; 343:618–624.
240. Iacono RP, Guthkelch AN, Boswell MV. Dorsal root entry zone stimulation for deafferentation pain. Stereotact Funct Neurosurg 1992; 59:56–61.
241. Ahmed HE, Craig WF, White PF, et al. Percutaneous electrical nerve stimulation: an alternative to antiviral drugs for acute herpes zoster. Anesth Analg 1998; 87:1–4.
242. Ghoname EA, White PF, Ahmed HE, Hamza A, Craig WF, Noe CE. Percutaneous electrical nerve stimulation: an alternative to TENS in the management of sciatica. Pain 1999; 83:193–199.
243. Hamza MA, White PF, Craig WF, Ghoname ES, et al. Percutaneous electrical nerve stimulation: A novel analgesic therapy for diabetic neuropathic pain. Diabetes Care 2000; 23:365–370.
243a. Boswell MV, Rosenberg SK, Chetimsky TC. Neuropathic pain: Mechanisms and management. Chapter 6. Weiner R: Pain Management. Florida: CRC Press, Boca Raton.
244. Goli V. A mechanistic approach to the treatment of neuropathic pain: Symposium, Dannemiller Foundation, 2002.
245. Gracely RH, Lynch SA, Bennett GJ. Painful neuropathy: Altered central processing, maintained dynamically by peripheral input. Pain 1992; 51:175–194.
246. Price DD, Mao J, Mayer DJ. Central neural mechanisms of normal and abnormal pain states. In: Fields HL, Liebskind JC, eds. Pharmacological approaches to the treatment of chronic pain: New concepts and critical issues. Progress in pain research and management. Vol. 1, Seattle: IASP Press, 1994:61–84.
247. Kovelowski CJ, Ossipov MH, Sun H, Malan TP, Porecca F. Supraspinal cholecystokinin may drive tonic descending facilitation mechanisms to maintain neuropathic pain in the rat. Pain 1992; 87:265–273.
248. Wessel K, Vieregge P, Kessler C, Kompf D. Thalamic stroke: correlation of clinical symptoms, somatosensory evoked potentials and CT findings. Acta Neurol Scand 1994; 90:167–173.
249. Caudle RM, Mannes AJ. Dynorphin, friend or foe? Pain 2000; 87:235–239.

250. Hart RG, Easton JD. Carbamazepine and hematological monitoring. Ann Neurol 1982; 11:309–312.
251. Sotgiu ML, Lacerenza M, Marchettini P. Effect of systemic lidocaine on dorsal horn neuron hyperactivity following chronic peripheral nerve injury in rats. Somatosens Mot Res 1992; 9:227–233.
252. Vanderah TW, Gardell LR, Burgess SH, et al. Dynorphin promotes abnormal pain and spinal opioid antinociceptive tolerance. J Neurosci 2000; 20:7074–7079.
252a. McCleane GJ. Intragvenous infusion of phenytoin relieves neuropathic pain: a randomized double-blinded, placebo controlled, crossover study. Anesth analg 199; 89:985.
253. Blom, S. Trigeminal neuralgia: Its treatment with a new anticonvulsant drug G-32883. Lancet 1962; 1:839–840.
254. Brodie MJ, Dichter MA. Antiepileptic drugs. N Engl J Med 1996; 334:168–175.
255. Matthew NT, Saper JR, Silberstein SD, et al. Migraine prophylaxis with divalproex. Arch Neurol 1995; 52:281–286.
256. Raskin P, Donofrio PD, Rosenthal NR, et al. Topiramate vs. placebo in painful diabetic neuropathy: analgesic and metabolic effects. Neurology 2004; 63:865–873.
257. Tohen M, Castillo J, Baldessarin RJ, Zarate C, Kando JC. Blood dyscrasias with carbamazepine and valproate: a pharmacoepidemiological study of 2,228 patients at risk. Am J Psychiatry 1959; 152:413–418.
258. Jun JH, Yaksh TL. The effect of intrathecal gabapentin and 3-isobutyl gamma-aminobutyric acid on the hyperalgesia observed after thermal injury in the rat. Anesth Analg 1998; 86:348–354.
259. Chapman V, Suzuki R, Chamarette HLC, Rygh LJ, Dickenson AH. Effects of systemic carbamazepine and gabapentin on spinal neuronal responses in spinal nerve ligated rats. Pain 1998; 75:261–272.
260. Abdi S, Lee DH, Chung JM. The anti-allodynic effects of amitriptyline, gabapentin, and lidocaine in a rat model of neuropathic pain. Anesth Analg 1998; 87:1360–1366.
261. Shimoyama M, Shimoyama N, Inturrisi CE, Elliott KJ. Gabapentin enhances the antinociceptive effects of spinal morphine in the rat tail-flick test. Pain 1997a; 72:375–382.
262. Sindrup SH, Gram LF, Brosen K, Eshj O, Morgensen EF. The selective serotonin reuptake inhibitor paroxetine is effective in the treatment of diabetic neuropathy symptoms. Pain 1990; 42:135–144.
263. Backonja MM, Beydoun A, Edwards KR, et al. Gabapentin for the symptomatic treatment of painful neuropathy in patients with diabetes mellitus. A randomized controlled trial. JAMA 1998; 280:1831–1836.
264. Morello CM, Leckband SG, Stoner CP, Moorhouse DF, Sahagian GA. Randomized double-blind study comparing the efficacy of gabapentin with amitriptyline on diabetic peripheral neuropathy. Arch Int Med 1999; 159:1931–1937.
265. Mattia C, Coluzzi F. Tramadol: focus on musculoskeletal and neuropathic pain. Minerva Anestesiol 2005; 71:565–584.
266. Sindrup SH, Jensen TS. Efficacy of pharmacological treatments of neuropathic pain: an update and effect related to mechanism of drug action. Pain 1999; 83:389–400.
267. Sindrup SH, Jensen TS. Pharmacological treatment of pain in polyneuropathy. Neurology 2000; 55:915–920.
268. Rowbotham M, Harden N, Stacey B, Bernstein P, Magnus-Miller L. Gabapentin for the treatment of postherpetic neuralgia. A randomized controlled trial. JAMA, 280:1837–1842.
269. Beydoun A, Uthman BM, Sackellares JC. Gabapentin: Pharmacokinetics, efficacy, and safety. Clin Neuropharmacol 1995; 18:469–481.
270. Zareba G. Pregabalin: a new agent for the treatment of neuropathic pain. Drugs TodayBarc. 2005; 41(8):509–516.
271. Freynhagen R, Stojek K, Griesing T, et al. Efficacy of pregabalin in neuropathic pain evaluated in a 12-week, randomised, double-blind, multicenter, placebo-controlled trial of flexible- and fixed-dose regimens. Pain 2005; 115(3):254–263.
272. Lesser H, Sharma U, LaMoreaux L, Poole RM. Pregabalin relieves symptoms of painful diabetic neuropathy: a randomized controlled trial. Neurology 2004; 63(11):2104–2110.
273. Richter RW, Portenoy R, Sharma U, et al. Relief of painful diabetic peripheral neuropathy with pregabalin: a randomized, placebo-controlled trial. J Pain 2005; 6(4):253–260.

274. Frampton JE, Scott LJ. Pregabalin: in the treatment of painful diabetic peripheral neuropathy. Drugs 2004; 64(24):2813–2820.
275. Rosenstock J, Tuchman M, LaMoreaux L, Sharma U. Pregabalin for the treatment of painful diabetic peripheral neuropathy: a double-blind, placebo controlled trial. Pain 2004; 110(3):628–638.
276. Hadj Tahar A. Pregabalin for peripheral neuropathic pain. Issues Emerg Health Technol 2005; 67:1–4.
277. Max M. Antidepressants as analgesics. In: Fields HL, Liebskind JC, eds, Pharmacological approaches to the treatment of chronic pain: New concepts and critical issues. Progress in pain research and management, Vol. 1, Seattle: IASP Press, 1994:229–246.
278. Onghena P, van Houdenhove B. Antidepressant-induced analgesia in chronic non-malignant pain: a meta-analysis of 39 placebo controlled studies. Pain 1992; 49:205–220.
279. Glassman A, Roose S, Bigger J. The safety of tricyclic antidepressants in cardiac patients. Risk-benefit reconsidered. JAMA 1993; 269:2673–2677.
280. American Medical Association 1993. Drugs used in mood disorders. AMA Drug Evaluations Annualpp. 277–306. Chicago: American Medical Association.
281. Sobotka JL, Alexander B, Cook BL. A review of carbamazepine's hematologic reactions and monitoring recommendations. DICP 1990; 24:1214–1219.
282. Rani PU, Naidu MUR, Prasad VBN, Rao TRK, Shobha JC. An evaluation of antidepressants in rheumatic pain conditions. Anesth Analg 1996; 83:371–375.
283. Siegfried J. Long term results of electrical stimulation in the treatment of pain my means of implanted electrodes. In: Rizzi C, Visentin TA, eds, Pain Therapy. Amsterdam: Elsevier, 1983:463–475.
284. Galer BS. Neuropathic pain of peripheral origin: advances in pharmacologic treatment. Neurology, 1995; 45(suppl 9):S17–S25.
285. Rowbotham MC, Goli V, Kunz NR, Lei D. Venlafaxine extended release in the treatment of painful diabetic neuropathy: a double-blind, placebo controlled study. Pain 2004; 110(3):697–706.
286. Wernicke JF, Gahimer J, Yalcin I, et al. Safety and adverse event profile of duloxetine. Expert Opin Drug Saf 2005; 4(6):987–993.
287. Kirwin JL, Goren JL. Duloxetine: a dual serotonin-norepinephrine reuptake inhibitor for treatment of major depressive disorder. Pharmacotherapy 2005; 25(3):396–410.
288. Maizels M, McCarberg B. Antidepressants and antiepileptic drugs for chronic non-cancer pain. Am Fam Physician 2005; 71(3):483–490.
289. DuloxetineCymbalta for diabetic neuropathic pain. Med Lett Drugs Ther 2005; 47(1215–1216):67–68.
290. Raskin J, Pritchett YL, Wang F, et al. A double-blind, randomized multicenter trial comparing duloxetine with placebo in the management of diabetic peripheral neuropathic pain. Pain Med 2005; 6(5):346–356.
291. Goldstein DJ, Lu Y, Detke MJ, et al. Duloxetine vs. Placebo in patients with painful diabetic neuropathy. Pain 2005; 116(1–2):109–118.
292. Arnold LM, Lu Y, Crofford LJ, et al. A double-blind, multicenter trial comparing duloxetine with placebo in the treatment of fibromyalgia patients with or without major depressive disorder. Arthritis Rheum 2004; 50(9):2974–2984.
293. Offenbaecher M, Ackenheil M. Current trends in neuropathic pain treatments with special reference to fibromyalgia. CNS Spectr 2005; 10(4):285–297.
294. Sindrup S, Otto M, Finnerup N, Jensen T. Antidepressants in the treatment of neuropathic pain. Basic Clin Pharm Toxicol 2005; 96(6):399–409.
295. Coluzzi F, Mattia C. Mechanism-based treatment in chronic neuropathic pain: the role of antidepressants. Cur Pharm Design 2005; 11(23):2945–2960.
296. Grond S, Sablotzki A. Clinical pharmacology of tramadol. Clin Pharmacokinet 2004; 43(13):879–923.
297. Desmeules JA. The tramadol option. Eur J Pain 2000; 4(suppl A):15–21.
298. Dworkin RH, Backonja M, Rowbotham MC, et al. Advances in neuropathic pain. Arch Neurol 2003; 60:1524–1534.
299. Stacey BR. Management of peripheral neuropathic pain. Am J Phys Med Rehabil 2005; 84(suppl 3):S4–S16.

300. Marchettini P, Teloni L, Formaglio F, Lacerenza M. Pain in diabetic neuropathy case study: whole patient management. Eur J Neurol 2004; (suppl 1):12–21.
301. Mullins CR, Wild TL. Pain management in a long-term care facility: compliance with JCAHO standards. J Pain Palliat Care Pharmacother 2003; 17(2):63–70.
302. Sindrup SH, Andersen G, Madsen C, et al. Tramadol relieves pain and allodynia in polineurpathy: a randomised, double-blind, controlled trial. Pain 1999; 83:85–90.
303. Waikakul S, Waikakul W. Penkitti P, et al. Comparison of analgesics for pain after brachial plexus injury: tramadol vs. paracetamol with codeine. Pain Clinic 1998; 11:119–124.
304. Harati Y, Gooch C, Sweenson M, et al. Double-blind randomized trial of tramadol for the treatment of the pain of diabetic neuropathy. Neurology 1998; 50:1842–1846.
305. Duhmke RM, Cornblath DD, Hollingshead JR. Tramadol for neuropathic pain. Cochrane Database Syst Rev 2004; 2:CD003726.
306. Cook RJ, Sackett DL. The number needed to treat: a clinically useful measure of treatment effect. BMJ 1995; 310:452–454.
307. Chabal C, Jacobson L, Mariano A, Chaney E, Britell CW. The use of oral mexiletine for the treatment of pain after peripheral nerve injury. Anesthesiology 1992; 76:513–517.
308. Abram SE, Yaksh TL. Systemic lidocaine blocks nerve injury-induced hyperalgesia and nociceptor-driven spinal sensitization in the rat. Anesthesiology 1994; 80:383–391.
309. Swerdlow M. Anticonvulsant drugs and chronic pain. Clin Neuropharmacol 1984; 7:51–82.
310. Burchiel KJ, Chabal C. A role for systemic lidocaine challenge in the classification of neuropathic pains. Pain Forum 1995; 4:81–82.
311. Chaplan SR, Flemming BW, Shafer SL, Yaksh, TL. Prolonged alleviation of tactile allodynia by intravenous lidocaine in neuropathic rats. Anesthesiology 1995; 83: 775–785.
312. Jaffe RA, Rowe MA. Subanesthetic concentrations of lidocaine selectively inhibit a nociceptive response in the isolated rat spinal cord. Pain 1995; 60:167–174.
313. Galer BS, Miller KV, Rowbotham MC. Response to intravenous lidocaine infusion differs based on clinical diagnosis and site of nervous system injury. Neurology 1993; 43:1233–1235.
313a. Rowbotham MC, Davies PS, Verkernpinck C, Galer BS. Lidocaine patch; double-blind, controlled study of a new treatment method for post-herpetic neurologia. Pain 1996; 65:39–44.
314. Saal JS, Franson RC, Dobrow R, Saal JA, White AH, Goldthwaite N. High levels of inflammatory phospholipase A2 activity in lumbar disc herniations. Spine 1990; 15:674–678.
315. Fromm GH, Terrence CF, Chattha AS. Baclofen in the treatment of trigeminal neuralgia: double-blind study and long-term follow-up. Ann Neurol 1984; 15:240–244.
316. Caternia MJ, Schumacher MA, Tominga M, et al. The capsaicin receptor: a heat-activated ion channel in the pain pathway. Nature 1997; 389:816–824.
317. Kamel J, Mizoguchi H, Narita M, Tseng LF. Therapeutic potential of PKC inhibitors in painful diabetic neuropathy. Exp Opin Invest Drugs 2001; 10(9):1653–1664.
318. Haslbeck M. New options in the treatment of various forms of diabetic neuropathy. MMW Fortschr Med 2004; 146(21):47–50.
319. Vinik AI, Bril V, Kempler P, et al. Treatment of symptomatic diabetic peripheral neuropathy with the protein kinase C beta-inhibitor ruboxistaurin mesylate during a 1-year, randomized, placebo controlled, double-blind clinical trial. Clin Ther 2005; 27 (8):1164–1180.
320. Khedr EM, Kotb H, Kamel NF, et al. Longlasting antalgic effects of daily sessions of repetitive transcranial magnetic stimulation in central and peripheral neuropathic pain. J Neurol Neurosurg Psychiatry 2005; 76(6):833–838.
321. Finnerup NB, Otto M, McQuay HJ, et al. Algorithm for neuropathic pain treatment: an evidence based proposal. Pain 2005; Epub ahead of print.

12 Tension-Type Headache

Tension-type headache (TTHA), with or without secondary medication overuse headache (MOH), is probably the most common primary headache disorder seen by primary care physicians and neurologists, and, when chronic, by headache specialists. It has been estimated that about 80% of the general population may suffer from episodic TTHA, with 3% having chronic TTHA (1). TTHA is typically not as disabling as migraine, but chronic TTHA (CTTHA) can significantly impair patient function (2). In spite of this, much less research has been done on this, possibly the most common form of primary headache, compared to migraine or even cluster headache.

While the relatively recent understanding of the presence of peripheral and central sensitization, as well as peripheral myogenic nociceptive input has given more impetus for research, it has only recently begun to give some benefit to TTHA and CTTHA sufferers.

The diagnostic criteria of TTHA, according to the International Headache Society (3,4) indicate that episodic TTHA is recurrent headache occurring fewer than 15 days a month, lasting from 30 minutes to seven days. The pain characteristics include two of four of the following: pain with a pressing/tightening (nonpulsating) quality; pain which is mild to moderate in intensity and may inhibit, but not prohibit activities; pain which is always bilateral; and pain which is not aggravated by walking stairs or doing other routine physical activity. These criteria also state that both of the following are true: no nausea or vomiting, but anorexia may occur, and photophobia and phonophobia are absent, or one but not the other is present.

All other organic diagnoses must be ruled out first, as well as other primary headache diagnoses, including migraine and cluster headache. In spite of diagnostic differences along with treatment differences, there remains, to some, the question of the presence of TTHA and migraine on the same pathophysiologic spectrum (5).

Additionally, TTHA has six entities: episodic, frequent episodic and chronic, with each entity subdivided into being with or without pericranial muscle tenderness.

In TTHA, the pain is typically described as aching or pressure like, or "like there is a vice around my head." The pain has also been described as feeling like a tight band around the head. The pain is typically bilateral, although it may be unilateral. It may include various areas, some or all of: occipito-nuchal, bifrontal, bitemporal, suboccipital, at the vertex (crown) of the head, as well as extend into the neck and shoulders.

The pain intensity may wax and wane depending on a number of factors including movement, activity level, stress, and others. Emotional/psychologic aspects may increase pain.

There is a female preponderance.

Unlike migraine headache patients, TTHA patients can typically carry on with their activities. Most take some form of analgesic, frequently on a daily basis.

Without question, TTHA patients may also have migraine, as well as analgesic rebound or MOH.

The CTTHA patient has headache 15 or more days a month. This is also a diagnostic exercise, as most frequently, nosologically, TTHA may be one of several headache diagnoses all of which are part of a chronic daily headache differential, which would include MOH, at a minimum. CTTHA differs from episodic TTHA in frequency, a poor response to many treatment strategies, increased incidence of analgesic overuse (MOH), and a poorer quality of life (6).

The TTHA patient frequently has headache daily or every other day. The headache is typically there when they awaken, and remains until they go to sleep. The intensity of the pain varies, decreasing for several hours after analgesics are taken.

The majority of TTHA patients, if seen early on, will have associated pericranial muscle spasm or pain, while others will not, yet still complain of pain.

Episodic TTHA appears to have more input from peripheral pain mechanisms, while abnormalities in central pain mechanisms appear to be more important in CTTHA (7).

Patients with TTHA will also endure elements of depression and anxiety. There is a "chicken and egg" aspect to this, in terms of which problem comes first. In many cases, central neurochemical changes begin concurrent to an injury and manifest as both pain and affective disturbances (see subsequent text).

When one understands the pathophysiology of TTHA, it should be understood that the history and physical examination must be done quite specifically. Knowing what questions to ask and what, on occasion can be fairly subtle, physical findings to look for on examination are obviously important.

PATHOPHYSIOLOGY OF TTHA

Pathologic changes in the musculoskeletal system may initiate, modulate, or perpetuate TTHA. Episodic and CTTHA are, at least at first, secondary to a muscle-induced pain syndrome that is typically associated with the aforementioned myofascial pain syndrome (MPS) (see Chapters 4–6).

The continuous input to the CNS of peripheral myogenic nociception may in fact be responsible for transforming episodic TTHA into CTTHA (8).

The CNS controls muscle tone via systems that influence the gamma efferent neurons in the anterior horn cells of the spinal cord, which act on the alpha motor neurons supplying muscle spindles. The Renshaw cells, apparently via the inhibitory neurotransmitter gamma aminobutyric acid (GABA) will influence this synaptic system. There is also supraspinal control from cortical, subcortical, and limbic afferent and efferent systems. Physiologic and emotional inputs interact in the maintenance or flux of muscle tone. Adverse influences from both localized and regional myofascial nociception, with or without limbic (affective) stimulation, may produce significant muscle spasm, which, if prolonged, will become tonic with the additional aspects of increased anxiety or a maintained muscle contraction-pain cycle (9,10). This helps to differentiate acute versus CTTHA, to a degree.

Tonic or continued muscle contraction may induce hypoxia via compression of small blood vessels. Ischemia, the accumulation of pain-producing metabolites (bradykinin, lactic acid, serotonin, prostoglandins, etc.) may increase and potentiate muscle pain and reactive spasm. These nociception-enhancing or algetic chemicals may stimulate central mechanisms that, through continued stimulation, may induce continued reactive muscle spasm/contraction and maintenance of the myogenic nociceptive cycle (11–13).

The MPS was, for a long while, ignored in the pathophysiology of headache of any type. Some researchers found a causal relationship between muscle spasm and headache (14–16) while others have felt that muscle spasm associated with headache is an epiphenomenona, not the etiology of headache (17–22), but a reflexive response. Other authors have indicated that muscle activity/spasm or increased tone may be more pronounced in migraine than in TTHAs (23,24).

Unfortunately, this research, which was obtained via electromyographic (EMG) studies, appears to be problematic, as the various authors evaluated different groups of muscles in different types of patients, many of whom had poorly defined diagnoses (15,23,25,26). Other authors defined CTTHA as an entity with or without associated pericranial muscle disorder (27). The concept of muscle fatigue was not taken into consideration, that is, metabolically spent muscles which may become relatively flaccid, losing aspects of increased tonus or spasm.

One study found a positive correlation between pericranial muscle tenderness and headache intensity, with the former felt to be a source of nociception (28). Another study (29) found that pressure pain thresholds in patients with CTTHA were highly dependent on myofascial factors. This study indicated that the generally lower pain thresholds in the CTTHA patients suggested a dysmodulation of central nociception. A lower pain threshold in CTTHA patients, when compared to normal volunteers, was also noted (30).

Scalp muscle tenderness and sensitivity to pain in both migraine and TTHA patients were measured in another study, and the author indicated that the pathophysiology of TTHA may involve a diffuse disruption of central pain-modulating mechanisms (31). Lower pain thresholds were also found in patients diagnosed with MPSs, including lower back pain (32,33).

In another study, lower pain thresholds in muscle and skin of the cephalic regions but not in lower limb muscle and skin were demonstrated in patients with CTTHA as compared to healthy controls (34). Furthermore, TTHA patients were found to be more liable to develop shoulder and cervical pain in response to static exercise as compared to normal, healthy controls (35). When looking at deep pain and surface EMG responses to stress in migraineurs during headache-free periods, TTHA patients and healthy controls, TTHA patients were found to have delayed recovery from pain in all muscle regions as compared with controls, while the migraine patients had delayed pain recovery in a much more restricted area (trapezius and temporalis musculature), indicating the presence/importance of central sensitization of pain pathways in TTHA patients (1).

Increased pericranial muscle tenderness in patients with TTHA during headache-free periods has at least implied that the tenderness is not just correlated with the presence of headache (36).

While the absolute origin of increased muscle tenderness in TTHA is not known, it is felt that the nociceptors around blood vessels in striated muscle and their tendonous insertions and fascia may be sources of pain (37).

CTTHA patients frequently have a stereotypic posture, with their shoulders raised and their heads flexed forward. This tightly held posture, or muscular splinting, is effective in preventing unconscious head movement that may induce pain. The continued splinting, by maintaining tonic muscle contraction, also works to increase myogenic nociception and perpetuate this cycle. The potential role of this forward head posture in association with decreased cervical mobility has a possible role in the origin or maintenance of TTHA (38).

The pericranial muscles are innervated by sensory fibers in nerves from the second or third cervical roots and in the trigeminal nerve (39). The functions of these muscles contribute to the maintenance of posture and the stabilization of the head, as well as withdrawal and protection of the head.

Muscle fatigue occurs, both metabolic and neurochemical in nature, and typically follows prolonged or tonic muscle spasm. It may be secondary to "sympatheticopenia" or the depletion of epinephrine and norepinephrine (NEP), the peripheral sympathetic transmitters (40). The muscle spindle is directly affected by the sympathetic nervous system via these neurotransmitters, particularly NEP. Prolonged and sustained peripheral sympathetic activity may lead to the depletion of NEP at the synaptic receptors. Continued afferent sympathetic input from myogenic nociception, at least in part from buildup though ischemia of nociceptive metabolites, may result in sympatheticopenia (40,41). There are also significant sympathetic aspects of myofascial pain, which will not be dealt with in this chapter (42) (see Chapter 5).

Tenderness of the cervical, thoracic, and lumbar paravertebral muscles is also positively correlated with pericranial muscle tenderness (43). It has also been noted that the contraction of shoulder and cervical muscles as well as emotional arousal contribute to TTHA (44).

Three mechanisms of muscle pain are thought to be relevant to acute, but more often CTTHA; myogenic nociception may be induced by: (*i*) low-grade inflammation associated with the release of algetic, or pain-inducing substances, rather than signs of acute inflammation, (*ii*) short- or long-lasting relative ischemia, and (*iii*) tearing of ligaments and tendons secondary to abnormal sustained muscle tension (39).

MYOFASCIAL PAIN SYNDROME (MPS)

Travell and Rinzler identified the contribution of musculoskeletal factors in the etiology of acute and CTTHA (45). They demonstrated that there are consistent patterns of referred pain from trigger points within specific muscle and defined perpetuating factors that convert acute myofascial pain into a chronic pain syndrome (46).

The MPS is a localized or regional pain problem associated with small zones of hypersensitivity within skeletal muscle called trigger points. With palpation of these points, pain is referred to adjacent or even distant sites. Trigger points in the head, neck, and upper back may elicit headache, as well as tinnitus, vertigo, and lacrimation, all features noted in patients with PTTHA as well as CTTHA (47) (Figs. 1–8).

Trigger points may be active, with consistently reproducible pain on palpation, or latent, with no clinically associated complaints of pain, but with associated muscle dysfunction. Trigger points may shift between active and latent states. Clinically, continuous myogenic nociception from active trigger points appears to be a prime instigator of the central neurochemical nociceptive dysmodulation found in patients with CTTHA.

Increased stiffness, weakness, and fatigue as well as a decreased range of motion are typically found in muscles in which trigger points are identified. These muscles may be shortened, with increased pain perceived on stretching. Patients may protect these muscles by adapting poor posture with sustained contraction, as noted above (39,48). The resulting muscular restrictions may perpetuate existing trigger points and aid in the development of others.

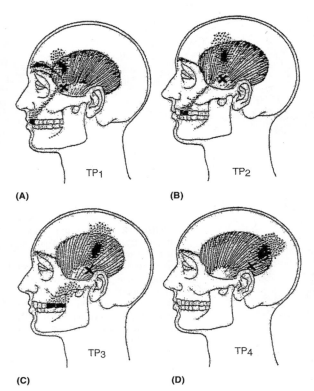

(A)   (B)

(C)   (D)

FIGURE 1 Referred pain patterns from trigger points in the left temporalis muscle. Dark areas show essential zones; spillover zones are stippled. (**A**) Anterior "spokes" of pain arising from the anterior fibers, trigger point 1 region. (**B**) and (**C**), middle spokes, trigger point 2 and 3 regions. (**D**) Posterior supra-auricular spoke, trigger point 4 region. *Source*: Ref. 170. Reprinted with permission.

Another author (49) found that a large percentage of patients suffering from a MPS of the head and neck were found to have significant postural problems, with forward head tilt and rounded shoulders, as well as poor standing and sitting posture, all findings frequently seen in both CTTHA patients.

A MPS of the head and neck, via myofascial trigger point referred pain, may mimic other conditions, including migraine headache, temporomandibular joint (TMJ) dysfunction, sinusitis, and cervical neuralgias, as well as various otologic problems including tinnitus, ear pain, and dizziness (48).

The onset of an acute, single muscle MPS may be associated with trauma, such as an acceleration/deceleration injury, a slip and fall, or even a direct blow. It may also come on insidiously, for example, in patients who work multiple hours typing or at the computer.

The MPS may show a spontaneous regression to a latent status, with continued muscular dysfunction, but with significant diminution of the initial pain complaints. In other patients, the MPS may "metastasize" and involve associated musculature, becoming regional, or even involving multiple muscular regions.

Migraine, a neurovascular disorder, has associated scalp tenderness and referred pain. Trigger points were found in one study in 93.9% of migraineurs compared to controls (29%) (50). The presence of central sensitization in migraineurs with frequent attacks and long duration of disease may be assumed, as pericranial and extracephalic allodynia can be found in these patients.

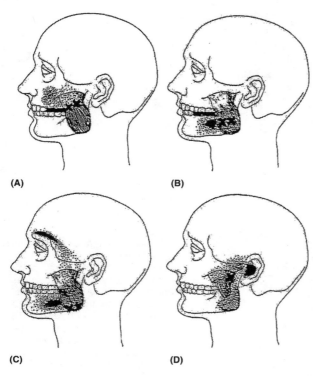

(A)   (B)

(C)   (D)

FIGURE 2 Each *X* indicates a trigger point in various parts of the masseter muscle. Dark areas show essential zones; spillover zones are stippled. (**A**) Superficial layer, upper portion. (**B**) Superficial layer, mid-belly. (**C**) Superficial layer, lower portion. (**D**) Deep layer, upper part, just below the temporomandibular joint. *Source*: Ref. 170. Reprinted with permission.

OTHER CLINICAL ASPECTS

After the onset of CTTHA, emotional/psychological factors including stress, anxiety, and depression may become important in the maintenance or perpetuation of the headache.

A major difficulty in the literature is the fact that determinations of depression, anxiety, and other affective components are found to occur in patients with

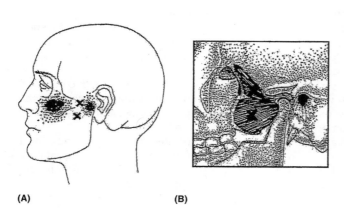

(A)   (B)

FIGURE 3 (**A**) Referred pain pattern (*shaded area*) of trigger points (*X*) in the left lateral psterygoid muscle (**B**). *Source*: Ref. 170. Reprinted with permission.

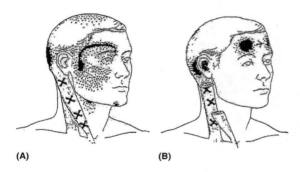

FIGURE 4 Referred pain patterns with location of corresponding trigger points (*X*) in the right sternocleidomastoid muscle. Dark areas show essential zones; spillover zones are stippled. (**A**) The sternal (superficial) division; (**B**) the clavicular (deep) division. *Source*: Ref. 170. Reprinted with permission.

CTTHA. Without premorbid psychologic analyses, it is very difficult to state with any certainly whether these patients were depressed or anxious prior to the onset of their headache problems. It is therefore possible that the neurochemical changes associated with CTTHA, such as probable central serotonergic dysfunction, initiate depression as a response to these pain-induced neurochemical changes (see subsequently).

Some authors have thought that the "conversion V" found in the hypochondriasis, depression, and hysteria scales of the Minnesota Multiphasic Personality Inventory is a marker for CTTHA as well as PTTHA. However, similar responses are found in chronic non-headache pain patients (51–53).

Altered brain stem reflexes have suggested that limbic system control of the descending antinociceptive systems may be abnormal in patients with CTTHA (54). TTHA can be precipitated by stress, anxiety, or mental tension; a correlation has been made between headache and stress in patients with TTHA (55). It has also been demonstrated that depression increased the "vulnerability" of patients to develop TTHA which was associated with increased pericranial muscle pain (56,57). Anxiety

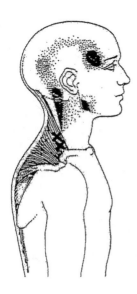

FIGURE 5 Referred pain pattern and location of trigger point (*X*) in the upper trapezius muscle. Dark areas show essential zones; spillover zones are stippled. *Source*: Ref. 170. Reprinted with permission.

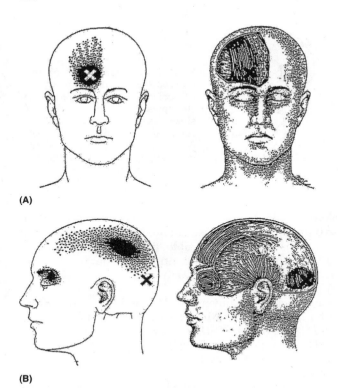

(A)

(B)

FIGURE 6 Pain patterns (*shaded areas*) referred from trigger points (*X*) in the occipitofrontalis muscle, commonly associated with unilateral, supraorbital, or ocular headache. **(A)** Right frontalis belly; **(B)** left occipitalis belly. *Source*: Ref. 170. Reprinted with permission.

and depression may contribute to increased excitability in the central nociceptive pathways, possibly via limbic system input (58,59).

ASSOCIATED SLEEP DISORDERS

There appears to be an important relationship between sleep, headache, and the muscle-pain syndromes. Central biogenic amines, particularly serotonin and NEP, are important to sleep physiology as well as to the central pain-modulating systems. Both human and animal research indicate that central serotonin metabolism plays a role in pain modulation, affective states, and the regulation of non–rapid eye movement (REM) sleep (60).

A high incidence of sleep difficulties has been found in CTTHA patients (61). Different sleep disorders appear to be associated with different headache entities. Migraine has been found to occur in association with REM sleep, as well as have an association with excessive stages three, four, and REM sleep (62). CTTHA has been found to be associated with frequent awakenings and decreased slow wave sleep, as well as an alpha-wave intrusion into stage four sleep (63).

Moldofsky et al. (64) noted a disturbance in stage four sleep to be the first laboratory-based abnormality found in fibromyalgia. They induced a similar alpha non-REM pattern of alpha-wave intrusion in delta (stage four) sleep in

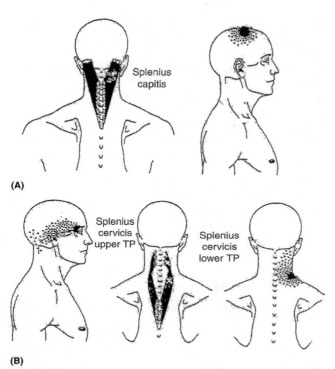

(A)

(B)

FIGURE 7   Trigger points (*X*) and referred pain patterns (*shaded areas*) for the right splenius capitis and splenius cervicis muscles. (**A**) Splenius capitis trigger point that overlies the occipital triangle; (**B**) left, the upper splenius cervicis trigger point (TP) refers pain to the orbit. The dashed arrow represents pain shooting from the inside of the head to the back or pain shooting from the inside of the head to the back of the eye. Right, another site of pain referral. *Source*: Ref. 170. Reprinted with permission.

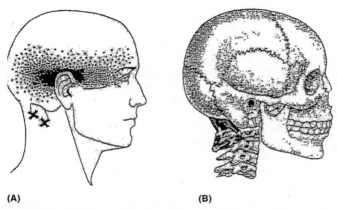

(A)   **(B)**

FIGURE 8   (**A**) Referred pain pattern (*shaded area*) of trigger points (*X*) in the right suboccipital muscles (**B**). *Source*: Ref. 170. Reprinted with permission.

normal subjects by stage four sleep deprivation. These subjects developed musculoskeletal pain and affective changes comparable to those seen in fibromyalgia
patients. Small doses of serotonergic tricyclic antidepressant (TCA) medications,
which reduced the alpha intrusions into stage four sleep (amitriptyline), were
utilized to ameliorate the symptoms.

Alpha-wave intrusions into deep sleep have also been found in patients with
other chronic pain syndromes, including rheumatoid arthritis (65). The alpha non-
REM disturbance has also been seen in asymptomatic people as well as in those
who experience severe emotional stress, such as combat veterans (60). In the latter
group, the veterans with this sleep disorder also complained of chronic headaches,
diffuse pain, and emotional distress.

Sleep disturbance is also associated with increased pain severity. As noted
above, chronic headache patients seem to have a higher incidence of sleep abnormalities than do normal, pain-free subjects. Etiologic aspects of chronic headache
may be linked to sleep abnormalities as an initiating event or as the result of the
underlying pathologically dysmodulated neurochemical factors inducing a sleep
disorder.

OTHER POSSIBLE ASSOCIATED FACTORS

There are several possible mechanical etiologies of CTTHA. First is cervical spondylosis, which is defined as a degenerative disease affecting intervertebral discs and
apophyseal joints of the cervical spine. While several authors indicated a possible
correlation between cervical spondylosis and TTHA (2,3,13), others concluded the
contrary (47) suggesting that the basis of existing headache is secondary to muscle
contraction and/or central neurochemical dysmodulation.

Cervicogenic headache, from referred pain perceived in any region of the head
which was referred by a primary nociceptive source in the musculoskeletal tissues
innervated by cervical nerves, is a second suggestive diagnosis (67–69).

Finally, the dental literature has been most active in reporting a possible correlation between TMJ dysfunction and acute and CTTHA (70,71). The relationship
appears to be dependent mainly on tenderness of the masticatory muscles, which
may have other etiologies and induce TMJ dysfunction, when it exists, on a secondary basis (43,72,73). Clinically, in the presence of direct trauma to the TMJ, the
incidence of anatomical dysfunction is increased.

NEUROPHYSIOLOGIC CHANGES

Fewer than 50% of acute and CTTHA patients complain of mild associated autonomic symptoms such as lack of appetite, hyperirritability, dizziness, and increased
light sensitivity (photophobia) (74). Notably, some of these symptoms may be
secondary to autonomic changes associated with active myofascial trigger points
located in the head and neck.

While muscle contraction and tenderness may be interpreted as primary
symptoms of CTTHA, EMG activity, and muscle tenderness increase, in some
studies more often during migraine than TTHA (75–77).

Differences have been found in the pain threshold of TTHA patients, which
were different in ETTHA versus CTTHA. The patients with ETTHA had normal pain
thresholds (78). Extending upon this, the pressure, thermal, and electrical pain thresholds in the head have been found to be lower in patients with CTTHA than controls or

patients with ETTHA (79–83). The question of the primary source of this increased pain remains: pain hypersensitivity as the source or a source of pericranial muscle tenderness. It appears that central sensitization may account for much of the difference (84,85). The data appear to indicate that patients with CTTHA have central sensitization, as is discussed below, while this is not found in patients with ETTHA.

In research comparing TTHA with common migraine patients exposed to auditory stimulation, TTHA patients showed a lower heart-rate reactivity than migraine patients (86). It was shown that TTHA patients exhibited the greatest cardiovascular arousal during headache (87). In another study (23) both migraine and TTHA patients decreased pulse velocity. In a psychophysiologic comparison of migraine and TTHA, it was found that migraine patients are vasodilated and TTHA patients are vasoconstricted both during and between headache episodes (75). During another study, administration of ergotamine tartrate, a vasoconstrictor, increased the pain of TTHA, while amyl nitrate, a vasodilator, yielded only transient pain relief (88).

Greater sympathetic arousal was found in TTHA patients as compared to controls (44). Another study reported that both TTHA and migraine patients demonstrated cardiovascular sympathetic hypofunction, indicated by low basal levels of NEP, as well as orthostatic hypotension (89). It has been suggested that TTHA patients have phasic hypersympathetic activity, while migraineurs do not differ from controls during psychogalvanic response testing (90).

Evidence of pupillary sympathetic hypofunction and subtle anisocoria has been found in both TTHA and migraine patients (91). It was suggested that this may have reflected a central bioaminergic system dysfunction. Another study suggested a pupillary sympathetic system imbalance in CTTHA patients, who showed asymmetric mydriasis after tyramine instillation and in the physiologic pupillary tests (92). Oculomotor dysfunction in the amplitude and number of corrective saccades during testing of TTHA patients has also been found (93).

Drummond (94) has reported increased photophobia in TTHA patients as compared to controls. He hypothesized that changes in central neurotransmitter modulation may induce increased sensitivity or hyperexcitability-induced photophobia.

Episodic platelet abnormalities with associated serotonergic dysfunction have been well documented in migraine (95,96). Nonepisodic decreased platelet serotonin in CTTHA patients has also been documented (97).

NEUROANATOMY AND NEUROCHEMISTRY

The central modulation of pain appears to originate in the brainstem and involves at least two systems. The "descending" inhibitory analgesia system appears to regulate the "gating" mechanisms of the spinal cord. This system includes the midbrain periaquaductal gray region, the medial medullary raphe nuclei, and the adjacent reticular formation, as well as dorsal horn neurons in the spinal cord (98). The "ascending" pain modulation system originates in the midbrain and is projected to the thalamus (99). Both systems utilize biogenic amines, opiod peptides, and nonopiod peptides (198–100).

The ascending system appears to show more relevance to headache disorders. This system has projections from the brainstem to the medial thalamus, which include large number of serotonergic and opiate receptors. The midbrain dorsal raphe nucleus, a serotonergic nucleus, projects to the medial thalamus and is associated with pain perception. Serotonergic projections to the forebrain are implicated in the regulation of the sleep cycle, mood changes, pain perception, and the hypothalamic regulation of hormone release (101).

The endogenous opiate system (EOS) within the CNS may act as a nociceptive "rheostat" or "algostat," setting pain modulation to a specific level. As this level changes, an individual's pain tolerance may also change. Fluctuations in pain intensity may be interpreted as being secondary to fluctuations in the function of antinociceptive pathways (102,103). Headache, along with other "nonorganic" or idiopathic central pain problems are thought to be the most common expression of impairment of the antinociceptive systems (104).

The EOS modulates the neurovegetative triad of pain, depression, and autonomic disturbances that are found in only two conditions—CTTHA and acute morphine abstinence (104). The EOS is also implicated as a primary protagonist in idiopathic headadche (104,105). Reduced plasma concentrations of beta-endorphin have been found in idiopathic headache patients, including those with CTTHA (106–109). Cerebral spinal fluid met-enkephalin was determined to be increased in patients with CTTH (110). Dysfunction in the EOS may exist and be one of the contributing intrinsic issues in the development of CTTHA.

A primary relationship also exists between the EOS and the biogenic amine systems that are intrinsic to both the pathophysiology of pain modulation and its treatment. Clinical and neuropharmacologic information indicates that dysmodulated serotonergic neurotransmission probably generates chronic headache and head pain. It has also been noted that the ordinary, acute, or periodic headache may be the "noise" of serotonergic neurotransmission (107).

Decreased levels of serotonin (111–113) (with good indications of an impairment of serotonergic metabolism in patients with CTTHA), substance P, an excitatory neuropeptide (114,115) and plasma NEP (116) are found in CTTHA patients. The latter is also indicative of peripheral sympathetic hypofunction, which may also participate in the etiology or maintenance of central opiod dysfunction (109). A negative correlation was found between plasma serotonin and headache frequency in patients with CTTHA (110) Neurophysiologically, there may be, in CTTHA patients, an impaired ability to increase plasma serotonin as well as synaptic serotonin levels, possibly secondary to increased nociceptive peripheral stimulation. Looking at this at levels below the supraspinal regions, the serotonergic dysfunction would induce or contribute to central sensitization at the level of the spinal cord dorsal horn and, cervically, the trigeminal nucleus and hypothetically may contribute to a patient's change from episodic to CTTHA.

Platelet GABA levels are significantly increased in CTTHA patients. This may also act as a balance mechanism to deal with neuronal hyperexcitability and may also be associated with depression (117).

The opioid receptor mechanisms appear to be very susceptible to desensitization, or the development of tolerance. In CTTHA patients, opiod receptor hypersensitivity is marked, secondary to the chronically diminished secretion of neurotransmitters. This "empty neuron syndrome" may involve both autonomic and nociceptive afferent systems, as well as being latent, subpathologic, or pathologic with spontaneous manifestations (118).

The EOS modulates the activity of monoaminergic neurons. A chronic EOS deficiency can provoke transmitter leakage, of both opiod and bioaminergic neurotransmitters, and lead to neuronal exhaustion and "emptying," as well as compensatory effector cell hypersensitivity. The poor release of neurotransmitter along with cell/receptor hypersensitivity appears to be one of the most important phenomena of the hypoendorphin syndromes. It has also been concluded that CTTHA may result from dysmodulation of nociceptive impulses, with associated sensitized receptors in the CNS (119). This EOS dysmodulation is in effect the sign of dysfunctional EOS/antinociceptive pathways in CTTHA.

CTTHA may be, along with other chronic idiopathic headache, a "pain disease" directly linked to central dysmodulation/dysfunction of the nociceptive and antinociceptive systems, either latent or pathologic in nature. Research indicates that at least two arms of the main endogenous antinociceptive systems, the EOS and the serotonergic systems, are involved in the pathogenesis of CTTHA. This problem appears to be progressive, and the dysfunctions may result from neuronal exhaustion secondary to continuous activation of these systems (108,118).

An impairment of pain inhibitory systems has been noted in CTTHA patients, in a manner possibly similar to patients with anatomically generalized pain-like fibromyalgia (120).

Some try to place the pathophysiology of TTHA in accordance with the information previously presented dealing with the changes seen at the spinal cord level. They may try to place the problem in the realm of what is known about central sensitization secondary to peripheral nociception, in a manner that speaks more for a neurophysiologic etiology than may be seen, as described in this chapter, when TTHA is clinically evaluated and treated.

For example, other neurotransmitter systems are possibly also involved, but questionably to a lesser degree. Calcitonin gene-related peptide (CGRP) is known to be involved in the pathophysiology of migraine and cluster headache. While patients with TTHA have normal plasma levels of CGRP, the interictal plasma level of the neuropeptide was found to be increased in patients with a pulsatile quality to their headache pain (121). The CSF levels of CGRP in CTTHA patients was found to be normal (122). Glutamate, an excitatory amino acid, was found to be normal in the plasma of TTHA patients in one study and increased in platelets in CTTHA patients in another (123,124).

Nitric oxide (NO) also plays an important role in migraine and cluster headache. As noted in previous chapters, NO plays a role in sensory transmission in both the peripheral and CNS (125). Ashina et al. (126) demonstrated that glyceryl trinitrate, a NO donor, induced more headaches for CTTHA patients than for controls, with both an immediate headache and a delayed TTHA. It was suggested that the immediate headache was secondary to the direct effect of NO on the perivascular sensory afferents of trigeminal nerve, or NO-induced arterial dilatation. The delayed headache was felt to be secondary to central sensitization at the spinal and trigeminal level. As noted previously, the activation of N-methyl-D-aspartate (NMDA) receptors is associated with the production of NO, which may lead to changes as a result of potentiation of synaptic transmission that could effectively induce hyperalgesia, an expansion of receptive fields, central sensitization, and/or wind-up. The use of a NO synthase inhibitor [NG-monomethyl-L-arginine hydrochloride (L-NMNA)] effectively reduced pain and muscle hardness (127,128).

In previous chapters, we have discussed in detail the peripheral activity of the excitatory neurotransmitters substance P (SP), glutamate and Neurokinin A (NA), and their role in increasing, at the spinal cord dorsal horn level, the responsiveness of second order neurons, and the apparent structural reorganization including the development of novel synapses between A-beta fibers inputs to nociceptive dorsal horn neurons. Once sensitized by the excitatory neurotransmitters, the previously non-nociceptive A-beta fiber inputs to nociceptive dorsal horn neurons become effective, allowing nociceptive input by the low-threshold A-beta fibers that can manifest themselves as allodynia (129). These glimpses into peripheral activity may or may not have definitive activity regarding TTHA.

Levels of SP, neuropeptide Y, and vasoactive intestinal polypeptide were not found to be different when looking at controls or TTHA patients in either the intracranial or peripheral circulation: their levels were not related to either headache or between headache, interictal state (130)

Further evidence of failure or dysmodulation of the central nociceptive/ antinociceptive systems was noted by Mazzotta et al. (131), who found higher levels of SP in platelets corresponded to lower levels of beta-endorphin in peripheral blood mononuclear cells (PBMCs) in patients with episodic TTHA compared with controls. PBMCs are thought to reflect cerebral beta-endorphin modulation and possibly mirror the central EOS (132). The study found a positive correlation between beta-endorphin levels and the pressure pain threshold, as well as a negative correlation between SP in platelets and the pressure pain threshold in patients and control subjects (131). This also suggests that the antinociceptive pathways, including the EOS, are dysfunctional in TTHA patients even during inter-ictal periods.

CTTHA patients have been found to have significant decreases in the gray matter of the brain in regions known to be associated with pain processing, including the dorsal rostral and ventral pons, anterior cingulate cortex, anterior and posterior insular cortex, right posterior temporal lobe, orbitofrontal cortex, the bilateral para hippocampus, and the right cerebellum, when using MRI and voxel-based morphometry (6,133). These findings are not seen in subjects with medication-overuse headache (MOH) or in healthy controls, raising the question of the specificity of these findings to CTTHA patients.

PATHOPHYSIOLOGY

On a neurophysiologic basis, having more basic knowledge of the peripheral and spinal-level pathoetiologic aspects of pain and sensitization, authors have determined that TTHA would fit into this paradigm (134). Basically, painful stimuli from pericranial myofascial tissue would provide prolonged nociceptive input in predisposed patients who would then develop sensitization of nociceptive second-order neurons in the spinal cord dorsal horn and trigeminal nucleus. This may be secondary to dysfunctional inhibition (see Chapter 1) or serotonergic system dysmodulation/dysfunction. When thus sensitized, afferent A-beta fibers that normally would inhibit A-delta and C-fibers by the "gating effect" in the dorsal horn would stimulate nociceptive second-order neurons. Continued A-delta and C-fiber stimulation would be potentiated and expanded receptive fields of the dorsal horn neurons would occur (135), with NMDA receptors and NO playing an important role in the resulting central sensitization. This would increase the excitability of supraspinal neurons and induce dysfunctional inhibition, or increased facilitation of nociceptive transmission in the spinal dorsal horn, inducing generalized pain hypersensitivity (136). The resulting neuroplastic changes could then increase excitation in motor neurons at supraspinal segmental levels and induce increased muscle activity and increased muscle tonus (137). Neurochemical changes in the spinal cord dorsal horn may then induce the release of algetic neurochemicals such as SP from the sensory afferents in the myofascial tissue and create an ongoing cycle of peripheral nociception induced and promulgated central sensitization.

Looking at this problem on an anatomical/physiologic basis, the hyperalgesia/increased pain sensitivity seen in patients with CTTHA may be secondary to disinhibition of the descending antinociceptive systems versus solely disturbed central pain modulation. Willer et al. (138) looked at the spinally organized nociceptive flexion reflex, a withdrawal reflex in human subjects secondary to supraspinal influence, and which can be decreased (with an increased threshold) by diffuse noxious inhibitory control. This diffuse noxious inhibition is triggered by the peripheral nociceptive fibers A-δ and C-fibers and may be caused by the activation of brain structures thought to be involved in descending inhibition (139). Langemark et al. (140) found that patients with CTTHA had a decreased nociceptive flexion reflex thresholds compared to controls, indicating central dysfunction of antinociceptive systems.

While it appears that central sensitization may take place, it also appears that the central neurochemical changes in the EOS, serotonergic, and noradrenergic systems could take place without this: one would question whether central sensitization is needed, if peripheral nociception is continuous. This would raise the question of the possibility of an intermediate state secondary to this continuous peripheral nociception from soft tissue: a state between acute peripheral nociception and central sensitization. While research indicates the formation of central sensitization as noted above, it remains a question as to the necessity of this pain state to create the central neurochemical dysmodulation/dysfunction described in this chapter.

Clinically, looking at the upper portion of Figure 9, most of the basics have been mentioned: continuous peripheral stimulation from myofascial nociceptive input from a MPS, with or without trigger points, may effectively trigger a change in the central pain "rheostat" associated with nociceptive input, secondary to the continuous need for pain-modulating antinociceptive neurotransmitters. The affective aspects of pain, including depression, anxiety, and fear, are secondary to changes in neurotransmitters such as serotonin and NEP, directly influence myofascial nociception, as well as further reinforce central neurochemical changes.

After a period of between 4 to 12 weeks or so, changes in the CNSs central modulation of nociception can occur. Secondary to continuous peripheral nociceptive stimulation, in association with affective changes, the central modulating mechanisms will assume a primary rather than a secondary or reactive role in pain perception, as well as antinociception, shifting the initiating aspects of pain perception from the peripheral regions to the CNS; a direct consequence can be central sensitization.

This intrinsic shift may make innocuous stimuli more aggravating to the pain-modulating systems, the "irritable everything syndrome." The already dysmodulated internal feedback mechanisms may react until central neurochemical mechanisms dominate, secondary to neurotransmitter exhaustion, and receptor hypersensitivity and abnormal biogenic amine metabolism/exhaustion occurs. These neurochemical changes may induce and/or exacerbate a sleep disorder (serotonergic in nature, from the nucleus raphe magnus), which by itself can perpetuate the central neurochemical dysmodulation, which is primarily responsible for CTTHA.

EVALUATION AND TREATMENT OF CTTHA

The neurologic examination of migraine patients is, in the absence of complicated aura, negative. The examination of the cluster headache patient may yield signs of

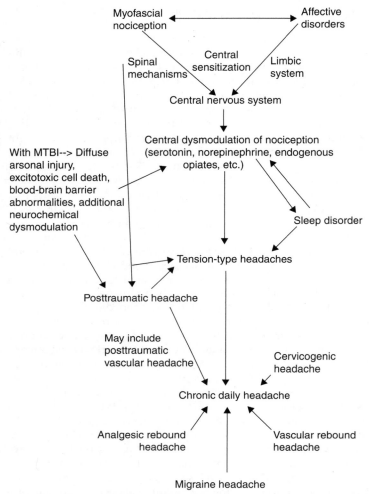

FIGURE 9 Pathophysiology of acute and chronic tension-type headache.

a partial Horner's syndrome. The examination of the patient with acute or CTTHA may yield a great deal of information.

Typically, the neurologic examination is negative. It is the musculoskeletal evaluation that will give you the facts. Begin by observing the patient's shoulders. In the vast majority of cases, there is an asymmetry of the acromioclavicular joints, with one being higher than the other secondary to greater ipsilateral muscle spasm. The large muscles, and others, should be carefully palpated both for general tenderness and the presence of trigger points. These include the trapezius muscles, the deltoids, the scalenes, the rhomboids, the levaeter scapulae, and all associated muscles, including the pericranial musculature. Pay careful attention to the sternocleidomastoid muscles, particularly in patients complaining of dizziness and tinnitus. Palpate the bioccipital and bitemporal insertions. Look for true pericranial muscle tenderness, as well as masseter pain or tenderness. Ask the patient to open their mouth: look for the amount of space between the teeth and see if the jaw deviates.

Perform a passive as well as active cervical range of motion.

Observe the patient's head: is it flexed forward? Is it tilted to one side? What about the shoulders: are they rounded? Rolled forward?

Evaluate the presence and degree of muscle spasm found in the paravertebral muscles over the entire length of the spine.

If the patient is a CTTHA sufferer, post-traumatic or otherwise, or if there is a complaint of upper extremity or hand numbness, perform an axillary stretch maneuver as well as the Adson's maneuver to evaluate for a myogenic thoracic outlet syndrome.

And these are just the basics.

Until you know what you are dealing with physiologically, it is impossible to determine an appropriate treatment plan. Once you know, and are positive about your diagnosis reached by the history and physical/neurologic examination, you can begin to formulate a treatment plan.

TREATMENT OF ACUTE TTHA

The medical management of acute or episodic TTHA is relatively simple. Remember that the older nomenclature titled these headaches as "acute muscle contraction headache" or "tension headache." This form of headache is the most common, as previously indicated, accounting for up to 80% of all idiopathic forms of headache. It has been estimated that over 90% of Americans experience an acute TTHA at some time in their lives. The majority of these headaches are self-treated with over-the-counter medications and therefore never come to the attention of a physician. This indicates that the statistics are probably low, in that a fairly large number go unnoticed by physicians.

The greatest problem in the treatment of acute TTHA is the avoidance of the development of MOH, which can easily occur if a patient is overmedicated. This is one step into the development of chronic or daily TTHA. MOH is now thought to be the third most common form of headache after TTHA and migraine (141).

Physicians should be particularly familiar with the various types of medications that can be utilized for patients complaining of acute posttraumatic TTHA.

The old adage, that less is better, certainly applies here. Many patients deal with the pain and discomfort by taking two aspirin and relaxing. Exercise is useful, as is a simple glass of wine, on an occasional basis. Any type of relaxation, which distracts the patient from their headache is useful.

Dealing with the medication management, physicians have a more than ample supply to choose from. It may be therefore tempting to overtreat a minor headache with medications, which have a significant risk of dependency.

The simple analgesics are easily chosen by the patient, if not the physician. They are inexpensive and easy to obtain. They include aspirin and acetaminophen. Like the other nonsteroidal anti-inflammatory drugs (NSAIDs), aspirin appears to work by inhibiting the synthesis of prostaglandin by blocking the action of cyclooxygenase, an enzyme that enables the conversion of arachidonic acid to prostaglandin to occur. Prostoglandins are synthesized from cellular membrane phospholipids after activation or injury, and sensitize pain receptors.

Aspirin, the prototypical NSAID, has anti-inflammatory and antipyretic properties, along with its pain relieving properties. The recommended adult dose for treatment of acute TTHA is 650 mg every six hours. Taking the aspirin with milk or food may decrease gastric irritation. Aspirin can also double bleeding time for four to seven days after taking 0.65 g. Peak blood levels are found after 45 minutes. The plasma half-life is two to three hours.

Acetaminophen usage is common. It provides about the same amount of analgesia as aspirin, but does not have the gastrointestinal side effects. That acetaminophen may work by inhibition of prostaglandin synthesis in the CNS has been suggested. It has much weaker anti-inflammatory activity than aspirin. Peak plasma levels occur between 30 to 60 minutes. Its plasma half-life is two to four hours. Recent evidence indicates the elevation of liver enzymes (aminotransferase) in healthy patients receiving 4 g/day, typically within two weeks (142).

Ibuprofen, an NSAID, is also available over-the-counter in doses of 200 mg per tablet. It can cause significant GI distress. It has a half-life of two to four hours, with peak plasma levels attained in one to two hours. The adult dosage is 200 to 400 mg every four to six hours, with a maximum of 1200 mg/day.

These medications are frequently sold in combination with other drugs such as caffeine, which exerts no specific analgesic effects, but may potentiate the analgesic effects of aspirin and acetaminophen. There are aspirin-caffeine combination drugs (Anacin®) and aspirin, acetaminophen and caffeine combinations (Excedrin Extra-Strength®, Excedrin Migraine®, and Vanquish®). The recommended dosage is two tablets every six hours as needed.

The biggest problem is that taking aspirin, acetaminophen, or combination tablets daily or even every other day for a week or more (possibly less) can induce the problem of MOD (which will be discussed later).

As with birth control pills, when you ask a patient what medications they are taking, they may forget that nonprescription medications such as aspirin or acetaminophen are "medications," and forget to tell you, or even be too embarrassed to tell you because they are taking a large number of pills each day, so you must be certain to ask specifically.

There are a number of NSAIDs that are prescribed. Because of the variability in their efficacy, pharmacokinetics and side effects, patients may need to be tried on more than one, sequentially, not in combination, to determine the best one for them.

The NSAIDs work, as noted before, by interfering with the action of cyclooxygenase in the synthesis of prostoglandins. GI side effects are common, in up to 15% to 20% of patients, and may include epigastric pain, nausea, heartburn, and abdominal discomfort. A history of GI bleeding or ulcerations should indicate that great caution must be used, if these medications are used at all.

The most frequently prescribed NSAIDs include:

Naproxen sodium (Anaprox®), which reaches peak plasma levels in one to two hours, and has a mean half-life of 13 hours. It can be taken at 275 or 550 mg every six to eight hours, with a top dosage of 1375 mg/day. This NSAID is useful in prophylactically treating hormonally related migraine.

Ibuprofen (Motrin®) is prescribed in dosages of 600 and 800 mg per tablet. The suggested dosage for mild to moderate pain is 400 mg every four to six hours as needed.

Ketoprofen (Orudis®) is a cyclooxygenase inhibitor, but also stabilizes lysosomal membranes and possibly antagonizes the actions of bradykinin. Its peak plasma level is reached in one to two hours and has a two-hour plasma half-life. It is now over the counter (12.5 mg tablets), but is best used at 50 to 75 mg capsules. The recommended daily dosage is 150 to 300 mg a day in three or four divided doses. GI side effects are generally mild. Care should be taken when given to a patient with impaired renal function.

Keterolac tromethamine (Toradol®) can be given orally or parentally for moderate to severe acute headache pain. Peak plasma levels occur after intramuscular injection in about 50 minutes. Its analgesic effect is considered to be roughly equivalent to a 10 mg dose of IM morphine. The typical injectable dose is 60 mg. Because of its potentially significant hepatic/renal side effects, the FDA has stated that Toradol should be given orally, after an IM injection of 60 mg, at 10 mg, every eight hours, for a maximum of five days.

The COX 2 inhibitor celecoxib is a nonsteroidal anti-inflammatory agent that also has analgesic properties without, for most patients, the typical gastrointestinal problems associated with NSAIDs. Newer research may not support this. These medications appear to work by inhibiting prostaglandin synthesis, via inhibition of cyclooxygenase-2, which corresponds to its improved GI side effect profile, while not affecting the cyclooxygenase-1 isozyme, responsible for its anti-inflammatory functions. Celecoxib may be taken twice a day, 100 to 200 mg bid. Rofecoxib and valdecoxib have at the present time been taken off of the market secondary to the potential for cardiovascular problems.

Muscle relaxants are given for acute TTHA by some clinicians. They are probably best utilized during the first three weeks post injury related headache. They are useful in patients with significant muscle spasm and pain, which may be seen in acute post-traumatic TTHA, but which is not usually seen with an episodic TTHA. They are used appropriately after the development of muscle spasm after injury such as a slip and fall, motor vehicle accident, work and athletic injuries or over stretching.

These medications work via the development of a therapeutic plasma level. Their exact mechanism of action is unknown, but they do not directly affect striated muscle, the myoneural junction, or motor nerves. They produce relaxation by depressing the central nerve pathways, possibly through their effects on higher CNS centers, which modifies the central perception of pain without effecting the peripheral pain reflexes or motor activity.

Carisoprodol (Soma®) is a CNS depressant which metabolizes into a barbiturate, which makes it both addictive and particularly inappropriate to use for patients with pain from muscle spasm in addition to minor traumatic brain injury. It acts as a sedative and it is thought to depress polysynaptic transmission in interneuronal pools at the supraspinal level in the brainstem reticular formation. It is short lived, with peak plasma levels in one to two hours and a four to six hour half-life. Dosage is 350 mg every six to eight hours. It should not be mixed with other CNS depressants. It is also marketed in two other combined forms (with aspirin as Soma Compound) and with Codeine, for additional analgesic effects.

Chlorzoxazone (Parafon Forte® DSC) is a centrally acting muscle relaxant with fewer sedative properties. It inhibits the reflex arcs involved in producing and maintaining muscle spasm at the level of the spinal cord and subcortical areas of the brain. It reaches its peak plasma level in three to four hours, and duration of action is three to four hours. It is well tolerated, and side effects are uncommon. Dosage is 500 mg three times a day.

Metaxalone (Skelaxin®) is a centrally acting skeletal muscle relaxant, which is chemically related to mephenaxalone, a mild tranquilizer. It is thought to induce muscle relaxation via CNS depression. Onset of action is about one hour, with peak blood levels in two hours, and duration of action is four to six hours. The recommended dose is 2,400 to 3,200 mg a day in divided doses (tablets are 400 mg each). It should be used carefully in patients with impaired liver function, and should not be used at all in patients with significant renal or liver disease as well as a history of drug-induced anemias. Side effects include nausea, vomiting, GI upset, drowsiness, dizziness, headache, nervousness, and irritability as well as rash or pruritis. Jaundice and hemolytic anemia are rare.

Methocarbamol (Robaxin®) is a centrally acting skeletal muscle relaxant. It may inhibit nerve transmission in the internuncial neurons of the spinal cord. It has a 30-minute onset of action. Peak levels are found in about two hours, and its duration of action is four to six hours. It comes as 500 and 750 mg tablets. Tablets containing methocarbamol and aspirin (Robaxisal®) are also available. The recommended dose of Robaxin is 750 mg three times a day. As with all of these medications, it should be taken for 7 to 10 days. It is well tolerated, with initial side effects which resolve over time, including lightheadedness, dizziness, vertigo, headache, rash, GI upset, nasal congestion, fever, blurred vision, urticaria, and mild muscular incoordination. In situations of severe, seemingly intractable muscle spasm, Robaxin may be given intravenously in doses of about a gram every 8 to 12 hours.

Orphenedrine Citrate (Norflex®, Norgesic®) is a centrally acting skeletal muscle relaxant with anticholinergic properties thought to work by blocking neuronal circuits, the hyperactivity of which may be implicated in hypertonia and spasm. It is available in injectable and oral formulations. The IM dose of Norflex is 2 mg, while the intravenous dosage is 60 mg in aqueous solution. The oral formulation (Norflex) is given in 100 mg tablets—one tablet every 12 hours. Norgesic is a combination form, including caffeine and aspirin and should be given one or two tablets every six to eight hours. Norgesic Forte®, a stronger combination, is given one half to one tablet every six to eight hours. Because of its anticholinergic effects, it should be contraindicated in patients with glaucoma, prostatic enlargement, or bladder outlet obstruction. Its major side effects are also secondary to its anticholinergic properties, and include tachycardia, palpitations, urinary retention, nausea, vomiting, dizziness, constipation, and drowsiness. It may also cause confusion, excitation, hallucinations, and syncope.

Many of these medications are given in combination with other drugs, including barbiturates (butalbatal and meprobamate) and narcotics (codeine, oxycodone, propoxyphene, etc.). This is probably not a good idea, as the barbiturates and narcotics can easily help develop patient dependence.

For patients with extreme pain on an acute basis, the use of tramadol hydrochloride (50–100 mg every 4–6 hours) may be helpful. This medication appears to bind to the opioid receptors as well as inhibit reuptake of serotonin and NEP. Other patients may need an opioid such as codeine or hydrocodone. These medications should be given for up to 7 to 10 days, if necessary. One published rule of thumb noted that immediate-relief analgesic medication of any kind should be taken no more than two days a week.

Again, narcotic medications should not be used, if they can be avoided, for the patient with acute TTHA, as the risk of dependence, as well as analgesic rebound headache, is too great.

Further information on these medications is available in appropriate pharmacology textbooks (143).

MEDICATION MANAGEMENT OF CTTHA

The medication treatment of choice is the TCAs, or the specific serotonergic reuptake inhibitors, the SSRIs.

A meta-analysis reviewing 38 published, randomized, placebo-controlled studies found that patients who received TCAs were twice as likely to report headache improvement whether they had CTTHA or migraine (144).

The TCA medication of choice is amitriptyline, a sedating TCA. Like all of the tricyclics, it works in the synapse to decrease re-uptake of serotonin and (depending on the individual medication) NEP. Amitriptyline, unlike the other TCAs, also works to repair the damage in stage 4 sleep architecture. It is the most sedating tricyclic. The typical dosage is between 10 and 50 mg at night. The author has found it rare for more than 20 or 30 mg to be required at night.

Amitriptyline potentiates the effects of endogenous opioids and may act as an NMDA receptor antagonist, possibly inducing a reduction in central sensitization (145). Amitriptyline may also induce pain relief by an effect on the segmental action in the CNS, possibly at the level of the spinal cord dorsal horn and trigeminal nucleus (146). It also appears to block α_1 adrenergic receptors, muscarinic cholinergic receptors, and Na^+, Ca^{2+}, and K^+ ion channels (147). Its peripheral analgesic effects may be secondary to its ability to block Na^+ ion channels as well as serotonin $(5-HT)_{2A}$ receptors (148).

Doxepin is also a very good TCA. Anticholinergic side effects such as sedation are reduced (but not by much) when compared to amitriptyline. It does not work on the sleep architecture. It is used at the same dosage levels of amitriptyline.

The tricyclics are not used in their antidepressant dosages, anywhere from 100 to 350 mg a day. Even though the doses are low, their effectiveness in the treatment of CTTHA is marked.

The SSRIs include Prozac®, Paxil®, Zoloft®, and Celexa®. These medications are not typically sedating (although for some patients they may be) and with the exclusion of those patients, they may be energizing. They should be given in the morning. Prozac and Paxil should start at 10 to 20 mg a day and they can be increased to 60 to 80 mg. Zoloft should be given at 25 to 50 mg in the morning, up to 150 mg in divided doses. Doses should be divided, giving one when the patient gets up in the morning (around 7:00 am) and one at noon. Celexa should be utilized at dosages of 20–40 mg a day. Explain to the patients that taking these medications later than noon can, in many cases, give them problems sleeping.

It is certainly possible to safely combine 10 to 40 mg of Prozac or Paxil, or 50 mg of Zoloft or 20 to 40 mg of Celexa with a small dose of amitriptyline or doxepin (10 to 30 mg) at night. Inappropriate dosages of these two forms of medications can, rarely, induce the serotonin syndrome.

There are other excellent antidepressants such as Wellbuterin, Serzone, and Effexor. These should be considered as needed.

These medications should not be combined with MAO inhibitors.

Another excellent medication is Clonazepam®, a fifth generation form of benzodiazepine. It is GABAnergic in effect. It works at the level of the internuncial neurons of the spinal cord to enhance muscle relaxation. It helps, a bit, with anxiolysis. It has a side effect of sedation. In doses of 4 to 12 mg a day, it works as an anticonvulsant. At smaller doses, 0.5 to 1 mg given at night, it is very useful in the treatment of patients with CTTHA. The sedation lasts for a shorter time than the sedation from tricyclics, and this itself is useful.

If the acute use of muscle relaxant medications is not enough to end the problem, Tizanidine is a good choice of medication after the first three weeks or so has gone by and the patient is still exhibiting painful neuromuscular spasm. Tizanidine is an alpha$_2$ noradrenergic agonist (149,150). It has supraspinal effects by inhibiting the facilitation of spinal reflex transmission by the descending noradrenergic pathways, as it decreases firing of the noradrenergic locus ceruleus (151). It acts presynaptically in the spinal cord inducing a polysynaptic reduction in released excitatory transmitters (152). It also decreases hyperexcitability of the muscle without acting on the neuromuscular junctions or muscle fibers (153). Short acting, its maximum plasma concentrations are reached within one to two hours (153). It has a large first pass metabolism, with a half-life of 2.1 to 4.2 hours (154). Dosages should be slowly increased, starting at 1 to 2 mg at night and slowly increasing to 20 to 24 mg. Maximum dosage is 36 mg in divided dosages, typically found in patients who need an antimyotonic. Interestingly, this medication appears to decrease muscle pain while providing its antimyotonic effects.

Finally, treating patients with CTTHA with tricyclics, physical therapy, psychotherapy, and so on, will not work if the patient is taking daily or four times a week analgesic medications of any type! In the presence of medication overuse headache, nothing will show long-lasting effectiveness until the chronic analgesics are stopped.

TREATMENT OF CTTHA

Treatment of CTTHA is best accomplished via an interdisciplinary rehabilitation approach, the main purpose of which is NOT to "teach the patient to live with the headache," but to properly diagnose and effectively ameliorate or stop the patient's headache.

Drug detoxification/weaning is the necessary first step, whether the patient is over utilizing simple, over the counter analgesics, or narcotics or barbiturates. Chronic daily analgesics appear to prevent appropriate functioning of the EOS (possibly via negative neurochemical feedback loops) and other associated antinociceptive systems, inducing MOSs, which are secondary problems from the medications that induce headache secondary to purely neurochemical/neurophysiologic changes. Vascular rebound headaches from over utilization of vasoconstrictors may also occur and must be stopped before other treatment is applied. Clinically, an effective way to detoxify CTTHA patients is with the repetitive DHE-45 protocol described by Raskin (155). Concurrently, prophylactic medications should be started. The use of prophylactic medications, as well as physical therapy and other treatments given while a patient is enduring MOAs is an ineffectual waste of time and money.

After detoxification, an outpatient interdisciplinary headache rehabilitation program utilizing neuropharmacological therapy (to restore neurochemical homeostasis), physical therapy (156), psychotherapy, and stress management (including biofeedback-enhanced neuromuscular re-education and muscle relaxation) is the most time and cost-effective treatment. Optimal psychotherapy or physical therapy regimes by themselves will not resolve myofascial difficulties or depression if the affective, sleep, and CNS neurochemical dysmodulation affecting them is not concurrently and appropriately treated. The interdisciplinary treatment paradigm also enables fine-tuning of diagnosis and possible determination of a secondary or "hidden" etiology for a patient's headaches (157).

In patients with recalcitrant soft tissue pain problems the use of botulinum toxin A or B to decrease muscle spasm and pain has increased significantly (158,159). However, several randomized, placebo-controlled studies do not support the effectiveness of botulinum toxin in the treatment of headache (160,161). In one randomized study (161) no improvement of primary or secondary pain endpoints were found after six weeks. Similar findings were found in a study of episodic TTHA (121). Other abstracts touted more successful results; however, few patients were noted to have CTTHA (163–165).

The continued contradictory results for the efficacy of botulinum toxin in randomized, double-blind, placebo-controlled studies for the treatment of TTHA continues even more recently (166).

De Tommaso et al. (167) looked at the effects of amitriptyline and intraoral appliances on the clinical and laser-evoked potentials in CTTHA. Their study indicated that pericranial tenderness is primarily a phenomenon that can initiate a self-perpetuating circuit, at the level of the cortical nociceptive areas which are also involved in attention and emotional components of pain, with both interventions being able to "interrupt this reverberating circuit" and improve the CTTHA.

Future use of NO synthase inhibitors may promise to bring headache relief (168,169). These studies indicate that the locus for nociception for CHHTA may be found in the brain stem, not the peripheral nervous system. NO is found in the nociceptive neurons in the trigeminal nucleus caudalis, and possibly higher in the CNS (169).

Regardless of the possible future treatments, at this time failure to treat the CTTHA patient with an interdisciplinary, whole-person approach (Fig. 9) may be responsible for multiple treatment failures as well as monetary waste, as long-term response—headache remediation—is most often not achieved.

REFERENCES

1. Leistad RB, Sand T, Westgaard RH, et al. Stress-induced pain and muscle activity in patients with migraine and tension-type headache. Cephalalgia 2006; 26(1):64–73.
2. Lenaerts ME. Pharacoprophylaxis of tension-type headache. Curr Pain Headache Rep 2005; 9(6):442–447.
3. Headache Classification Committee of the International Headache Society. The international Classification of headache disorders. Cephalalgia 1988; 8(suppl 7):1–96.
4. Headache Classification Committee of the International Headache Society. The international Classification of headache disorders, edn 2. Cephalalgia 2004; 24(suppl 1):9–160.
5. Anttila P. Tension-type headache in childhood and adolescence. Lancet Neurol 2006; 5(3):268–274.
6. Mathew NT. Tension-type headache. Curr Neurol Neurosci Rep 2006; 6(2):100–105.
7. Araki N. Tension-type headache. (Abst.) Nippon Rinsho 2005; 63(10):1742–1746.
8. Ashina S, Bendtsen L, Ashina M. Pathophysiology of tension-type headache. Curr Pain Headache Rep 2005; 9(6):415–422.
9. Speed WG. Muscle contraction headaches. In Saper JR ed. Headache Disorders. Boston: John Wright, 1983:115.
10. Diamond S, Dalessio DJ. The Practicing Physicians Approach to Headache. 3d Ed. Baltimore: Williams and Wilkins, 1980.
11. Dorpat TL, Holmes TH. Mechanisms of skeletal muscle pain and fatigue. Arch Neurol Psychiatry 1955; 74:628.
12. Perl S, Markle P, Katz LN. Factors involved in the production of skeletal muscle pain. Arch Intern Med 1934; 53:814.
13. Hong S, Kniffki K, Schmidt R: Pain Abstracts. Second World Congress on Pain 1978; 1:58.
14. Rodbard S: Pain associated with muscle contraction. Headache 1970; 10:105.
15. Martin PR, Mathews AM. Tension headaches: psychophysiological investigation and treatment. J Psychosom Res 1978; 22:389.
16. Sakuta M: Significance of flexed posture and neck instability as a cause of chronic muscle contraction headache. Rinsho Shinkeigato 1990; 30:254.

17. Riley TL. Muscle-contraction headache. Neurol Clin 1983; 1:489.
18. Philips C. Tension headache: theoretical problems. Behav Res Ther 1978; 16:249.
19. Philips C, Hunter MS. A psychophysiological investigation of tension headache. Headache 1982; 22:173.
20. Simons DJ, Day E, Goodell H, Wolff HG. Experimental studies on headache: muscles of the scalp and neck as sources of pain. Assoc Res Nerv Ment Dis Proc 1943; 23:228.
21. Robinson CA. Cervical spondylosis and muscle contraction headaches. In: Dalessio DJ ed. Wolff's Headache and other Head Pain. 4th ed. New York: Oxford University Press 1980; 362.
22. Haynes SN, Cuevas J, Gannon L. The psychophysiological etiology of muscle—contraction headache. Headache 1982; 22:122.
23. Bakal DA, Kaganov JA. Muscle contraction and migraine headache: psychophysiologic comparison. Headache 1977; 17:208.
24. Cohen MJ. Psychological studies of headache: is there a similarity between migraine and muscle contraction headaches? Headache 1978; 18:189.
25. Anderson CD, Franks RD. Migraine and tension headache: is there a physiological difference? Headache 1981; 21:63.
26. Pozniak-Patewicz E. Cephalgic spasm of head and neck muscles. Headache 1976; 15:261.
27. Shoenen J, Pasqua VD, Sianard-Gainko J. Multiple clinical and paraclinical analyses of chronic tension-type headache associated or unassociated with disorder of the pericranial muscles. Cephalalgia 1991; 11:135.
28. Langemark M, Olesen J. Pericranial tenderness in tension headache. A blind controlled study. Cephalalgia 1987; 7:249.
29. Langemark M, Jensen K, Jensen TS, Olesen J. Pressure pain thresholds and thermal nociceptive thresholds in chronic tension-type headache. Pain 1989; 38:203.
30. Borgeat F, Hade B, Elie R, Larouche LM. Effects of voluntary muscle tension increases in tension headache. Headache 1984; 24:199.
31. Drummond PD. Scalp tenderness and sensitivity to pain in migraine and tension headache. Headache 1987; 27:45.
32. Yang JC, Richlin D, Brand L, Wagner J, Clark WC. Thermal sensory decision theory indices and pain threshold in chronic pain patients and healthy volunteers. Psychol Med 1985; 47:461.
33. Malow RM, Grimm L, Olsen RE. Differences in pain perception between myofascial pain dysfunction and normal subjects: a signal detection analysis. J Psychosom Res 1980; 24:303.
34. Ashina S, Babenko L, Jensen R, et al. Increased muscular and cutaneous pain sensitivity in cephalic region in patients with chronic tension-type headache. Eur J Neurol 2005; 12(7): 543–549.
35. Christensen MB, Bendtsen L, Ashina M, Jensen R. Experimental induction of muscle tenderness and headache in tension-type headache patients. Cephalalgia 2005; 25(11): 1061–1067.
36. Jensen R. Pathophysiological mechanisms of tension-type headache: a review of epidemiological and experimental studies. Cephalalgia 1999; 19:602–621.
37. Ashina M. Neurobiology of chronic tension-type headache. Cephalalgia 2004; 24:61–172.
38. Fernandez-de-las-Penas C, Alonso-Blanco C, Cuadrado ML, Pareja JA. Forward head posture and neck mobility in chronic tension-type headache: a blinded, controlled study. Cephalalgia 2006; 26(3):314–319.
39. Langemark M, Jensen K. Myofascial mechanisms of pain. In: Olesen J, Edvinsson L, eds. Basic Mechanisms of Headache. Amsterdam: Elsevier Science Publishers B.V., 1988:321.
40. Cailliet R. Pain: Mechanisms and Management. Philadelphia: F.A. Davis, 1993:83.
41. Jay GW. The autonomic nervous system: Anatomy and pharmacology. In Raj P ed. Pain Medicine-A Comprehensive Review. St. Louis: Mosby, 1996:461:465.
42. Jay GW. Sympathetic aspects of myofascial pain. Pain Digest 1995; 5:192–194.
43. Langemark M, Olesen J, Poulsen DP, Bech P. Clinical characterization of patients with chronic tension headache. Headache 1988; 28:590.

44. Murphy AI, Lehrer PM: Headache versus nonheadache state: a study of electrophysiological and affective changes during muscle contraction headache. Behav Med 1990; 16:23.
45. Travell J, Rinzler SH. The myofascial genesis of pain. Postgrad Med 1952; 11:425–434.
46. Travell JG, Simons DG. Myofascial pain and dysfunction: The trigger point manual. Baltimore: Williams and Wilkins, 1983.
47. Jay GW. Chronic daily headache and myofascial pain syndromes: pathophysiology and treatment. In Cady RK, Fox AW eds. Treating the Headache Patient. New York: Marcel Decker, 1995:211–233.
48. Fricton JR. Myofascial pain syndrome. In: Fricton JR, Awad E, eds. Advances in Pain Research and Therapy, Vol. 17. New York: Raven Press, 1990:107.
49. Fricton JR, Kroening R, Haley D, Siegart R. Myofascial pain syndrome of the head and neck: a review of clinical characteristics of 164 patients. Oral Surg 1985; 60:615.
50. Calandre EP, Hidalgo J, Garcia-Leiva JM, Rico-Villademoros F. Trigger point evaluation in migraine patients: an indication of peripheral sensitization linked to migraine predisposition? Eur J Neurol 2006; 13(3):244–249.
51. Kudrow L. Muscle contraction headaches. In: Rose FC ed. Handbook of Clinical Neurology, Vol. 48. Amsterdam: Elsevier Science Publishing, 1986:343.
52. Martin MJ, Rome HP. Muscle contraction headache: therapeutic aspects. Res Clin Stud Headache 1967; 1:205.
53. Jay GW, Grove RN, Grove KS. Differentiation of chronic headache from non-headache pain patients using the Millon Clinical Multiaxial Inventory (MCMI). Headache 1987; 27:124.
54. Schoenen J. Depression in tension-type headache suffers: bystander or villain? Pain 2004; 111:225.
55. Rasmussen BK. Migraine and tension-type headache in a general population: precipitating factors, female hormones, sleep pattern and relation to lifestyle. Pain 1993; 53: 65–72.
56. Clark GT, Sakai S, Merrill R, et al. Cross-correlation between stress, pain, physical activity and temporalis muscle EMG in tension-type headache. Cephalalgia 1995; 15:511–518.
57. Holroyd KA. Behavioral and psychological aspects of the pathophysiology and management of tension-type headache. Curr Pain Headache Rep 2002; 6:401–407.
58. Lipchik GL, Holroyd KA, O'Donnell FJ, et al. Exteroceptive suppression periods and pericranial muscle tenderness in chronic tension-type headache: effects of psychopathology, chronicity and disability. Cephalalgia 2000; 20:638–646.
59. Janke EA, Holroyd KA, Romanek K. Depression increases onset of tension-type headache following laboratory stress. Pain 2004; 111:230–238.
60. Goldenberg DL. Fibromyalgia and chronic fatigue syndrome: are they the same? J Musculoskel Med 1990; 7:19.
61. Mathew NT, Glaze D, Frost J. Sleep apnea and other sleep abnormalities in primary headache disorders. In: Rose C, ed. Migraine. Proceedings of the 5th International Migraine Symposium, London, 1984. Basel: Karger, 1985:40.
62. Shahota PK, Dexter JDS. Sleep and headache syndromes: a clinical review. Headache 1990; 30:80.
63. Drake ME, Pakalnis A, Andrews JM, Bogner JF. Nocturnal sleep recording with cassette EEG in chronic headaches. Headache 1990; 30:600.
64. Moldofsky H, Scariabrick P, England R, et al. Musculoskeletal symptoms and non-REM sleep disturbances in patients with fibrositis syndrome and healthy subjects. Psychosom Med 1975; 37:341.
65. Goldenberg DL. Diagnostic and therapeutic challenges of fibromyalgia. Hosp Pract 1989; 9:39.
66. Iansek R, Heywood J, Karnaghan J, Nalla JI. Cervical spondylosis and headaches. Clin Exp Neurol 1987; 23e:175.
67. Jay GW. Post-traumatic Headache: Diagnosis, pathophysiology and treatment. In: Boswell MV, Cole BE, eds. Weiner's Pain Management, 7th edn. Boca Raton: CRC Press, 2006:333–360.
68. Bogduk N. The anatomical basis for cervicogenic headache. J Manip Physiol Ther 1992; 15:67–70.

69. Sjaastad O, Fredriksen TA, Pfaffenrath V. Cerviocgenic headache diagnostic criterion. Headache 1992; 30:725–726.
70. Forsell H. Mandibular dysfunction and headache. Proc Finn Dent Soc 1985; 81(suppl II):591.
71. Mikail M, Rosen H. History and etiology of myofascial pain-dysfunction syndrome. J Prosthet Dent 1980; 44:438.
72. Magnusson T, Carlsson GE. Comparison between two groups of patients in respect to headache and mandibular dysfunction. Swed Dent J 1978; 2:85.
73. Magnusson T, Carlsson GE. Recurrent headaches in relation to temporomandibular joint pain-dysfunction. Acta Odontol Scand 1978; 36:333.
74. Olesen J. Clinical Characterization of tension headache. In: Olesen J, Basic Mechanisms of Headache. Amsterdam: Elsevier Science, 1988, p. 9.
75. Tfelt-Hansen P, Lous I, Olesen J. Prevalence and significance of muscle tenderness during common migraine attack. Headache 1981; 21:49.
76. Olesen J. Some clinical features of the acute migraine attack. An analysis of 750 patients. Headache 1978; 18:268.
77. Ellertsen B, Norby H, Sjaastad O. Psychophysiological response patterns in tension headache: effects of tricyclic antidepressants. Cephalalgia 1987; 7:55.
78. Jensen R, Rasmussen BK, Pedersen B, et al. Muscle tenderness and pressure pain thresholds in headache: a population study. Pain 1993; 52:193–199.
79. Bendtsen L, Jensen R, Olesen J. Decreased pain detection and tolerance thresholds in chronic tension-type headache. Arch Neurol 1996; 53:373–376.
80. Langemark M, Olesen J. Pericranial tenderness in tension-type headache: a blind, controlled study. Cephalalgia 1987; 7:249–255.
81. Schoenen J, Bottin D, Hardy R, et al. Cephalic and extracephalic pressure pain thresholds in chronic tension-type headache. Pain 1991; 47:145–149.
82. Ashina S, Babenko L, Jensen R, et al. Increased muscular and cutaneous pain sensitivity in cephalic region in patients with chronic tension-type headache. Eur J Neurol 2005; 12:543–549.
83. Ashina S, Bendtsen L, Ashina M. Pathophysiology of tension-type headache. Curr Pain and Headache Reports 2005; 9:415–422.
84. Bendtsen L. Central sensitization in tension-type headache: possible pathophysiological mechanisms. Cephalalgia 2000; 20:486–508.
85. Bendtsen L, Jensen R, Olesen J. Qualitatively altered nociception in chronic myofascial pain. Pain 1996; 65:259–264.
86. Haynes SN: Muscle contraction headache- a psychophysiological perspective. In: Haynes SN, Gannon LR, eds. Psychosomatic Disorders: a Psychophysiological Approach To Etiology and Treatment. New York: Praeger Press, 1981.
87. Tunis MM, Wolff HG. Studies on headache: cranial artery vasoconstriction and muscle contraction headache. Arch Neurol Psychiatry 1954; 71:425.
88. Mikamo K, Takeshima T, Takahashi K. Cardiovascular sympathetic hypofunction in muscle contraction headache and migraine. Headache 1989; 29:86.
89. Covelli V, Ferrannini E. Neurophysiologic findings in headache patients. Psychogalvanic reflex investigation in migraineurs and tension headache patients. Acta Neurol 1987; 9:354.
90. Takeshima T, Takao Y, Takahashi K. Pupillary sympathetic hypofunction and asymmetry in muscle contraction headache. Cephalalgia 1987; 7:257.
91. Shimomura T, Takahashi K. Pupillary functional asymmetry in patients with muscle contraction headache. Cephalalgia 1986; 6:141.
92. Rosenhall U, Johansson G, Orndahl G. Eye motility dysfunction in patients with chronic muscular pain and dysesthesia. Scand J Rehab Med 1987; 19:139.
93. Drummond PD. A quantitative assessment of photophobia in migraine and tension headache. Headache 1986; 26:465.
94. Hanington E, Jones RJ, Amess JAL, Wachowicz B. Migraine: a platelet disorder. Lancet 1981; ii:720.
95. D'Andrea G, Toledo M, Cortelazzo S, Milone FF. Platelet activity in migraine. Headache 1982; 22:207.

96. Rolf LH, Wiele G, Brune GG. 5-Hydroxytryptamine in platelets of patients with muscle contraction headache. Headache 1981; 21:10.
97. Basbaum AI, Fields HL. Endogenous pain control systems: Brainstem spinal pathways and endorphin circuitry. Ann Rev Neurosci 1984; 7:309.
98. Andersen E, Dafny N. An ascending serotonergic pain modulation pathway from the dorsal raphe nucleus to the parafascicularis nucleus of the thalamus. Brain Res 1983; 269:57.
99. Raskin NH. On the origin of head pain. Headache 1988; 28:254.
100. Raskin NH. Headache. 2nd ed. New York: Churchill Livingstone, 1988.
101. Fields HL. Sources of variability in the sensation of pain. Pain 1988; 33:195.
102. Wall PD. Stability and instability of central pain mechanisms. In: Dubner R, Bond MR, eds. Proceedings of the Fifth World Conference on Pain. Amsterdam: Elsevier Science, 1988:13.
103. Sicuteri F. Natural opiods in migraine. In: Critchley M, Friedman AP, Gorini S, et al. eds, Vol. 33. Advances in Neurology. New York: Raven Press, 1982:65.
104. Sicuteri F, Spillantini MG, Fanciullacci M. "Enkephalinase" in migraine and opiate addiction. In: Rose C ed. Migraine: Proceedings of the Fifth International Migraine Symposium, S. Karger, Basel, 1985:86.
105. Mosnaim AD, Diamond S, Wolf ME, et al. Endogenous opiod-like peptides in headache: An overview. Headache 1989; 29:368.
106. Genazzani AR, Nappi G, Gacchinetti F, et al. Progressive impairment of CSF B-EP levels in migraine sufferers. Pain 1984; 18:127.
107. Facchinetti F, Genazzani AR. Opiods in cerebrospinal fluid and blood of headache sufferers. In: Olesen J, Edvinsson L, eds. Basic Mechanisms of Headache. Amsterdam: Elsevier Science, 1988:261.
108. Nappi G, Gacchinetti G, Legnante G, et al. Impairment of the central and peripheral opiod system in headache. Paper presented at the Fourth International Migraine Trust Symposium, London, 1982.
109. Rolf LH, Wiele G, Brune GG. 5-Hydroxytryptamine in platelets of patients with muscle contraction headache. Headache 1981; 21:10.
110. Langmark M, Bach FW, Ekman R, et al. Increased cerebrospinal fluid met-enkephalin immunoreactivity in patients with chronic tension-type headache. Pain 1995; 63: 103–107.
111. Giacovazzo M, Bernoni RM, Di Sabato F, Martelletti P. Impairment of 5HT binding to lymphocytes and monocytes from tension-type headache patients. Headache 1990; 30:20.
112. Shimomura T, Takahashi K. Alteration of platelet serotonin in patients with chronic tension-type headache during cold pressor test. Headache 1990; 30:581.
113. Pernow B. Substance P. Pharmacol Rev 1983; 35:85.
114. Almay BGL, Johansson F, von Knorring L, et al. Substance P in CSF of patients with chronic pain syndromes. Pain 1988; 33:3.
115. Takeshima T, Takao YU, Urakami K, et al. Muscle contraction headache and migraine. Platelet activation and plasma norepinephrine during the cold pressor test. Cephalalgia 1989; 9:7.
116. Kowa H, Shimomura T, Takahashi K. Platelet gamma-amino butyric acid levels in migraine and tension-type headache. Headache 1992; 32:229.
117. Sicuteri F, Nicolodi M, Fusco BM. Abnormal sensitivity to neurotransmitter agonists, antagonists and neurotransmitter releasers. In: Olesen J, Edvinsson L, eds. Basic Mechanisms of Headache. Amsterdam: Elsevier Science, 1988:275.
118. Langemark M, Jensen K, Jensen TS, Olesen J. Pressure pain thresholds and thermal nociceptive thresholds in chronic tension-type headache. Pain 1989; 38:203.
119. Ashina M, Bendtsen L, Jensen R, et al. Plasma levels of calcitonin gene-related peptide in chronic tension-type headache. Cephalalgia 2000; 20:292.
120. Pielsticker A, Haag G, Zaudig M, Lautenbacker S. Impairment of pain inhibition in chronic tension-type headache. Pain 2005; 118(1–2): 215–223.
121. Aley KO, McCarter G, Levine JD. Nitric oxide signaling in pain and nociceptors sensitization in the rat. J Neurosci 1998; 18:7008.

122. Bach FW, Langemark M, Ekman R, et al. Effect of sulpiride or paroxetine on cerebrospinal fluid neuropeptide concentrations in patients with chronic tension-type headache. Neuropeptides 1994; 27:129–136.
123. Alam Z, Coombes N, Waring RH, et al. Plasma levels of neuroexcitatory amino acids in patients with migraine or tension headache. J Neurol Sci 1998; 156:102–106.
124. Sarchielli P, Alberti A, Floridi A, et al. L-Arginine/nitric oxide pathway in chronic tension-type headache: relation with serotonin content and secretion and glutamate content. J Neurol Sci 2002; 198:9–15.
125. Ashina M, Bendtsen L, Jensen R, et al. Nitric oxide-induced headache in patients with chronic tension-type headache. Brain 2000; 1123:1830.
126. Ashina M, Bendtsen L, Jensen R, et al. Possible mechanisms of action of nitric oxide synthase inhibitors in chronic tension-type headache. Brain 1999; 122:1629.
127. Ashina M, Lassen LH, Bendtsen L, et al. Effect of inhibition of nitric oxide synthase on chronic tension-type headache. Lancet 1999; 353:287.
128. Woolf CJ, Thompson SW. The induction and maintenance of central sensitization is dependent on N-methyl-D-aspartic acid receptor activation; implications for the treatment of post-injury pain hypersensitivity states. Pain 1991; 44:293.
129. Ashina M, Bendtsen L, Jensen R, et al. Plasma levels of substance P, neuropeptide Y, and vasoactive intestinal polypeptide in patients with chronic tension-type headache. Pain 1999; 83:541.
130. Mazzotta G, Sarchielli P, Gaggioli A, et al. Study of pressure pain and cellular concentration of neurotransmitters related to nociception in episodic tension-type headache patients. Headache 1997; 37:565.
131. Sacerdote P, Rubboli F, Locatelli L, et al. Pharmacologic modulation of neuropeptides in peripheral mononuclear cells. J Neuroimmunol 1991; 32:35.
132. Vandenheede M, Shoenen J. Central Mechanisms in tension-type headache. Cur Pain Headache Reports 2002; 6(5):392.
133. Schmidt-Wilcke T, Leinisch E, Straube A, et al. Gray matter decrease in patients with chronic tension-type headache. Neurology 2005; 65(9):1483–1486.
134. Olesen J. clinical and pathophysiologic observations in migraine and tension-type headache explained by integration of vascular, supraspinal, and myofascial inputs. Pain 1991; 46:125.
135. Coderre TJ, Katz J, Vaccarino AL, et al. Contribution of central neuroplasticity to pathological pain: review of clinical and experimental evidence. Pain 1993; 52:259.
136. Wall PD, Devor M. The effect of peripheral nerve injury on dorsal root potentials and on transmission of afferent signals into the spinal cord. Brain Res 1981; 23:95.
137. Woolf CJ. Evidence for a central component of post-injury pain hypersensitivity. Nature 1983; 15:686.
138. Willer JC, De Broucker T, Le Bars D. Encoding of nociceptive thermal stimuli by diffuse noxious inhibitory controls in humans. J Neurophysiol 1989; 62:1028–1038.
139. Le Bars D. The whole body receptive field of dorsal horn multireceptive neurones. Brain Res Rev 2002; 40:29–44.
140. Langemark M, Bach FW, Jensen TS, et al. Decreased nociceptive flexion reflex threshold in chronic tension-type headache. Arch Neurol 1993; 50:1061–1064.
141. Obermann M, Bartsch T, Katsarava Z. Medication overuse headache. Expert Opin Drug Saf 2006; 5(1):49–56.
142. Watkins PB, Kaplowitz N, Slattery JT, et al. Aminotransferase elevations in healthy adults receiving 4 grams of acetaminophen daily: a randomized controlled trial. JAMA 2006; 296(1):87–93.
143. Professional's Handbook of Drug Therapy for Pain. Springhouse, Pennsylvania, 2001.
144. Tomkins GE, Jackson JL, O'Malley PG, et al. Treatment of chronic headache with antidepressants: a meta-analysis. Am J Med 2001; 111:54.
145. Eisenach JC, Gebhart GF. Intrathecal Amitriptyline acts as an N-methyl-D-aspartate receptor antagonist in the presence of inflammatory hyperalgesia in rats. Anesthesiology 1995; 83:1046.
146. Bendtsen L, Jensen R. Amitriptyline reduces myofascial tenderness in patients with chronic tension-type headaches. Cephalalgia 2000; 20:603.
147. Sawynok J, Esser MJ, Reid AR. Antidepressants as analgesics: an overview of central and peripheral mechanisms of action. J Psychiatry Neurosci 2001; 26:21–29.

148. Blier P, Abbott FW. Putative mechanisms of action of antidepressant drugs in affective and anxiety disorders and pain. J Psychiatry Neurosci 2001; 26:37–43.
149. Sayers AC, Burki HR, Eichenberger E. The pharmacology of 5-chloro-4-(2-imidazolin-2gamma-1-amino)-2, 1, 3-benzothiadiazole (DS 103 282), a novel myotonic agent. Arzneimittelforschung 1980; 30:793–803.
150. Coward DM, Davies J, Herrling P, Rudeberg C. Pharmacological Properties of Tizanidine (DS 103–282). New York, NY: Springer-Verlag NY Inc. 1984:61–71.
151. Palmeri A, Wiesendanger M. Concomitant depression of locus coeruleus neurons and of flexor reflexes by an alpha$_2$-adrenergic agonist in rats: a possible mechanism for an alpha$_2$-mediated muscle relaxation. Neuroscience 1990; 34:177–187.
152. Davies J, Johnson SE, Lovering R. Inhibition by DS 103-282 of D-(^{3}H) aspartate release from spinal cord slices. Br J Pharmacol 1983; 78:2P.
153. Wagstaff AJ, Bryson H. Tizanidine. A review of its pharmacology, clinical efficacy and tolerability in the management of spasticity associated with cerebral and spinal disorders. Drugs 1997; 53:435–452.
154. Koch P, Hirst DR, von Wartburg BR. Biological fate of sirdalud in animals and man. Xenobiotica 1989; 19:1255–1265.
155. Raskin NH. Headache. 2nd ed. New York: Churchill Livingstone, 1988.
156. Jay GW, Brunson J, Branson SJ. The effectiveness of physical therapy in the treatment of chronic daily headaches. Headache 1989; 29:156.
157. Jay GW. Headache Handbook: Diagnosis and Treatment. Boca Raton: CRC Press, 1999:17–32.
158. Gobel H, Heinze A, Heinze-Kuhnk A, Jost WH. Evidence-based medicine: botulinum toxin A in migraine and tension-type headache. J Neurol 2001; 248(suppl 1):34–38.
159. Argoff C. successful treatment of chronic daily headache with Myobloc. Poster presented at the 21st Annual Scientific Meeting of the American Pain Society, Baltimore, MD, March 14–17, 2002.
160. Smuts JA, Baker MK, Smuts HM, et al. Botulinum toxin-type A as prophylactic treatment in chronic tension-type headache. Cephalalgia 1999; 19:454.
161. Gobel H, Lindner V, Krack P, et al. Treatment of chronic tension-type headache with botulinum toxin. Cephalalgia 1999; 19:455.
162. Rollnik JD, Tanneberger O, Schubert M, et al. Treatment of tension-type headache with botulinum toxin-type A: a double-blind, placebo-controlled study. Headache 2000; 40:300.
163. Eros EJ, Doric DW: The effects of botulinum toxin-type A on disability in episodic and chronic migraine [abstract]. Presented at the American Headache Society Meeting. June 21–23, 2002. Seattle, WA.
164. Troost B: Botulinum toxin-type A (Botox, Allergan, Irvine, CA) therapy for intractable headaches [abstract]. Presented at the American Headache Society Meeting, June 21–23, 2002. Seattle, WA.
165. Miller T: Retrospective cohort analysis of 48 chronic headache patients treated with botulinum toxin-type A (Botox) in a combination fixed injection site and follow-the-pain protocol [abstract]. Presented at the American Headache Society Meeting, June 21–23, 2002. Seattle, WA.
166. Rozen D, Sharma J. Treatment of tension-type headache with botox: a review of the literature. Mt Sinai J Med 2006; 73(1):493–498.
167. de Tommaso M, Shevel E, Libro G, et al. Effects of amitriptyline and intra-oral appliance on clinical and laser-evoked potentials features in chronic tension-type headache. Neurol Sci 2005; 26(suppl 2):S152–S154.
168. Ashina M, Lassen LH, Bendtsen L, et al. Effect of inhibition of nitric oxide synthase on chronic tension-type headache: a randomized crossover trial. Lancet 1999; 353:287.
169. Ashina M, Bendtsen L, Jensen R, et al. Possible mechanisms of action of nitric oxide synthase inhibitors in chronic tension-type headache. Brain 1999; 122:1629.
170. Simons DG, Travell JG, Simons LS, Cummings BD. Travell and Simons Myofascial Pain and Dysfunction: The Trigger Point Manual. Lippincott Williams and Wilkins. 2nd Ed. 1999.

13 | Medications

The purpose of this chapter is to go over the various types of medications that can be used for the treatment of pain. Many of the medications have been discussed previously, but this chapter attempts to consolidate these various medications.

There are two more pain states that need to be discussed: chronic pain, which persists for three to six months or more, and breakthrough pain, or acute-on-chronic pain.

There is no one way to use medications. It really depends on the patient with chronic non-cancer pain, and what they need. As will be noted, there are some better methods of providing pain medication for the chronic non-cancer pain patient, with specific reasons for both how and why. The use of adjunctive medication is also extremely important.

While opioids are discussed within this chapter, the next chapter will deal with some narcotic-specific issues: things that should be done to protect both the patient taking the opioids and the physician who prescribes opioids.

When a patient is initially seen, most physicians will follow the World Health Organization (WHO) three-step ladder (1), which divides pain into mild, moderate, and severe categories. It is felt that mild pain should be treated with aspirin, acetaminophen, and nonsteroidal anti-inflammatory drugs (NSAIDs), with or without the use of adjuvant medication.

For moderate pain, the WHO indicates the use of mild narcotics (for the most part). These include codeine, hydrocodone, oxycodone, dihydrocodeine, and tramadol, with or without adjuvant medications.

Severe pain would mandate the use of the traditional opioids: morphine, hydromorphone, methadone, levorphanol, fentanyl, and oxycodone, with or without adjuvant medication.

Adjuvant medications include anticonvulsants, membrane stabilizers, NMDA antagonists, alpha2 agonist,; GABAnergic medications, and other agents, including the antidepressants and neuroleptics. When used with opioids, NSAIDs may also be considered adjuvant medications.

An important concept is multimodal (or balanced) analgesia, which is beneficial to both acute and chronic pain. This entails a rational combination of several analgesics that have differing mechanisms of action to obtain improved efficacy and/or tolerability and safety when compared to similar or equianalgesic doses of a single drug (2).

For many years NSAIDs have been used for treatment or management of mild to moderate pain, frequently in combination with acetaminophen, which acts centrally and inhibits brain cyclo-oxygenase (COS) and nitric oxide (NO) synthase. New information has determined that acetaminophen dosages of 4 g/day or more can induce hepatic abnormalities. NSAIDs can cause gastrointestinal symptoms and can potentially induce gastric bleeding. The selective COX-2 inhibitors were developed to deal with this problem, but they are now known to have potentially serious cardiovascular problems. New guidelines or statements from both the American (FDA) and European (EMEA) agencies indicate that when using NSAIDs, the smallest effective dose should be used for the shortest period of time (3). These reasons, among others, show the advantages of combining drugs at decreased dosages to give a better risk-benefit ratio for pain management. Weak opioids combined with acetaminophen may be more beneficial, as more than one mechanism of action (MOA) are utilized (3,4).

Studies have shown that combinations of NSAIDs and patient-controlled morphine analgesia offer advantages over morphine alone, another example of multimodal analgesia (5).

Multimodal analgesia is also used for out-patient surgery. These regimens should include nonopioid analgesics (i.e., local anesthetics, NSAIDs, COS inhibitors, acetaminophen, ketamine, and alpha-2 agonists, for example) to supplement opioid analgesics. As this procedure may give good opioid sparing effects, this may lead to a reduction in nausea, vomiting, constipation, urinary retention, sedation, and respiratory depression (6).

NONOPIOIDS
Acetaminophen (Called Paracetamol in the United Kingdom)
This medication is used fairly universally for mild to moderate pain of all forms, including musculoskeletal pain, neuropathic pain, and even osteoarthritis. An aniline derivative (coal tar analgesic), it is an antipyretic (with possible effects in the hypothalamic thermoregulatory center) and is very commonly used in combination drugs for pain and many other uses including combination cold (URI) preparations. Acetaminophen appears to work centrally; its MOA is not known, but it has been hypothesized that it may involve the serotonin system, substance P (SP), and even (COS) COX-1 and 3 (a COX-2 variant).

Naloxone (an opiate receptor antagonist) can prevent acetaminophen's activity; acetaminophen may be involved with the dynorphin system, as dynorphins interact with kappa receptors, and if they are blocked, the acetaminophen-induced antinociceptive effects are reversed (7).

Acetaminophen is used for mild to moderate pain. Some physicians use it instead of NSAIDs. It has few adverse effects except for hepatic toxicity, most typically found at dosages of 4 g a day or more, especially in patients with hepatic problems secondary to chronic alcohol abuse. Newer research finds the same problem (elevations in aminotransferase) in healthy adults taking 4 g of acetaminophen a day for 14 days (8).

It is important to take a very specific history from patients regarding their acetaminophen intake. While they may tell you the amount of the medication they take as Tylenol®, they may not tell you of other over-the-counter medications that they take with acetaminophen in it, as they may not even be aware of its presence.

Its recommended dosage is 325 to 650 mg every four hours or 325 to 500 mg every three hours, with a maximum of 4 g (4000 mg) a day. The author tries to limit his patients' acetaminophen to 2500 to 3000 mg a day, maximum. For moderate pain, a gram may need to be given for optimal effectiveness, three (no more than four) times a day.

Acetaminophen is not extensively bound to proteins (only 10–25%). It has a high bioavailability (85–98%), a two hour plasma half-life and easily crosses the blood-brain barrier with a peak concentration in the cerebrospinal fluid (CSF) in two to three hours.

Nonsteroidal Anti-inflammatory Drugs

NSAIDs are anti-inflammatory, analgesic, and antipyretic agents. They decrease prostaglandin production by inhibiting COS (COX-1 and 2) enzymes. They are the drugs of choice for use in osteoarthritis (OA) and rheumatoid arthritis for pain.

There are over 20 different NSAIDs available in the United States in ten different chemical classes:

1. Propionic acids (ibuprofen, naproxen, ketoprofen, ketorolac)
2. Indoleacetic acids (indomethacin, sulindac, etodolac)
3. Salicylic acids (nonacetylated)—sodium salsalate, choline magnesium, trisalicylate. Aspirin is acetylated
4. Phenylacetic acid (diclofenac)
5. Naphthylalkanone (nabumetone)
6. Oxicam (piroxicam)
7. Anthranilic acid (enolic)—(mefenamic acid, meclofenamate)
8. Pyrroleacetic acid (tolmetin)
9. Pyrazolone (phenylbutazone)
10. COX-2 inhibitors (celecoxib—rofecoxib and valdecoxib have been withdrawn from the market secondary to cardiovascular concerns)

The importance of the different chemical classes is simple: not every NSAID will help every patient. If a patient does not receive relief from ibuprofen, the clinician should not try naproxen, which is in the same drug class, but another NSAID from another class should be utilized.

NSAIDs are extensively bound to serum albumin (95%). They are metabolized by the cytochrome P-450 system (the CYP2C0 isoform) in the liver and excreted in the urine. Therefore their use in patients with renal or hepatic dysfunction may be problematic. The half-lives of the NSAIDs vary greatly, ranging from an hour to longer than 55 hours.

NSAIDs may induce problems including: constipation, confusion, headaches, and the aforementioned renal and hepatic toxicity, as well as gastrointestinal (GI) ulcerations. They should be avoided in the elderly and those patients with congestive heart failure, coronary artery disease, hypertension, cirrhosis, and renal insufficiency. NSAIDs do have drug interactions, including: ACE inhibitors, anticoagulants, beta-blockers, and loop diuretics.

The selective COX-2 inhibitors have less risk of GI toxicity and have no effect on platelets/coagulation.

Risk factors for nonselective NSAID GI toxicity include combinations of NSAIDs; concomitant use of glucocorticoids and a past history of peptic ulcer disease, bleeding, or perforation. Again, their use in the older patient increases possible problems.

The idiosyncratic adverse effects of NSAIDs are also important to note, and include:

- Rash
- Photosensitivity
- Tinnitus
- Aseptic meningitis
- Psychosis
- Cognitive dysfunction (especially in the elderly treated with indomethacin)

- Possible infertility
- Pulmonary infiltrates with eosinophilia
- Possible hypertension from naproxen and ibuprofen

Finally, long-term use of some NSAIDs appears to have accelerated cartilage damage in osteoarthritis and some question the appropriateness of the use of NSAIDs in OA.

Some prescribing information:

Ibuprofen (Motrin®)-half-life is 2–2.5 hours after multiple dosing. Typical adult dose is 1200–2400 mg/day.

Naproxen is highly protein bound with a half-life of 12 to 15 hours. May use naproxen sodium 275 mg and 550 mg tabs twice a day.

Ketoprofen (Orudis®) is 99% protein bound; its half-life is between 1.4 and 3.3 hours. It is available in 25, 50, and 75 mg and an extended release 200 mg capsule. It can be taken three times a day.

Oxaprozin (Daypro®): The elimination half-life is between 50 and 60 hours after repeated doses—adult dose is 600 to 1200 mg/day. Patients can begin with a loading dose of 1800 mg.

Etodolac (Lodine®): The elimination half-life is six to seven hours. Maximum analgesia n one hour after oral dose. Doses range, in the adult, from 400 to 1200mg/day.

Indomethacin (Indocin®): The elimination half-life is 2 to 11 hours. Adult dose is 75 to 150 mg/day.

Diclofenac [Cataflam® (potassium salt), Voltaren® (enteric coated)] has a 75-minute half-life. The adult dose is 75 to 225 mg/day.

Nabumetone (Relafen®): A prodrug, metabolized to active metabolite with half-life of 24 hours. Adult dose is 1000–2000 mg/day.

Ketorolac (Toradol®): The only NSAID with parenteral usage; its half-life is 4–6 hours. Oral dosing is 10 mg three or four times a day. If given via IM or IV route, typically oral dosing is limited to four to five days.

When using NSAIDs in the elderly, dosages should be decreased, in many cases, by 50%.

Celecoxib (Celebrex®): 11 hours half-life; adult dose is 100–400 mg a day.

Finally, it may be safe to give COX-1 or COX-2 to patients with asthma and aspirin intolerance (9).

ANTICONVULSANTS

Neuropathic pain is defined as pain secondary to a dysfunction of the nervous system without active ongoing neural damage. While the most common treatments for nociceptive pain include anti-inflammatory and opioid medications, anticonvulsant medications (ACMs) are the first-line drugs for neuropathic pain (see Chapter 11).

Both older (conventional) and newer ACMs may be used in patients with neuropathic pain, migraine, essential tremor, spasticity, restless legs syndrome, and several psychiatric disorders including bipolar disorder and schizophrenia (6,10).

There remains a relative paucity of randomized clinical trials of ACMs in the treatment of neuropathic pain. Published studies (RCTs) do show that carbamazepine and gabapentin had favorable results. In spite of this, the use of gabapentin for neuropathic pain (and the majority of ACMs) is considered off-label use. However, there is no consensus regarding the use of ACMs in the treatment of neuropathic pain.

For one thing, there is not a great deal of knowledge regarding the MOA of most ACMs. Generally, there are some proposed mechanisms of action:

1. sodium-current blockade—carbamazepine, oxcarbazepine, lamotrigine, sodium valproate, and phenytoin,
2. calcium-current blockade—Gabapentin, oxcarbazepine,
3. increased GABA—gabapentin, topiramate, valproic acid, clonazepam, and pregabalin,
4. reduced-excitatory amino acids—topiramate, lamotrigine, and phenytoin, and
5. anti-inflammatory effects—gabapentin and lamotrigine.

Of note here is the multiple proposed MOA of multiple drugs, indicative of the uncertainty of the MOA.

Some clinical pearls to take into consideration, as there are no specific rules of thumb in the use of ACMs for neuropathic pain:

1. Always start low and go slow when titrating an ACM.
2. Understand the pharmacokinetic as well as the mechanistic differences between the ACMs.
3. In treatment-resistant patients (poor effectiveness) it is useful to combine two ACMs, if necessary, but be certain to use drugs with different modes of action.
4. All too frequently a patient will state that they have tried and failed an ACM, or many of them. Be certain to find out exactly what happened. Most commonly, a patient took a very low dose of an ACM for a very short period of time (less than would be necessary to develop a steady state or clinical efficacy) and claimed lack of effectiveness, at which point, instead of insisting that the titration be continued appropriately, a different ACM is used, and the same problems persist. If an ACM is not titrated appropriately, the drug was really not used, as clinically there would not have been any effectiveness. Stopping a drug secondary to adverse effects is absolutely appropriate.
5. Push the ACM dosages until you see clinical effectiveness or you have to stop it secondary to side effects.
6. In many patients, maximal effectiveness is found with ACMs given at 50% to 100% of their antiepileptic dosages.

Carbamazepine and gabapentin are the most commonly used first-line drugs for chronic neuropathic pain. A listing of which neuropathic pain disorders would have which ACMs as first-line treatment can be found in Chapter 11.

As a form of multimodal analgesia, oral gabapentin has been used perioperatively for adjunctive management of postoperative pain, as a supplement to opioids and other analgesics (11).

The most commonly used ACMs and their typical are listed in Table 1:

Some other pertinent information:

Carbamazepine—check liver enzymes and CBC routinely to rule out (possibly aplastic) anemia and hepatic dysfunction.

Oxcarbazepine—an analog of carbamazepine—typically no blood dyscrasias seen, nor hepatic problems.

Topiramate—used and approved for migraine prophylaxis—may be associated with weight loss, cognitive dysfunction.

Valproate—also approved for migraine prophylaxis—associated with weight gain, multiple drug interactions, check hepatic enzymes, may be associated with

TABLE 1   Anti-convulsant Medications Used to Treat Neuropathic Pain

Name	Half-life (hours)	Dosing (mg/day)/regimen
Carbamazepine (Tegretol®)	10–20	200–400 mg TID
Gabapentin (Neurontin®)	5–9	300–1200 mg TID
Phenytoin (Dilantin®)	12–36	300–400 mg/day QD–TID
Oxcarbazepine (Trileptal®)	8–10	300–1200 mg BID
Topiramate (Topamax®)	18–30	50–200 mg BID or QHS
Lamotrigine (Lamictal®)	15–30	50–200 mg BID
Valproate (Depakote®)	6–16	250–500 mg TID
Clonazepam (Klonopin®)	18–36	0.5–6 mg QHS
Levetiracetam (Keppra®)	6–8	500–1500 mg BID
Zonisamide (Zonegran®)	25–60	100–300 mg BID
Tiagabine	5–10	32–56 mg BID–QID
Pregabalin (Lyrica®)	6.3	150–300 mg/BID–TID

Note: Check renal and hepatic function.
Abbreviations: BID, twice a day; QHS, at night; TID, three times a day.

pancreatitis and hepatic injury as well as hair loss. There is a "fetal valproate syndrome," so it should not be used in pregnant women.

Gabapentin—may be associated with confusion, dizziness, possible weight gain.

Lamotrigine—can be associated with Stevens-Johnson syndrome/toxic epidermal necrolysis; visual blurring with long-term use.

Levetiracetam—caution if used with carbamazepine; may have typical GI and CNS side effects (nausea, ataxia, headache, dizziness, and sedation).

Zonisamide—contraindicated in patients with sulfonamide hypersensitivity, can be associated with renal calculi.

See Chapter 11 for more specific information on ACMs.

ANTIDEPRESSANTS

Generally, the tricyclic antidepressants (TCAs) are associated with pain relief/anti-nociception (particularly amitriptyline) when compared to the selective serotonin reuptake inhibitors (SSRIs). A newer class of medications, the selective noradrenergic reuptake inhibitors (SNRIs) are also associated with antinociception.

TCAs, along with ACMs are considered first-line drugs for the treatment of neuropathic pain, and migraine (12). As indicated, while they work centrally, there also appears to be peripheral activity (10). Several mechanisms may account for this including inhibition of monoamine transporters and the subsequent facilitation of descending pain inhibition systems (10). ADMs, aside from decreasing pain, may also be effective for the treatment of sleep disturbance, depression, and anxiety, all commonly seen problems in chronic pain patients (12).

Amitriptyline is associated with significant sedation. There may also be cardiac toxicity in susceptible patients from TCAs. They should not be used in individuals with heart block, or prolonged QTc intervals. Use lower dosages of drug, not approaching the antidepressant level. Overdosage with TCAs is particularly difficult to treat.

Venlafaxine may be used, off label, for neuropathic pain, as it has a dual MOA (serotonin and norepinephrine reuptake inhibitor).

Duloxetine has been approved for the treatment of diabetic peripheral neuropathy. It is an SNRI.

Side effects are typically present in all forms of ADMs. The TCAs are associated with weight gain and anticholinergic side effects (dry mouth, blurred vision, urinary hesitancy, and retention, as well as constipation). The SSRIs are associated with sexual dysfunction (lowered libido, erectile dysfunction, anorgasmia) as well as weight gain.

See Chapters 6 and 11 for more specific information regarding ADMs.

OTHER ADJUNCTIVE MEDICATIONS

Other possible forms of adjunctive medications include N-Methyl-D-Aspartate (NMDA) receptor antagonists. There are no NMDA receptor antagonists approved for pain-one, memantine is approved for treatment of Alzheimer's disease. The NMDA receptor antagonists include ketamine, dextromethorphan, amantadine, magnesium, and methadone, an opiate that is considered to have 10% NMDA effectiveness. These medications may, in the future be very beneficial, particularly antagonists at the glycine-site NR2B sites, at which weak-binding channel blockers have shown an improved side effect profile in animal models of pain (13). Ketamine is used as an adjunctive therapy in the hospice setting when opioid therapy is not sufficient (14). Ketamine alone, or with midazolam, have long been used for sedating children undergoing minor operative procedures or painful procedures such as changing dressings for burn patients (15,16).

Alpha-2-agonists include clonidine and tizanidine. Clonidine is widely used, orally, transdermally, epidurally, and intrathecally, for the treatment of pain secondary to cancer, postoperative pain, neuropathies, postherpetic neuralgia, headaches, labor and complex-regional pain syndrome (CRPS), restless leg syndrome, and orofacial pain.

Tizanidine has been used for painful conditions involving spasticity, myofascial pain, tension-type headache, acute low-back pain, and fibromyalgia. This medication is very sedating, but it works well when given at HS, rather than TID. Also, the generic forms of tizanidine are very frequently found to have side effects of hallucinations and vivid dreams, much more frequently than the nongeneric form (Zanaflex®).

Vistaril®, an antihistamine, can also be used in combination with narcotics as an adjunctive medication to prolong and possibly amplify their effects.

Skeletal muscle relaxants as an alterenative are discussed in Chapter 11.

OPIOIDS

The antinociceptive pain pathways have been described in detail in Chapter 1. The descending pathways are opioid and monoaminergically based. The opioid analgesics appear to produce analgesia by inhibiting the ascending pain pathways (which carry nociceptive information to the brain), and activate the descending pain control pathways, which go from the CNS down the ventromedial medulla and down to the spinal cord dorsal horn. Opioids act in the periaqueductal gray (via mu receptors) to decrease GABAnergic inhibition of the descending pathways.

The basic mode of opioid action is to inhibit the release of EAAs such as glutamate from peripheral nociceptors and postsynaptic neurons in the spinal cord dorsal horn.

After acute pain, algetic or pain-inducing chemicals are released from the nociceptors terminals, including substance P, glutamate, calcitonin gene-related

peptide, neurokinins, and more. These chemicals will enable nociceptive information to reach the dorsal horn (via the substantia gelatinosa) and move rostrally via
the ascending pain pathways. Locally, these algetic chemicals induce a neurogenic
or sterile inflammation, the presence of which continues to feed nociceptive
information centrally.

Glutamate will anneal to the NMDA receptor as well as the alpha-amino-3-
hydroxy-5-methyl-4-isoxazole proprionic acid (AMPA) receptor.

The AMPA receptor has a low threshold and quickly fluxes sodium and potassium through it. The NMDA receptor has a voltage-gated magnesium "plug."
Typically, in acute pain this is not dislodged and the NMDA receptor provides only
minimal stimulation.

As a consequence of chronic pain, the magnesium is forced out of the NMDA
receptor (secondary to continuous stimulation, in part) and calcium fluxes through
the receptor and into the cell, where it reacts with protein kinase C and NO synthase, which enables the formation of NO. The NO leaves the cell and reacts with
guanyl synthase, which closes the sodium channel. This enables the development of
pain that will not respond to opioids, as opioids can only work on the terminal if the
sodium channel is open. A major goal is to prevent this from occurring by treating
pain earlier rather than later.

Continued nociceptive stimulation will produce other phenomena including,
"windup" secondary to continuous C-fiber stimulation to the dorsal horn which
will enable the wide-dynamic range neurons, which are essentially "on–off" cells, to
turn on and not go off, producing, with the help of the NMDA receptors, central
sensitization with changes in perception inducing hyperalgesia, mechanical hypersensitivity, and allodynia. When this occurs, simple analgesics, even strong opioids
may not be able to diminish the pain.

As noted, the NMDA receptors contribute significantly to these problems.
They help effectuate wind-up; they stimulate apoptosis (along with the increase
of EAAs such as glutamate), and one can see the induction of cell death by
"hyperstimulation" by the EAAs.

Neuronal plasticity occurs—new neuronal connections are made, in the dorsal
root ganglia (DRG) as well as the spinal cord dorsal horn. One example is the
formation of new sympathetic neurons sprouting in the DRG. As noted earlier in
this text, the sympathetic nervous system responds to pain only during pathologic
conditions. This enables greater hypersensitivity in the DRG and the corresponding
areas of the dorsal horn.

When the sympathetic nerves sprout into the DRG's somatic nerves, this
interaction makes the pain more difficult to treat.

Does all chronic noncancer pain involve sympathetic nervous system input?
Probably yes, but to a lesser degree.

The use of opioids becomes important, as the majority of chronic noncancer
pain may not involve significant degrees of central sensitization. This is important,
in that the more significant the degree of central sensitization that exists, the less
likely the opioids will be very effective in stopping the pain.

Opioids are used for moderate to severe pain. They are agonists of opioid
receptors (mu—the most common; kappa, dealing with spinal cord and supraspinal
information and may contribute to nociception; and delta).

Evaluation of studies of long-term use of opioids on the quality of life of
patients with chronic noncancer pain identified both moderate/high and low-
quality evidence indicating long-term treatment with opioids can lead to significant

improvements in functional outcomes, including quality of life in patients with CNCP (17).

Opioids are considered safe drugs, in that they have been used for centuries and we know a fair bit about them. The most common adverse events (AEs) include constipation, dizziness, nausea, vomiting, somnolence, and confusion. The serious AEs include respiratory depression and death.

Addiction, a nonphysiologic reaction, is also considered a serious AE.

Opioid medications have multiple routes of administration, including oral, IV, IM, SQ, sublingual, intranasal, inhaled, transdermal, vaginal, rectal, intrathecal, and epidural.

Opioids are either hydrophilic—propoxyphene, codeine, morphine, hydrocodone and oxycodone, hydromorphone and methadone, which also has NMDA antagonistic properties—or lipophilic—fentanyl and sufentanil. The lipophilic drugs are more lipid-soluble and have greater mu receptor affinity.

Another way of evaluating opiates is looking at them as weak or strong. Going along with the WHO three-step process, this may make more sense.

Weak Opiates

- Codeine—has a weak affinity to mu opioid receptors; it is about 15% as potent as morphine (the opiate "gold standard"). It has a 2.5 to 3 hour half-life; major side effects include constipation and nausea; dosages greater than 65 mg every four to six hours are not appropriate.
- Hydrocodone (Vicodin®, Vicoprofen®, Lorcet®, Lortab®)—considered to be the most abused analgesic, per Drug Abuse Warning Network studies)—analgesic and antitussive; has active metabolites (hydromorphone, dihydrocodeine); renal dysfunction will be problematic; same half-life as codeine; typically found in combination with acetaminophen or an NSAID; use 1–2 Q 4–6 hours as needed. As with all PRN analgesics, limit use to seven or 10 days.
- Oxycodone (Percodan®, Percocet®, Roxicet®, Tylox®)—elimination half-life of 3 to 3.5 hours; no active metabolites; effectiveness is 7.7 times the potency of codeine; typically found in combination with acetaminophen; has fewer side effects than morphine when given orally; no ceiling effect for analgesia—typically given one to two orally every 4 to 6 hours. The combination tablets have different strengths of oxycodone, (2.5/325, 5/325, 7.5/325 and 500, 10/325 and 650) which should be monitored with appropriate dose escalation.
- Oxycontin®, extended release oxycodone, has many good characteristics: short half-life, long duration of action; no clinically active metabolites; easy titration, with a steady state found in 24 to 36 hours; no ceiling dose; minimal adverse effects; low first-pass effect; 60% to 87% bioavailability; no crushing/chewing. Comes in 10, 20, 40, 60, and 80 mg tablets. At least one review of studies on the use of controlled release oxycodone has found it to be a good alternative in the treatment of CNCP (18). Unfortunately, this drug is subject to multiple misconceptions and has been given the appellation "hillbilly heroin" by the news. It was considered a major drug of diversion. Of interest is a recent note that Oxycontin on the street is so expensive, addicts are going back to heroin (19). It is second on the DAWN list of medications associated with overdoses. This is a schedule II drug, and may be considered a strong opiate for that reason alone.
- Meperidine (Demerol®)—has 10% of the efficacy of morphine, has significant anticholinergic properties; has been associated with tachycardia, mydriasis; the

half-life is three hours; its metabolite normeperidine (half-life of 15 to 30 minutes) is considered neurotoxic, with the ability to induce seizures and myoclonus. It is rarely used at this time.

- Propoxyphene (Darvon®)—related to methadone; efficacy similar to codeine; half-life is 6 to 12 hours, but duration of effect is three to five hours; its demethylated metabolite norpropoxyphene has a very long half-life of 30–60 hours and can induce cardiotoxicity; it can induce seizures; it is also a weak competitive NMDA receptor antagonist. It should be used with care in the elderly if it should be used at all in this patient population.
- Tramadol (Ultram®)—a synthetic analog of codeine, with oral potency equal to codeine; it inhibits norepinephrine and serotonin (5-HT3) reuptake and has weak central opioid receptor activity (about 30%); half-life is 6.7 hours; peak plasma level in 2.3 hours; has active metabolite; analgesia from tramadol and its metabolite—typically used at 50–100 mg every six hours, maximum dose of 400 mg/day.
- Possible seizure risk with concurrent TCA, SSRI, monoamine oxidase inhibitor (MAOI), and opioid use.
- Ultracet® is tramadol (37mg) in combination with acetaminophen. The combination of these two drugs has been found to have a possibly significant role in multimodal analgesia (2).

Strong Opiates

- Morphine—the prototypical opiate; half-life of two hours, but an analgesic effect lasting 4 to 5 hours; 50% of oral morphine reaches the central compartment within 30 minutes; it has active metabolites morphine-6-glucuronide (M6G) and morphine-3-glucuronide (M3G). M6G is found to be more potent than morphine when given intrathecally as well as less potent than morphine when comparing central effects; M3G has no affinity for the mu and delta opioid receptors and appears to have no analgesic potency; it can induce allodynia and hyperalgesia and, with higher dosages, myoclonus and seizures—this appears to induce antinociceptive activity. It can also bring on a syndrome similar to opioid withdrawal. Renal impairment will enhance the buildup of M3G and M6G. When given anally, M6G is found in much higher concentrations than M3G.
- Has extended release formulations: Kadian® and MS-Contin®, given every 8 to 12 hours, and Avinza, given once daily.
- Kadian—peak level in 9 to 10 hours, lasts 6 to 7 hours; typical use is Q12 hours; consider QD use in the elderly; no crushing/chewing.
- MS-Contin—50% of oral dose reaches the central compartment within 1.5 hours and peaks at 2.5 to 4 hours; steady state is reached in 24 hours; no chewing/crushing.
- Avinza®—once a day—no crushing/chewing; equal mg doses over a 24-hour period with one Avinza and a six times a day immediate release morphine (MSIR).
- Hydromorphone (Dilaudid®)—an analog of morphine; given IV, 1.5 mg of hydromorphone is equivalent to 10 mg of morphine; duration of action is three to four hours; it is metabolized primarily to hydromorphone-3-glucuronide (H3G) and accumulation of the H3G, which is also not analgesically active, can induce neuroexcitatory side effects including allodynia, myoclonus, and seizures.
- Palladone, an extended release formulation was withdrawn secondary to overdosages when mixed with alcohol.

- Methadone, a synthetic mu opioid agonist with approximately 10% NMDA antagonistic activity; considered equipotent to morphine when given parenterally; terminal elimination half-life is 50 to 120 hours; 90% protein bound; undergoes N-demethylation in liver and is excreted in urine; duration of analgesia is four hours, given chronically every six to eight hours. Given in 5 and 10 mg tablets.

  Major problem is the half-life—clinically, one should wait at least five to seven days (longer is better) before adjusting methadone dose—if increased too soon, as steady state is not reached quickly, patient may develop significant sedation and/or overdosage—discordance between analgesic duration and half-life.

  If patient develops respiratory depression, long half-life necessitates at least a 36 to 48 hour observation period; multiple dosages of opiate antagonist may be necessary.

  Cipro inhibits CYP1A2 and 3A4 (of the P-450 system in the liver), thus increasing plasma levels of methadone.
- Fentanyl—oldest synthetic phenylpiperidine opioid agonist; 80 times more potent than morphine; it is very lipophilic; used IV for perioperative pain control; can be used epidurally or intrathecally. A buccal formulation has recently been approved.
- Duragesic transdermal therapeutic system—four dosages used for 72 hours per patch (25, 50, 75, and 100 mg patches); reaches steady state within 12 to 24 hours; can have end of dose failure; after the generic formulation of the patch, the DEA gave notice of increased overdosage.
- Actiq—given orally for transmucosal absorption—swallowed fentanyl has significant first pass (hepatic and intestinal) metabolism; fentenyl does have good buccal mucosal absorption—what is not absorbed here is swallowed; high lipid solubility means rapid transit to CNS.

CANNABINOIDS

It has been a relatively short period since cannabinoid receptors and their endogenous ligands, called endocannabinoids, have been identified. CB1 receptors appear to work in the CNS and are responsible for the psychoactive aspects of the use of cannabinoids. CB2 receptors appear to be found on immune cells and in the gut may be helpful in inflammatory and neuropathic pain (20,21). The endocannabinoid system appears to be involved in the effects of propofol, a widely used anesthetic (22). Low doses of cannabinoids may be useful as coanalgesics to inhibit neuroplasticity and central sensitization in the chronic pain patient, as higher dosages of cannabinoids are associated with significant side effects (22). One study noted that CB2 receptors may be found in the CNS, in addition to their presence in the immune system and spleen (23).

Sativex is an oromucosal spray containing tetrahydrocannabinol and cannabidiol. It has been used for the treatment of symptoms of multiple sclerosis (spasticity and neuropathic pain) as well as neuropathic pain secondary to other etiologies. It has been approved for use in neuropathic pain due to multiple sclerosis in Canada and England (24).

The medical use of marijuana in the United States remains a very sore point. It is illegal, generally, with some states fighting to enable the drug to be used for pain.

REFERENCES

1. World Health Organization. Cancer pain relieve, with a guide to opioid availability. 1996.
2. Schug SA. Combination analgesia in 2005- a rational approach: focus on paracetamol-tramadol. Clin Rheumatol 2006; June 2 [Epub ahead of print]
3. Langford RM. Pain management today- what have we learned? Clin Rheumatol 2006; 25(suppl 7): 2–8.
4. Schnitzer TJ. Update on guidelines for the treatment of chronic musculoskeletal pain. Clin Rheumatol 2006; 25(suppl 7):22–29.
5. Elia N, Lysakowski C, Tramer MR. Does multimodal analgesia with acetaminophen, nonsteroidal antiinflammatory drugs or selective cyclooxygenase-2 inhibitors and patient-controlled analgesia morphine offer advantages over morphine alone? Meta-analysis of randomized trials. Anesthesiology 2005; 103(6):1296–1304.
6. White PF. The changing role of non-opioid analgesic techniques in the management of postoperative pain. Anesth Analg 2005; 101(suppl 5):S5–S22.
7. Sandrini M, Romualdi P, Capobianco A. The effect of paracetamol on nociception and dynorphin A levels in the rat brain. Neuropeptides 2001; 35:110–116.
8. Watkins PB, Kaplowitz N, Slattery JT, et al. Aminotransferase elevations in healthy adults receiving 4 grams of acetaminophen daily: a randomized controlled trial. JAMA 2006; 296(1):87–93.
9. Szczeklik A, Murray JJ. Celecoxib in Aspirin-Intolerant Asthma Study Group. Celecoxib in patients with asthma and aspirin intolerance. The Celecoxib in Aspirin-Intolerant Asthma Study Group. N Engl J Med 2001; 344(2):142.
10. Mico JA, Ardid D, Berrocoso E, Eschalier A. Antidepressants and pain. Trends Pharmacol Sci 2006; 27(7):348–354.
11. Hurley RW, Cohen SP, Williams KA, et al. The analgesic effects of perioperative gabapentin on postoperative pain: a meta-analysis. Reg Anesth Pain Med 2006; 31(3):237–247.
12. Sullivan MD, Robinson JP. Antidepessant and anticonvulsant medication for chronic pain. Phys Med Rehabil Clin N Am 2006; 17(2):381–400.
13. Brown DG, Krupp JJ. N-methyl-D-aspartate Receptor (NMDA) antagonists as potential pain therapeutics. Curr Top Med Chem 2006; 6(8):749–770.
14. Legge J, Ball N, Elliott DP. The potential role of ketamine in hospice analgesia: a literature review. Consult Pharm 2006; 21(1):51–57.
15. Owens VF, Palmieri TL, Comroe CM, et al. Ketamine: a safe and effective agent for painful procedures in the pediatric burn patient. J Burn Care Res 2006; 27(2):211–216.
16. Cheuk DK, Wong WH, Ma E, et al. Use of midazolam and ketamine as sedation for children undergoing minor operative procedures. Support Care Cancer 2005; 13(12): 1001–1009.
17. Devulder J, Richarz U, Nataraja S. Impact of long-term use of opioids on quality of life in patients with chronic, non-malignant pain. Curr Med Res Opin. 2005; 21(10):1555–1568.
18. Stiehl M. Controlled release oxycodone—a new option in the treatment of severe and very severe pain. Review of studies on neuropathic, physical activity-related and post-operative pain. NNW Fortschr Med 2004; 145(suppl 2):61–69.
19. Tierney J. Handcuffs and Stethoscopes. Editorial. New York Times, July 23, 2005. http://www.nytimes.com.
20. Jonsson KO, Holt S, Fowler CJ. The endocannabinoid system: current pharmacological research and therapeutic possibilities. Basic Clin Pharmacol Toxicol 2006; 98(2):124–134.
21. Pertwee RG. The pharmacology of cannabinoid receptors and their ligands: an overview. Int J Obes (Lond) 2006; 30(suppl 1):S13–S18.
22. Azad AC, Rammes G. Cannabinoids in anaesthesia and pain therapy. Curr Opin Anaesthesiol 2005; 18(4):424–427.
23. CB2 receptor-mediated antihyperalgesia: possible direct involvement of neu ral mechanisms. Eur J Neurosci 2006; 23(6):1530–1538.
24. Barnes MP. Sativex: clinical efficacy and tolerability in the treatment of symptoms of multiple sclerosis and neuropathic pain. Expert Opin Pharacother 2006; 7(5):607–615.

14 Narcotic Therapy for Patients with Chronic Non-Cancer Pain

The use of narcotics in the management of chronic non-cancer pain (CNCP) is an important but extremely controversial subject. In 1991, Hardy noted that "there is no place for opiates in the treatment of chronic benign pain" (1). A year later, an American Pain Society survey of its physician members indicated that opioids are probably underutilized in CNCP (2).

TYPES OF PAIN

CNCP is a biological, psychological, and sociological phenomenon. All aspects of these problem areas must be appropriately diagnosed and treated. Not to do so will prevent a good outcome from treatment—secondary to lack of amelioration of pain and inability of the patient to regain function.

A major differentiating factor between acute-pain patients and those with CNCP is that the latter may not have significant physiologic, objective findings on examination that correlate to the patient's complaints. Some patients who have objective findings may not appear to have findings that would support the degree of their subjective complaints of chronic, severe pain.

These patients are quite numerous: statistics indicate the approximate numbers of such patients in the United States is upward of 70 million people.

The most common forms of CNCP include: myofascial pain syndromes; fibromyalgia; neuropathic (nerve related) pain; radiculopathies (chronic central nerve impingement by a disc in the spinal column); failed back syndromes (continued pain after one or more neck or mid- or low-back surgeries); sympathetically maintained pain—secondary to autonomic nervous system dysfunction; arthritis; and chronic headache.

The biological–psychological–sociological phenomenon that encompasses CNCP is most effectively treated, in terms of time, cost, and clinical considerations, within the framework of an interdisciplinary pain-management program (3). Such a program would consists of the following participants: a physician/medical director, typically a neurologist or physiatrist, who makes a diagnosis and deals with medical management including neuropharmacologic care; nurses, who act as both internal case managers and educators; psychologists, who deal with cognitive-behavioral therapy, biofeedback neuromuscular re-education, and other aspects of individual and group treatment; and rehabilitation professionals, including physical and occupational therapists. Other members of a pain-management team may include social workers, vocational specialists, and alternative medicine specialists such as acupuncturists. Published research, including evaluated evidence-based medicine with meta-analyses, has demonstrated the clinical effectiveness, along with the time- and cost-effectiveness, of these programs (4–8) (see Chapter 17).

Unfortunately, very few chronic-pain patients, possibly up to only 6%, obtain treatment in an interdisciplinary pain medicine program (9).

The typical pain patient is frequently seen first by their primary care physicians, a generalist or family physician. Tests are performed, probably including MRIs and/or CAT scans. If these clinicians are unable to help the patients, especially if any of these tests are positive, they are sent for consultation to an orthopedist or neurosurgeon, and more tests may be performed. It should be remembered that many people with no complaints of pain have an "abnormal MRI or CAT scan" of the cervical or lumbosacral spine (10). If surgery is not performed, the patient is typically sent to an interventional anesthesiologist, who will perform multiple treatments (epidural steroid injections, facet/medial branch nerve blocks, and radiofrequency neurolysis/rhizotomies). Many times these patients receive only a temporary decrement in their pain, which will soon return to baseline levels. The interventionalists may place the patients on narcotic pain medication or send them back to their referring physician for such pain medications.

USING NARCOTICS APPROPRIATELY

State and federal clinical practice guidelines do indicate that it is appropriate to ameliorate pain and that the use of pain medications to do so is not illegal (11,12). A set of so-called frequently asked questions (FAQ) was released by the Federal Drug Enforcement Agency (DEA) along with pain specialists from the University of Wisconsin, in August, 2004, the purpose of which was to indicate that physicians "cannot be arrested for properly prescribing narcotic pain killers that are the best treatment for millions of suffering patients" (13,14). Unfortunately, the FAQ was withdrawn by the DEA and many statements retracted. This is discussed in greater detail later.

The Joint Commission for Accreditation of Health Care Organization has determined that pain is the "Fifth Vital Sign" and mandated significant changes in hospital facilities to deal with this problem (15).

Undertreatment with opioid pain medication is becoming all too common for an estimated 40% to 70% of patients with chronic, intractable non-cancer pain (16).

Medically, there are significant adverse effects of undertreated pain:

- Physical
  - o Increased pulse, blood pressure, and respiration
  - o Increased risk of cardiac event in patients so predisposed
  - o Increased risk of atelectasis, pneumonia
  - o Decreased tissue oxygenation, leading to muscle breakdown, poor healing, and weakness
  - o Decreased activity, mobility leading to decreased recovery secondary to limited ambulation
  - o Increased risk of thromboembolic events
- Psychological
  - o Depression, anxiety disorders
  - o Sleep deprivation
  - o Anorexia
- Immunological
  - o Decreased immune response secondary to decreased nature killer cells

- Socioeconomic
  o Decreased productivity, loss of work
  o Increased use of health care resources
  o Familial breakdown

The treatment of the CNCP patient with only narcotics is problematic and most often leads to failure. The most appropriate treatment is within an interdisciplinary pain management program (4–8). An important issue here is that part of the typical interdisciplinary program is the use and then weaning off of chronic opioid medications, as tolerated by the patient, and reflected by their continued and improved functionality.

Kalso et al. (17) noted recommendations for the use of opioids in the CNCP patient. They indicated that the management of the patients' pain should be directed by the underlying cause of the pain. The prescribing physician should be aware of the patient's psychosocial status. Finally, they noted that opioid treatment should not be considered a lifelong treatment.

Opiates can have multiple routes of administration, including: oral, intramuscular, subcutaneous, intravenous, sublingual/buccal-transmucosal, rectal, inhaled, transdermal, vaginal and intrathecal, and epidural.

Opioids are basically either hydrophilic (propoxyphene, codeine, morphine, hydromorphone, hydrocodone, oxycodone, and methadone) or lipophilic, which are associated with greater mu receptor occupancy (fentanyl and sufentanil).

The use of opioids in the CNCP patient does not have a routine, nonindividualized answer. Clinically, many patients with CNCP with a very poor quality of life (QoL) can improve their function with the use of time release (around-the-clock) opioid pain medications. On the other hand, some patients may develop decreased functionality with chronic opioids. Therefore, FUNCTION is the most important issue when dealing with pain patients and chronic opioid medications. If these patients are not showing an improved functionality on these medications, they may need to be stopped.

Most importantly, prior to the use of chronic opioid medications, the CNCP patients must have received all conservative and/or appropriate surgical treatment and failed it—meaning, their pain was not ameliorated, and their functionality continued to be poor or show further decline.

For patients who have had and failed all appropriate treatment, the use of chronic narcotics may certainly be appropriate, on an individualized basis. There are several tenets, which should be followed. First, these patients should receive long-acting opioids on an around-the-clock basis to maintain an acceptable level of comfort. These medications provide a relatively flat dose-response curve, which engenders effective levels of analgesia without the peaks and valleys seen with short-acting pain medications, and therefore provide less risk for potential drug abuse.

There are four basic time-release medications:

- Duragesic patches® (Janssen)—percutaneous Fentenyl—used on the skin for, most typically, 72 hours at a time. This medication also enables the patient to stop taking pain pills multiple times a day, helping to extinguish a medication-related behavior. A generic patch with a different mechanism is now being used.
- Morphine sulphate—in different time-release formulations: MS Contin® (Purdue Pharma); Kadian® (Alpharma, Inc.); both formulations to be given, most typically

every 12 hours. Avinza® (Ligand Pharmaceuticals), once a day preparation.[a] There are also generic forms of MS Contin.

- Oxycontin® (Purdue Pharma)—time release oxycodone, typically taken every 12 hours. It was this medication, along with its nickname—"Hillbilly Heroin" and multiple stories of drug abuse and drug diversion and addiction that brought the current crises regarding the use of these medications to a head.
- Methadone (generic)—a very old medication, developed in the mid-20th century. This medication has a long half-life: it is not a "time release" medication. It may be given every 8 to 12 hours. The difficulty in its use is twofold: poor understanding by many physicians of its clinical attributes and use and the fact that it is also used in specific government approved heroin/opioid detoxification programs. Some pharmacies insist on having the words "for pain" on the prescription, or they would not fill it, another institutional problem for these patients—the stigma.

Even with a time release medication, the CNCP patients on occasion need to be given a "breakthrough pain" medication, typically a short acting, immediate release opioid, which may be needed to lower nociceptive pain brought about by an acute exacerbation of pain secondary to any number of factors such as overactivity.

There are three types of breakthrough pain: incident or episodic—patients know what can cause the pain and take a preemptive, fast acting pain medication. Next is idiopathic or spontaneous breakthrough pain, which comes on suddenly and not infrequently for no obvious reason. Lastly is end-of-dose failure, which is not as unusual as one would expect. Some patients will need to take MS Contin or even OxyContin two or three times a day. Some patients using transdermal fentanyl patches, which are labeled to last 72 hours, in some patients do not—they may only last 48 hours. The physician can see the end of dose failure by the marked increase in breakthrough pain that occurs when the time release medication has been metabolized and the blood level is dropping.

Breakthrough pain can be of moderate to severe intensity. It comes on quickly, typically in less than two to three minutes to maximal intensity. It can last, on average, 13 to 30 minutes. For these reasons, the goal of treatment would be to use a pain medication with fast onset, such as transmucosal fentanyl.

The typical immediate release medications used for breakthrough pain include:

- Darvocet (N-100)—propoxyphene, a mild narcotic, which should be avoided in the elderly.
- Ultram, Ultracet (Tramadol, with or without acetaminophen)—a medication which stimulates the mu-opioid receptors as well as effects serotonin and norepinephrine reuptake.
- Vicodin® (Abbott Pharmaceutical)—hydrocodone and acetaminophen given every four to six hours for breakthrough pain.
- Lorcet® (Forest Pharmaceuticals), Lortab® (UCB Pharma, Inc.), Norco® (Watson Pharmaceuticals)—hydrocodone and acetaminophen, to be used every four to six hours for breakthrough pain. Norco has the smallest dosages of acetaminophen,

---

[a]Many pharmacy formularies would not pay for the more expensive Oxycontin® or Durgesic® patches, leaving the morphine derived time release medications as well as methadone to be used. The problem here is natural selection. One of the breakdown products of morphine, morphine 3-glucuronide, is pronociceptive and can induce significant side effects in the elderly as well as (less frequently) the young, including increased pain.

making the acetaminophen load lowest, and is therefore the least hepatotoxic, depending on the number utilized each day.

- Percocet® (Endo Pharmaceuticals)—oxycodone and acetaminophen, given every four to six hours for breakthrough pain.
- Roxicodone® (Roxane Laboratories, Inc.)—oxycodone without acetaminophen, given every four to six hours for breakthrough pain.
- Actiq® (Cephalon, Inc.)—fentanyl oral transmucosal, an oralette or "lollypop" on a stick—allowed to dissolve in the mouth, with medication entering the system transmucosally; to be used every four to six hours for severe breakthrough pain. While labeled for breakthrough pain in cancer patients, it is now being used by many clinicians for moderate to severe breakthrough pain in the CNCP patients.

The use of immediate release narcotics given with acetaminophen and/or a nonsteroidal anti-inflammatory medication must be looked at carefully secondary to possible hepato- and nephro-toxicity.

In medical practice, physicians should use an extended release (around the clock-ATC) pain medication, for the chronic non-cancer pain (CNCP) patient, with attention being focused on analgesia and improved function, as well as the number of breakthrough pain episodes. The extended relief opioid typically enables an increased function, which may be responsible for the episodes of breakthrough pain that were not seen when the patient was bed/chair bound.

If the patient has more than three or four episodes of breakthrough pain, the ATC medications should be slowly increased, keeping an eye on continued improvement in function and the onset of drug-related problems such as sedation or poor cognitive function. If this occurs, the ATC medication should be decreased. Consideration of opioid rotation should be performed in such cases, as well as generally every four to six months as needed.

The use of breakthrough, instant/immediate release pain medication for breakthrough pain should be limited to three to five times a typical day for a patient.

The science is important. There is no one perfect opioid that will work for all patients. Typical side effects, such as constipation, should be treated at the same time an opioid is started.

Individual responses to opioids may vary, possibly secondary to genetic factors, but this must be recognized. If one opioid does not give good analgesia with a small number of side effects, it should be changed. The use of an adjuvant to help with pain management and possibly allow a smaller dosage of opiate should always be considered.

When prescribing an opiate, always follow established principles and the guidelines and laws applicable from the state and the federal levels; follow both, but particularly whichever is most strict.

Pain management physicians must always document (while monitoring) the four A's: Analgesia, activities of daily living, adverse effects, and aberrant drug taking behaviors (18).

By default, the pain management physician is responsible for identifying the rare drug abuser or drug diverter.

When concerned, get a consult from an addictionologist and even co-treat with this clinician.

The use of chronic opioids alone should only be done AFTER the patient has had, if needed, narcotic medication to help enable them to undergo appropriate rehabilitation. The initial use of chronic opioids is medically not indicated, However, there is a very common caveat to this: a patient's insurance company may not pay for rehabilitation. Many will pay for interventional pain medicine, where a patient may receive a series of epidural steroid medications, for example, and be placed on pain medications simultaneously, but all will pay for pain medications (sometimes only specific pain medications, for extended and immediate release).

The new reality is that the pain management physician must provide care while preventing misuse and drug diversion. Physicians are being turned into police, creating a significant problem in the older established patient/physician relationship. Physicians feel that they cannot always/just cannot trust a pain patient who may divert a pain medication and get the physician into trouble. Patients are afraid, possibly with good reason, that even in the presence of real pain, their pain management needs may not be met.

DEFINITIONS

There are several definitions that must be kept in mind. They are presented with only a little variation, as the concepts and definitions are very important:

Physical Dependence: Seen when the body has adapted to an opiate and there is a class-specific withdrawal syndrome that can be produced by the abrupt cessation, rapid dose reduction, and/or administration of an opiate antagonist. This is not addiction. It is associated with:

Tolerance: A state of adaptation in which exposure to a drug can induce changes that cause the body to enable a diminution of one or more of the drug's effects over time, with all other conditions/aspects of disease being the same. If the physical disorder is getting worse, or progressing, it may cause a need for more medication. If a patient's functional activity is continuing to progress, they may need more medication to make up for the tolerance induced, and an increase in breakthrough pain secondary to activity.

Pseudoaddiction: This is seen in pain patients who are seeking more pain medication, even doctor shopping to obtain these medications, secondary to the patient's real pain syndrome being undertreated. When the treatment enables the patient to achieve appropriate relief, all inappropriate behavior ends.

Addiction: A primary, chronic, neurobiologic disease associated with genetic, psychosocial, and environmental factors which significantly influence its development and how it manifests. It is specifically characterized by behaviors that are typified by impaired control over drug use, compulsive use, craving the drug, and compulsive use in spite of self-induced harm.

A consensus document regarding these definitions was published in 2001 as a joint effort of the American Academy of Pain Medicine, The American Pain Society, and the American Society of Addiction Medicine (19).

An important question is the risk of addiction and aberrant behavior. Portenoy and Savage (20) stated that addiction to opioids in the context of pain treatment is rare in those with no history of addictive behavior.

The Boston Collaborative Drug Surveillance Project looked at 11,882 inpatients who received an opioid while hospitalized; subsequently, only four cases of addiction could be identified (21).

Passik and Portenoy (22,23) worked to develop a model of aberrant drug taking behaviors. They felt that predictive behaviors included: selling prescription drugs; prescription forgery; stealing or borrowing another patient's drugs; injecting oral formulations; obtaining prescription drugs from nonmedical sources; concurrent abuse of related illicit drugs; multiple unsanctioned dose escalations; recurrent prescription losses. Behaviors felt to be less predictive included: aggressive complaining about a need for higher medication doses; drug hoarding during periods of reduced symptoms; requesting specific drugs; acquisition of similar drugs from other medical sources; unsanctioned medication dose escalation one to two times; unapproved use of the drug to treat another symptom; and reporting psychic effects not intended by the clinician.

TREATMENT PROCEDURES

CNCP patients should be seen monthly, at least for the first six months or more. If an escalation of the amount of breakthrough pain medication is seen, this may indicate a need to increase the time-release chronic narcotics.

In routine practice, the CNCP patients should be given a Pain Medication Agreement, which indicates the possible side effects of narcotic usage (including sedation, nausea, vomiting, itching, loss of sexual function, and immunologic problems, among others). Also, the patient must agree that only one physician will provide his/her narcotic pain medications, and the prescriptions will be taken to one (listed) pharmacy. Urine or blood tests may be performed at any time, and if an untoward substance (i.e., cocaine or narcotics not prescribed by the pain specialist) is found in the patient's urine or blood, or, if their blood/urine level of the prescribed pain medication is very inappropriate, the physician may wean the patient off of their opioid medications and treat them without further use of narcotics or discharge them. Other reasons for tapering and ending opioid maintenance include evidence of opioid hoarding; obtaining pain medications from other prescribers; obtaining drugs from others (diversion); and uncontrolled dose escalation or other aberrant behaviors (frequent loss of one's medication—"my dog ate it," reports of stolen medications without a proper police report, frequently calling in requesting medications earlier than should be indicated after being given a one month drug prescription). A past history of substance abuse may be considered a relative contraindication for the use of chronic opioids. However, it is not felt that it is infeasible to treat a chronic pain patient with a history of drug abuse. These patients, as noted above, may need to be treated while they are being seen by an addictionologist.

In some practices, urine testing is felt to be an important part of managing a chronic pain patient safely. Appropriate urine testing can help the prescriber determine if the patient is taking the prescribed medication, if they are taking the correct dosages, and if there is any other untoward drug in their system. Some clinicians do this routinely; some do not do it at all. Some clinicians will have consenting patients observed, to be certain that the urine is theirs. Rare practices may frisk a patient to be certain that they do not have a urine receptacle that they have used to transport "clean" urine. Both general class specific urine testing should be done in combination with gas chromatography/mass spectrometry to find the identity of, or confirm the presence or absence of a specific drug and/or its metabolites (24).

Another very useful tool is serial testing using drug-related questionnaires, such as the CAGE questionnaire (25), or the Pain Outcome Profile developed by the American Academy of Pain Management (26).

The Web site by former Federal Prosecutor Jennifer Bolen is an excellent resource for all physicians in pain management (93). Bolen has excellent examples of patient opioid medication agreements and informed consents for the use of opioids, as well as much more that is useful and should be mandatorily used, in one form or another by all pain management physicians.

Chronic Opioid Use in Patients with CNCP

Two interesting studies from Canada noted important facts, which would most likely be replicated if done in the United States.

A report in 2001 by Moulin et al. (27) found that 340 Canadian pain patients with an average pain intensity of 6.3 (on a 1–10 scale) were taking medication for pain. Eighty percent complained of moderate to severe pain. Their average pain history was 10.7 years. Only 22% of these patients were taking opioid medications and two-thirds of these patients were only taking codeine preparations.

A more recent report (2003) found that a cohort of 154 Canadian pain patients had a mean pain score of 7.7 on a Likert scale (0–10) with a mean duration of pain being 4.7 years. Over 40% of these patients had not used opioids and about 25% had not used any other antineuropathic pain medication in spite of these high levels of pain (28).

A number of authors felt that while the use of opioids may be helpful to treat the CNCP patient, there are no specific guidelines and therefore a greater degree of hesitancy and fear exists (29–37). The "correct" way to use opiates as noted in these various studies is described above. The most basic points being: make certain the patient is examined and documentation is excellent; symptom control leading to improved function and QoL is primary; chronic opioid therapy should be considered for both continuous nociceptive and neuropathic pain if all other appropriate therapies have been tried and failed, utilizing the proper time frame for the medications to work; know the psychosocial status of the patient; use ATC medications, with instant release opioids for breakthrough pain; monitor treatment including re-examinations, functional assessments and urine testing; the physician and the patient should have an appropriate Opioid Agreement which spells out the patients rights and responsibilities.

Opioid therapy can be enhanced via the use of adjunctive medications (see Chapter 13). These may include N-methyl-D-Aspartate (NMDA) antagonists, clonidine, calcium channel blockers, alpha 2-adrenergic agonists, nonsteroidal anti-inflammatory medications (NSAIDs), gabapentinoids, and Neurokinin-1 (NK-1) receptor antagonists (38,39).

The number of published opioid trials lasting longer than 6–12 weeks is very small. This leads to the concern regarding the safety of chronic narcotic usage. Reports show that there were 11 studies with 1025 patients that compared oral opioids with placebo and lasted for four days to eight weeks. Six trials had an open label follow-up of 6–24 months (40). The adverse events noted included constipation, nausea, and somnolence being the most common adverse events noted (at least one of the three) in 80% of patients. Also of interest is that only 44% of 388 patients placed in the open label trails were still taking opioids after therapy for between 7 and 24 months, showing a relatively small group of patients continuing with long-term opioid treatment (40).

Another study looked at the impact of opioid use on CNCP patients. The authors found 11 studies, which evaluated long-term opioid treatment for CNCP and also looked at QoL and included 2877 patients. Six were RCTs and five were observational studies. The authors concluded that there were both moderate/high- and low-quality evidence indicating that long-term treatment with opiates can help CNCP patients develop an increased QoL and significant improvements in function (41).

Maier et al. (42) looked at 121 patients with a three-year history of opioid use and found that the patients with long-term opioid use had significantly lower pain intensity and good improvements in QoL, global assessments, and physical status. During the five years of this study, 33% had no change in opioid dosage, 16% had their dosages decreased, and 27% had a slight overall increase and 19% had significant dose increase (secondary to loss of opioid efficacy). It was concluded that there was a very low frequency of withdrawal in CNCP patients taking long-term opiates, and no evidence for tolerance development, especially if the treatment was performed in a pain center.

Several controlled studies of opioids in CNCP have shown pain relief of 30% to 50% with chronic dosing, but no development of significant tolerance, except for side effects such as nausea and sedation (43).

A more recent meta-analysis of the effectiveness and side effects of opioids when used for CNCP found that both weak and strong opioids outperformed placebo for both pain and function in all types of CNCP (44). The authors of this review also noted that better functional outcomes were found with other drugs which were, for pain relief, only outperformed by strong opioids (44). They also found that in spite of the typically short time for opioid trials, more than one-third of participants withdrew from treatment (44).

The most common side effect/adverse event stemming from the use of opioids is constipation. Typically, when a patient is started on an opiate, a stimulant and stool-softening agent is stated at the same time. There are many patients who continue to have problems with significant constipation. The use of a peripheral opioid receptor antagonist, methylnaltrexone, for the treatment of severe constipation has been found to be useful in managing opioid-induced constipation without significant adverse events including opiate withdrawal (45,46). This drug, which is still in clinical development, can reverse morphine-induced gastrointestinal hypomotility (47–49).

It is also interesting to note that opioids have been ascribed anti-inflammatory properties (50).

Tolerance and Opioid-Induced Pain

Over time, continued opiate usage will induce "tolerance," a known effect, to the opioid analgesic effect (see above). It has been felt that most commonly, dose escalation is secondary to increasing pain, as a result of increasing nociception from ongoing disease processes. However, studies and additional clinical activity indicate that tolerance to different opioid effects can develop at different rates (selective tolerance); for example, one can rapidly develop tolerance to nausea and vomiting, sedation and respiratory depression, but little if any tolerance to constipation and miosis (51). Patient dose variability (genetic polymorphism) can occur as differences in opioid receptor synthesis and differences in various opioid affinities of ligands causing a wide margin of dose variability in patients (51). It is felt that once tolerance to analgesic effects of a specific opiate has developed, simultaneous use of analgesics which are mediated by different receptors may help avoid further tolerance; this concept, multimodal analgesia, is growing more common and involves techniques such as opioid switching/rotation and the use of adjuvant medications.

Two possible mechanisms have also been postulated regarding the development of drug tolerance. First, a with-in system mechanism involves opioid receptors downregulating at the highest affinity sites, and uncoupling from G-proteins. The between-systems mechanism is proposed, with the opiate activated opponent systems—the pain facility systems may be involved with the development of opioid tolerance (52). The first mechanism (with-in system) is the mechanism most often considered; other mechanisms indicate that chronic opiate treatment may also activate the pain facilitatory systems (NMDA receptors, nitric oxide (NO) production, and cyclooxygenase (COX) activation) during the development of opiate tolerance (52).

Data show that opioids can increase pain through activation of the bulbospinal facilitation from the rostral ventromedial medulla (RVM); increased pain can decrease spinal opioid antinociceptive potency and, finally, blockade of pain restores the antinociceptive potency (53).

Tolerance can also be induced by a state of hyperalgesia that results from opioid exposure. The paradoxical or abnormal pain secondary to opiate therapy may also be secondary to neuroplastic changes in the brain and spinal cord, including the activation of the descending pain facilitation mechanism from the RVM. This may be developed, at least in part, by the increased activity of cholecystokinin (CCK) in the RVM. This may induce more pronociceptive events including the upregulation of spinal dynorphin levels; increased calcitonin gene-related peptide (CGRP) and substance P (SP) expression in the dorsal root ganglia. It then appears that opioids can initiate pain due to descending facilitation, upregulation of spinal dynorphin, and increased evoked release of excitatory neurotransmitters from primary afferents (54,55). The neuroplastic changes secondary to chronic opioid utilization may be secondary to adaptive changes needed to promote increased pain transmission and induced tolerance (decreased antinociception) (55).

It has also been noted that chronic opioid use may be associated with the development of hyperalgesia (56). The use of chronic opiates does appear to induce the development of antinociceptive tolerance, which would necessitate increasing the doses of the opiate to maintain adequate analgesia. "Analgesic tolerance" has been associated with paradoxical pain in regions previously not affected by pain, as a result of sustained morphine utilization (57). Many neuropeptides and neurotransmitters (antagonists of algetic chemicals) have been able to block or reverse the antinociceptive tolerance (see below).

Chronic opioid use does upregulate SP and CGRP, which in turn increases the release of algetic, or pain-inducing substances from primary afferent nerve fibers after stimulation. This is correlated with the onset of the abnormal pain states and the opioid antinociceptive tolerance (57).

The descending pain modulatory pathway from the brainstem RVM occurs via the dorsolateral funiculus (DLF) and maintains changes in the spinal cord secondary to abnormal pain states, paradoxical pain, and antinociceptive tolerance. Lesioning the DLF in animals prevented increased evoked algetic neuropeptide release and the development of antinociceptive tolerance and abnormal pain secondary to chronic opiate exposure (57).

Microinjecting lidocaine or a CCK antagonist into the RVM blocks both thermal and touch hypersensitivity and antinociceptive tolerance. It is concluded that chronic opioid exposure will enhance a descending pain facilitatory pathway from the RVM that is mediated by CCK, among other neuropeptides, and is essential for the maintenance of antinociceptive tolerance (57,58). "Nociceptin," also called "orphanin FQ, or OFQ" is a ligand for the "opioid receptor-like1" receptor. When injected into the RVM, OFQ suppresses firing of all types of neurons and blocks opioid induced cell activation. In the medulla, OFQ can produce an antiopioid effect. It appears that depending upon in which region OFQ is placed, it may be able to produce either hyperalgesia or hypalgesia (59).

Chronic opioid administration induces increased expression of spinal dynorphin, which causes increased sensitivity to non-noxious and noxious stimuli: a decrease in spinal antinociceptive properties (60,61). Experimental use of a cannabinoid CB1 agonist to the spinal cord will also induce paradoxical/ abnormal pain, inducing increased spinal dynorphin (61). Continuous morphine use induces neuroplasticity in primary afferents and the spinal cord, and induces increased levels of CGRP and dynorphin (62). Dynorphin antiserum can block increased release of CGRP from rats given chronic morphine; so can lesions of the DLF (62).

NMDA receptor antagonists do decrease or prevent the development of tolerance to the antinociceptive effects of opioids (63,64). It is thought that a range of NMDA receptor antagonists potentiate morphine-induced antinociception (63).

Another study found that the mechanism of tolerance to receptor selective mu and delta opioids may be different compared to those associated with morphine tolerance (64). This would indicate that studies looking at paradoxical pain from chronic morphine utilization may not be generalizable to all opiates.

Specific neurons in the RVM include "off-cells," which are felt to inhibit nociceptive transmission, and "on-cells," which facilitate nociception. When these cells are tested with an NMDA antagonist, several things are noted: systemic morphine produces analgesia in part by involving an NMDA-mediated excitatory process to activate "off-cells" in the RVM. Secondly, activation of "on-cells" is mediated by a non-NMDA receptor, and this activation does not appear to be significant in regulating reflex responses to acute, noxious stimuli. Excitatory amino acid induced excitation appears to work several ways in the RVM, activating "off- cells" and "on-cells" under different conditions (65).

Algetic or pain-inducing neuropeptides are involved in both the development of tolerance and paradoxical/abnormal pain. Sustained morphine use increases SP and NK-1 receptor expression in the spinal cord dorsal horn. It also increases capsaicin-evoked SP release and internalization of NK-1 receptors in the presence of noxious stimuli. It appears that NK-1 receptors have an important role in the expression of chronic morphine-induced hyperalgesia. It may also indicate that chronic opiate usage can induce changes that are similar to those found in inflammatory pain (66).

As noted earlier, CGRP has been found to be increased in the spinal cord dorsal horn during morphine tolerance. The opiate receptors appear to be involved in upregulation of CGRP and SP following exposure to chronic opiates; protein kinase-C appears to have a role in this upregulation (67). Prostaglandins are also upregulated (68). Both CGRP and SP, which are co-localized and co-released, are involved with the development of tolerance to spinal antinociceptive effects of mu- and delta-related agonists. CGRP antagonists may be helpful in the prevention and reversal of opioid tolerance (69–71).

CCK, which is enhanced in the RVM during chronic opiate exposure, may also decrease spinal morphine antinociception by causing descending pain facilitatory mechanism to exacerbate spinal nociceptive activity. A CCK receptor antagonist may also be a useful tool in the prevention of paradoxical pain and analgesic tolerance (72).

Via the use of a serotonin 1A receptor (5-HT$_{1A}$) receptor agonist, it was determined that, as opioids produce bidirectional hypo- and pro-analgesic activity, the 5-HT$_{1A}$ receptor activation counteracts the various aspects of opioid-induced pain. An interesting point is made by the authors of this study that opioid addiction may be self-therapy of opioid-induced pathological pain (73).

Sexual Dimorphism

More evidence is being found that indicates anatomical and neuropsychologic differences exist between the nociceptive systems of males and females (74). Differences appear to exist between male and female perception of and response to pain (75). Women have been found to experience more severe and longer lasting pain than men (76).

Differences in analgesic responses to mu opioid agonists have been seen, but the findings have varied. One study found that women to have more and more robust response to morphine than men, in contrast to prior studies (77). Typically, the mu opioid antinociceptive response is greater in male rats than female rats (78). A recent study found that sexual dimorphism in the opioid effects was related to the opioid receptors on which a particular opioid predominately acts (78).

Studies have found that the analgesic effect of kappa partial agonists (pentazocine, butorphanol, nalbuphine) is much greater in women than men. This may be secondary to a naloxone-sensitive antinociceptive effect of these agonist/antagonists inducing decreased analgesia or increased pain (79,80).

Other studies suggest that it is estrogen receptors in trigeminal neurons which modulate nociceptive responses via serotonin and other neuropeptides. It was thought that the variation in estrogen receptor signaling and neuropeptide plasticity in the trigeminal neurons may have an inducing effect on menstrually related migraine (74).

Finally, inflammation and inflammatory disorders are thought to be sexually dimorphic, via neuro-immune mechanisms underlying sexual dimorphism in three possible aspects of the inflammatory process: plasma extravasation, neutrophil function, and inflammatory hyperalgesia (81).

Barriers to the Use of Opioids

There are patient and physician barriers to appropriate use of opioids: fears of addiction, medication dependence, and drug tolerance, with frequent lack of understanding of the differences between these issues.

Physicians are frequently afraid to prescribe opioids secondary to:

- an inadequate understanding of pain management principles
- inability to appropriately assess a patient's pain
- fear/concern about regulation of controlled substances
- fear that giving pain medication to one patient would make the physician a target of the DEA as well as other patients wanting/needing pain medications
- fears of patient addiction and other problems leading to liability
- concern about patients becoming tolerant to opioids, needing higher dosages, and needing them for extended periods of time (years)
- concern about side effects of opioids.

Patient barriers to appropriate opioid use include:

- fear that pain means a disease is worse

- concern that talking about pain would prevent a physician from dealing with a significant underlying disease
- wanting to be a good patient and not alienate the physician by reporting pain
- concerns about developing tolerance or addiction to pain medications
- fear of showing "weakness"
- embarrassment in going to the pharmacy for these medications; further embarrassment that they may be construed a "drug addict" even though they have no aberrant drug-related behavior and a physiologic reason for their pain.

Systemic/institutional barriers include:

- Restrictive regulation of controlled substances
- Poor access to treatment
- Poor access to Pain Management Specialists
- The most appropriate treatment would not be reimbursed
- The most appropriate treatment is too costly for the patient
- Lack of rehabilitation benefits—"Bad Insurance"
- Inability to obtain any rehabilitation—or even just physical therapy or psychologic care, as they are far more expensive than pain medications (an hour of physical therapy may bill at $150–200, while a single generic Tylenol #4 tablet—one grain of codeine—costs only pennies).

Other barriers to pain relief:

- Pharmacies do not stock adequate and/or appropriate opioids
- No continuity in patient care

Summary

The complexity of this subject is great—even though the medical aspects are fairly straightforward. It is the multitudes of other problems and barriers to appropriate pain management and opioid usage that make this problem so complex.

When one considers that the clinical definition of pain is simple—whatever the patient says it is—it is then up to the clinician to determine exactly what the patient means, utilizing a history, examination, and any necessary tests. Then appropriate treatment should be rendered. The utilization of chronic opioid analgesics is one very important treatment modality, which, when used appropriately, may help improve patients' function and ameliorate their pain.

THE GOOD, THE BAD, AND THE UGLY
The Good

The use of chronic narcotics to both decrease pain and improve function in the CNCP patient has become more widely accepted.

The Bad

An atmosphere of fear has grown and continues to fester regarding the use of Schedule II narcotics, as well as hydrocodone, a Schedule III narcotic. This fear has become so intense that in many places the majority of general practitioners, internists, and even rheumatologists have stopped giving patients more than a few days of hydrocodone, if they will give patients any narcotic analgesics at all.

Pain specialists will usually use opioids, but more recently the majority of pain specialists (who are, by number, interventional anesthesiologists) will start patients on Schedule II narcotics while they are doing interventional procedures, but once they are finished doing injections, they will chose to have other clinicians continue to prescribe the narcotics these patients are using.

Unfortunately, there are fewer and fewer physicians willing to do this, making the prescriptions of appropriate pain medication for the CNCP patient possibly very difficult to obtain.

The Very Bad

Patients who are involved in motor vehicle accidents with clinically obvious muscle spasm, even spasmodic torticollis, as well as headache and pain will receive enough mild narcotic to last a week or so, if they are lucky, and are then sent to the pain specialist for further treatment (i.e., pain medications). Typically, it will take several weeks or more to get in to see such a specialist, which means the patient will have long since run out of pain medications when they are seen.

The atmosphere of fear is becoming ubiquitous.

The Ugly

The major reason for this is physician fear of federal and state regulators. It would be nice to say that this fear is fallacious, but it does not appear to be so.

On August 11, 2004, the DEA published a document called "Prescription Medications: Questions and Answers."

On October 6, 2004, less than two months later, the DEA revoked the publication, claiming it contained misstatements.

Two important points here. First, speaking with one of the authors David Joranson, the Director, Pain & Policy Studies Group, University of Wisconsin-Madison Medical School (Private Communication) there had been a number of iterations of the document prior to its publication, between the DEA, Mr. Joranson, and Drs Russell Portenoy and Seven Passik.

Secondly, it has been noted that at the time the publication was pulled, there were arguments about its admissibility in the trial of William Hurwitz, a physician in Virginia, whose attorneys tried to place the publication in evidence to show that he did not go out of the "norm" in pain management. The Federal prosecutor argued that the DEA publication did not have the force of law behind it as it had not been published in the Federal Register, and the judge agreed. The publication was taken off of the DEA website, as well as that of the Pain & Policy Studies Group at the University of Wisconsin.

On November 16, 2004, the DEA issued the Interim Policy Statement in the Federal Register (26). This statement totally turned over several significant tenets that were in the earlier publication and had been accepted parts of pain management.

For example, the earlier pamphlet stated that it was legitimate for physicians to give patients a number of prescriptions for an opioid pain medication with "Fill On" dates. This, it was noted by Russell Portenoy, was something that had been discussed and recommended in training seminars and medical journals. All of a sudden, it was now illegal to do this, as it would be tantamount to "ordering refills of Schedule II pain medication," something which was acknowledged to be illegal. Thankfully, this problem appears to be fixing itself.

In the past, when a physician got to know a patient well and determined that there was no problem with addiction or diversion, and that their pain was decreased, with associated increased function, it was felt to be appropriate to see these patients every three months, for example, unless they had a problem and needed to be seen sooner. As it is illegal to "refill" a Schedule II drug, the different prescriptions, dated the day they were written and given a "fill-on" date were used so that these patients did not have to spend more money on co-pays for unnecessary physician visits. Then, when the DEA piece was pulled, in their answer published in the Federal Register, it was stated that it was "Illegal" to write multiple prescriptions with "fill-on" dates. This meant that the patients needed to be seen monthly to receive another prescription. Even if they were long-term patients with no existing medication problems. Even if they were unable to afford the copay amount.

This placed a major drain on Medicare and Medicaid and all other medical insurance. The DEA then stated that the physician did not need to actually see the patient, just give the prescription for Schedule II pain medications monthly. This, while now purportedly fulfilling the DEA mandates, did not necessarily follow individual State guidelines. So, physicians were again placed in a double-bind position of "damned if you do, and damned if you don't."

Specifically, the DEA stated in their clarification of August 26, 2005 (82) to their November 2004 interim policy statement: "What is required, in each instance where a physician issues a prescription for any controlled substance, is that the physician properly determine there is a legitimate medical purpose for the patient to be prescribed that controlled substance and that the physician be acting in the usual course of professional practice." For this reason, it was stated, "DEA wishes to make it clear that the Interim Policy statement did *not* state that such patients must visit their physician's office every month to pick up a new prescription" It went on to state that "the CSA and the DEA regulations contain no specific limit on the number of days worth of a schedule II controlled substance that a physician may authorize per prescription."

Then it notes that "Some states, however, do impose specific limits on the amount of schedule II controlled substance that may be prescribed. Any limitations imposed by state law apply in addition to the corresponding requirements under Federal requirements."

A bit of a quandary is found here, in that the various states are different. Some may argue that a physician must see/examine a patient prior to giving a Schedule II narcotic prescription. The best part of valor, in spite of the DEA's statement that it is fine with them to just give out a monthly prescription without seeing the patient, would be to bring the patient in on a monthly basis. If they have to come to the office anyway, they probably should get examined.

Just in case giving a Schedule II prescription to a patient without examining them becomes a crime.

Consider the original DEA publication said that the number of patients in a doctor's practice receiving prescription narcotics, the number of tablets they receive, and how long their therapy lasts "do not, by themselves, indicate a problem."

The DEA's interim statement two months later changed that point dramatically, stating, essentially, that all three of these factors "may be indicative of diversion." The Interim Statement also added, "it is a longstanding legal principle that the Government can investigate merely on suspicion that the law is being violated, or even just because it wants assurances that it is not" (26,82,83).

It was about at this point that physicians began to wonder, if the DEA can invade their practice just because it wants assurances that no law is being broken, then indeed, it can happen to them, or to anyone. If this is true, why should they risk their livelihood by prescribing narcotic pain medications at all?

Dr. Satel, in a piece published in *The New York Times* (84) quotes David Joranson as stating "Pain Management has become a crime story when it really should be a health care story." She notes that the Association of American Physicians and Surgeons has warned physicians against managing chronic pain, as they have to deal with "years of harassment and legal fees, even prison." She quotes the association as stating, "If you do (treat chronic pain) first discuss the risks with your family."

One survey in New York state (85) showed that of 1,300 physicians surveyed by the New York State Medical Society in 1998, 60% were either moderately or very concerned about the possibility of being investigated by regulatory authorities for prescribing opiates for non-cancer pain. About of third of these physicians also noted that they prescribed lower dosages and lower numbers of analgesic tablets because they were concerned about the possibly of being investigated.

The use of "triplicate prescriptions" in various states to monitor the use of Schedule II opiates also contributes to a lack of their use. This, along with a general fear of being investigated for the use of opioids in pain management, have had a long-term negative effect to the treatment of pain, both cancer- and non-cancer related (86–88).

In the last of his series of editorials in *The New York Times* dealing with these problems, John Tierney (89) wrote about "Handcuffs and Stethoscopes." He noted that having failed to win the country's so-called War On Drugs, the DEA and police departments began to "define deviancy up." He stated that, "As quarry for DEA. agents, doctors offered several advantages over crack dealers. They were not armed. They were listed in the phone book. They kept office hours and records of their transactions. And unlike the typical crack dealer living with his mother, they had valuable assets that could be seized and shared by the federal, state, and local agencies fighting the drug war." He accurately stated that doctors were not all blameless.

In his excellent policy analysis statement, Ronald Libby (90) went through the history of substance abuse problems in the United States, going back to the Harrison Act of 1914, which made it a crime for physicians (and pharmacists) to prescribe narcotics to an addict, which, since morphine and other opiates were freely available up to that time, made a quarter of a million people and their physicians into criminals. He described the later demonization of Oxycontin and essentially all narcotic analgesics, and described the DEA's "Oxycontin Action Plan" (91) a significant new antidrug campaign, which essentially made a legal prescription drug equivalent to cocaine.

According to Libby (90), the DEA stated that in the year 2000, physicians wrote 7.1 million prescriptions for oxycodone products without aspirin or Tylenol. They counted 146 "Oxycontin-verified deaths" and 318 "Oxycontin-related deaths," a total of 464 "Oxycontin-related deaths" This gave a risk of 0.00008%, or eight deaths in 100,000 Oxycontin prescriptions. Unfortunately, they made no determination on other forms of oxycodone that might have been in the blood, nor the presence of other drugs which may have contributed or caused death. Libby then contrasted these 464 deaths to the 16,500 deaths from nonsteroidal anti-inflammatory drug related deaths that year.

Libby's paper (90) is a frightening, factual account of the reasons physicians and patients are more at odds now, as are the physicians and regulatory bodies. It makes the dearth of pain management physicians understandable, and even more unfortunate.

An important note is that the majority of this information detailing the problems of pain patients and pain management physicians comes from sources who are neither, but who recognize the societal problem that exists.

In August, 2005, the National All Schedules Prescription Electronics Reporting Act (NASPER) of 2005 was passed into law (92). This bill, also called NASPER, enabled the establishment of a national prescription monitoring program, but at the state level. The purpose of the program was to enable pain specialists to see what drugs their patients, old and new, were obtaining, and from where. This bill has created significant concern from the physicians prescribing pain medications that it can be used to investigate them. Proponents of the bill indicate that the states may only disclose information to law enforcement personnel if it is related to furthering a specific investigation. Worry about erosion of medical privacy has grown, as have the fears of physicians, in spite of reported statements that physicians will monitor the DEA and state agencies to be certain that they are not profiling physicians.

Finally, Tierney noted (89) that a statement made in a field survey on drug use in Cincinnati read: "Because diverted Oxycontin is more expensive and difficult to purchase, users have switched to heroin."

REFERENCES

1. Hardy P. Use of opiates in treating chronic benign pain. Br J Hosp Med 1991; 45:257.
2. Turk D, Brody M, Okifuji EA. Physicians' attitudes and practices regarding the long-term prescribing of opioids for non-cancer pain. Pain 1994; 59:201–202.
3. IASP Taskforce: Desirable characteristics for pain treatment facilities, 1990. (http://www.iasp-pain.org/desirable.html)
4. Rosomoff HL, Rosomoff RS. Comprehensive multidisciplinary pain center approach to the treatment of low back pain. Neurosurg Clin N Am 1991; 2(4):877–890.
5. Cutler RB, Fishbain DA, Abdel-Moty E, et al. Does nonsurgical pain center treatment of chronic pain return patients to work? A review and meta-analysis of the literature. Spine 1994; 19:643–652.
6. Flor H, Fydrich T, Turk DC. Efficacy of multidisciplinary pain treatment centers: a meta-analytic review. Pain 1992; 49:221–230.
7. Chapman SL, Brena SF, Bradford LA. Treatment outcomes in a chronic pain rehabilitation program. Pain 1981; 11:255–268.
8. Turk DC, Loeser JD, Monarch ES. Chronic pain: purposes and costs of interdisciplinary pain rehabilitation programs. Trends in Evidence-Based Neuropsychiatry 2002; 4(2):64–69.
9. Pain management programs. A market analysis. Marketdata Enterprises, Inc., 1998, Tampa, FL.
10. Jensen MC, Brant-Zawadzki MN, Obuchowski N, et al. Magnetic resonance imaging of the lumbar spine in people without back pain. N Engl J Med 1994; 331(2):69–73.
11. Florida Administrative Code. Title 64, Department of Health, Board of Medicine, Chapter 64B8-9 Standards of Practice for Medical Doctors. 64B8-9.013 Standards for the Use of Controlled: Substances for Treatment of Pain. Available at: www.medsch.wisc.edu/painpolicy/domestic/fllaw.htm.
12. Federation of State Medical Boards of the United States. Model policy for the use of controlled substances for the treatment of pain. May, 2004. Available at www.fsmb.org
13. DEA issues new guidelines on pain drugs. Associated Press, Aug. 11. 2004. Available at www.msnbc.msn.com/id/5673456.
14. U.S. Department of Justice, Drug Enforcement Administration, with Pain & policy Studies Group, University of Wisconsin. "Frequently asked questions and answers for

Health Care Professionals and Law Enforcement Personnel." Available at http://www. deadiversion.usdoj.gov/

15. Joint Commission on Accreditation of Healthcare Organizations, Pain Assessment and Management: An Organizational Approach (Oakbrook Terrace, Illinois: JCAHO 2000):3.

16. Furrow BR. Pain management and provider liability: no more excuses. Journal of Law Medicine and Ethics 2001; 29(1):29–51.

17. Kalso E, Allan L, Dellemijn PLI, et al. Recommendations for using opioids in chronic non-cancer pain. Eur J Pain 2003; 7(5):381–386.

18. www.fda.gov/ohrms/dockets/ac/02/slides/3820s2_05_passik.ppt

19. Consensus document from the American Academy of Pain Medicine, The American Pain Society and the American Society of Addiction Medicine. Definitions related to the use of opioids for the treatment of pain. 2001. http://www.painmed.org/productpub/statements/pdfs/definition.pdf

20. Portenoy RK, Savage SR. Clinical realities and economic considerations: special therapeutic issues in intrathecal therapy—tolerance and addiction. J Pain Symptom Manage 1997; 14(suppl 3):S27–S35.

21. Porter J, Jick H. Addiction rare in patients treated with narcotics. N Engl J Med 1980; 302(2):123.

22. Passik SD, Portenoy RK, Ricketts PL. Substance abuse issues in cancer patients. Part 1: Prevalence and diagnosis. Oncology 1998; 12(4):517–521.

23. Passik SD, Portenoy RK, Ricketts PL. Substance abuse issues in cancer patients. Part 2: Evaluation and treatment. Oncology 1998; 12(5):729–734.

24. Heit HA, Gourlay D. Urine drug testing in pain medicine. J Pain Symptom Manage 2004; 27(3):260–267.

25. Fiellin DA, Reid MC, O'Connor PG. Outpatient management of patients with alcohol problems. Ann Intern Med 2000; 133(10):815–827.

26. Federal Register, November 16, 2004; 69(220):67170–67172.

27. Moulin DE, Clark AJ, Speechley M, Morley-Forster PK. Chronic pain in Canada. A patient survey. 10th World Congress on Pain. San Diego, California. USA. 2002; 93 (abstract).

28. Gilron I, Bailey JM. Trends in opioid use for chronic neuropathic pain: a survey of patients pursuing enrollment in clinical trials. Can J Anesth 2003; 50:42–47.

29. Nicholson B. Responsible prescribing of opioids for the management of chronic pain. Drugs 2003; 63(1):17–32.

30. Portenoy RK, Foley KM. Chronic use of opioid analgesics in non-malignant pain: report of 38 cases. Pain 1986; 25:171–186.

31. Portenoy RK. Opioid therapy for chronic nonmalignant pain: a review of critical issues. J Pain Symptom Manage 1996; 11(4):203–217.

32. Cowan DT, Allan L, Griffiths P. A pilot study into the problematic use of opioid analgesics in chronic non-cancer pain patients. Int J Nurs Stud 2002; 39(1):59–69.

33. Kalso E, Allan L, Dellemijn PL, et al. Recommendations for using opioids in chronic non-cancer pain. Eur J Pain 2003; 7(5):381–386.

34. Portenoy RK. Appropriate use of opioids for persistent non-cancer pain. Lancet 2004; 364(9436):739–740.

35. Breivik H. Opioids in chronic non-cancer pain, indications and controversies. Eur J Pain 2005; 9(2):127–130.

36. Reder RF. Opioid formulations: tailoring to the needs in chronic pain. Eur J Pain 2001; 5(suppl A):109–111.

37. Chou R, Clark E, Helfand M. Comparative efficacy and safety of long-acting oral opioids for chronic non-cancer pain: a systematic review. J Pain Symptom Manage 2003; 26(5): 1026–1048.

38. Kalso E. Improving opioid effectiveness: from ideas to evidence. Eur J Pain 2005; 9(2):131–135.

39. Christo PJ, Grabow TS, Raja SN. Opioid effectiveness, addiction, and depression in chronic pain. Adv Psychosom Med 2004; 25:123–137.

40. Kalso E, Edwards JE, Moore RA, McQuay HJ. Opioids in chronic non-cancer pain: systemic review of efficacy and safety. Pain 2004; 112(3):372–380.

41. Devulder J, RIcharz U, Nataraja SH. Impact of long-term use of opioids on quality of life in patients with chronic, non-malignant pain. Curr Med Res Opin 2005; 21(10):1555–1568.
42. Maier C, Schaub C, WIllweber-Strumpf A, Zenz M. Long-term efficiency of opioid medication in patients with chronic non-cancer-associated pain. Results of a survey 5 years after onset of medical treatment. Schmerz 2005; 19(5):410–417. (abstract)
43. Jovey JD, Ennis J, Gardner-Nix, et al. Use of opioid analgesics for the treatment of chronic noncancer pain- a consensus statement and guidelines from the Canadian Pain Society. Pain Res Manage 1998; 3:197–222.
44. Furlan AD, Sandoval JA, Mailis-Gagnon A, Tunks E. Opioids for chronic noncancer pain: a meta-analysis of effectivness and side effects. CMAJ 2006; 174(11):1589–1594.
45. Yuan CS, Foss JF, O'Connor M, et al. Methylnaltrexone for reversal of constipation due to chronic methadone use: a randomized controlled trial. JAMA 2000; 283(3):367–372.
46. Yuan CS, Foss JF. Oral methylnaltrexone for opioid-induced constipation. JAMA 2000; 284(11):1383–1384.
47. Yuan CS. Clinical status of methylnaltrexone, a new agent to prevent and manage opioid-induced side effects. J Support Oncol 2004; 2(2):111–117.
48. Greenwood-Van MB, Gardner CJ, Little PJ, et al. Preclinical studies of opioids and opioid antagonists on gastrointestinal function. Neurogastroenterol Motil 2004; 16(suppl 2): 46–53.
49. Yuan CS, Doshan H, Charney MR, et al. Tolerability, gut effects, and pharmacokinetics of methylnaltrexone following repeated intravenous administration in humans. J Clin Pharm 2005; 45(5):538–546.
50. Walker JS. Anti-inflammatory effects of opioids. Adv Exp Med Biol 2003; 521:148–160.
51. Freye E, Latasch L. Development of opioid tolerance- molecular mechanisms and clinical consequences. [Abstract]. Anasthesiol Intensivmed Notfallmed Schmerzther 2003; 38(1):14–26.
52. Hsu MM, Wong CS. The roles of pain facilitatory systems in opioid tolerance. Acta Aneaesthesiol Sin 2000; 38(3):155–166.
53. Vanderah TW, Suenaga NM, Ossipov MH, et al. Tonic descending facilitation from the rostral ventromedial medulla mediates opioid-induced abnormal pain and antinociceptive tolerance. J Neurosci 2001; 21(1):279–286.
54. Ossipov MH, Lai J, King T, et al. Underlying mechanisms of pronociceptive consequences of prolonged morphine exposure. Biopolymers 2005; 80(2–3):319–324.
55. Ossipov MH, Lai J, King T, et al. Antinocieptive and nociceptive actions of opioids. J Neurobiol 2004; 61(1):126–148.
56. Mao J, Price DD, Mayer DJ. Mechanisms of hyperalgesia and opiate tolerance: a current view of their possible interactions. Pain 1995; 62:259–274.
57. King T, Ossipov MH, Vanderah TW, Porreca F, Lai J. Is paradoxical pain induced by sustained opioid exposure an underlying mechanism of opioid antinociceptive tolerance? Neurosignals 2005; 14(4):194–205.
58. Ossipov MH, Lai J, Vanderah TW, Porreca F. Induction of pain faciliatation by sustained opioid exposure: relationship to opioid antinociceptive tolerance. Life Sci 2003; 73(6):783–800.
59. Heinricher MM, McGaraughty S, Grandy DK. Circuitry underlying antiopioid actions of orphanin FQ in the rostral ventromedial medulla. J Neurophysiol 1997; 78(6): 3351–3358.
60. Vanderah TW, Gardell LR, Burgess SE, et al. Dynorphin promotes abnormal pain and spinal opioid antinociceptive tolerance. J Neurosci 2000; 20(18):7074–7079.
61. Gardell LR, Burgess SE, Dogrul A, et al. Pronociceptive effects of spinal dynorphin promote cannabinoid-induced pain and antinociceptive tolerance. Pain 2002; 98(1–2): 79–88.
62. Gardel LR, Wang R, Burgess SE, et al. Sustained morphine exposure induces a spinal dynorphin-dependent enhancement of excitatory transmitter release from primary afferent fibers. J Neurosci 2002; 22(15):6747–6755.
63. Fischer BD, Carrigan KA, Dykstra LA. Effects of N-methyl-D-aspartate receptor antagonists on acute morphine-induced and l-methadone-induced antinociception in mice. J Pain 2005; 6(7):425–433.

64. Bilsky EJ, Inturrisi CE, Sadee W, et al. Competitive and non-competitive NMDA antagonists block the development of antinociceptive tolerance to morphine, but not to selective mu or delta opioid agonists in mice. Pain 1996; 68(2–3):229–237.

65. Heinricher MM, SHouten JC, Jobst EE. Activation of brainstem *N*-methyl-D-aspartate receptors is required for the analgesic actions of morphine given systemically. Pain 2001; 92(1–2):129–138.

66. King T, Gardell LR, Wang R, et al. Role of NK-1 neurotransmission in opioid-induced hyperalgesia. Pain 2005; 116(3):276–288.

67. Belanger S, Ma W, Chabot JG, Quirion R. Expression of calcitonin gene-related peptide, substance P and protein kinase C in cultured dorsal root ganglion neurons following chronic exposure to mu, delta and kappa opiates. Neuroscience 2002; 115(2):441–453.

68. Powel KJ, Quirion R, Jhamandas K. Inhibition of neurokinin-1-substance P receptor and protanoid activity prevents and reverses the developement of morphine tolerance in vivo and the morphine-induced increase in CGRP expression in cultured dorsal root ganglion neurons. Eur J Neurosci 2003; 18(6):1572–1583.

69. Menard DP, van Rossum D, Kar S, et al. A calcitonin gene-related peptide receptor antagonist prevents the development of tolerance to spinal morphine analgesia. J Neurosci 1996; 16(7):2342–2351.

70. Powell KJ, Ma W, Sutak M, et al. Blockade and reversal of spinal morphine tolerance by peptide and non-peptide calcitonin gene-related peptide receptor antagonists. Br J Pharmacol 2000; 131(5):875–884.

71. Menard DP, van Rossum D, Kar S, Quirion R. Alteration of calcitonin gene-related peptide and its receptor binding sites during the development of tolerance to mu and delta opioids. Can J Physiol Pharmacol 1995; 73(7):1089–1095.

72. Xie JY, Herman DS, Stiller CO, et al. Cholecystokinin in the rostral ventromedial medulla mediates opioid-induced hyperalgesia and antinociceptive tolerance. J Neurosci 2005; 25(2):409–416.

73. Colpaert FC, Deseure KR, Stinus L, Adriaensen H. High-efficacy 5-HT1A receptor activation counteracts opioid hyperallodynia and affective conditioning. J Pharmacol Exp Ther 2006; 316(2):892–899.

74. Lipozencic J. The 1st world congress on gender-specific medicine men, women and medicine in a new view of the biology of sex/gender differences and aging. Acta Dermatovenerol Croat 2006; 14(2):132–134.

75. Schwarz JB. Gender differences in response to drugs: pain medications. J Gend Specif Med 1999; 2(5):28–30.

76. Sun LS. Gender differences in pain sensitivity and responses to analgesia. J Gend Specif Med 1998; 1(1):28–30.

77. Fillingim RB, Ness TJ, Glover TL, et al. Morphine responses and experimental pain: sex differences in side effects and cardiovascular responses but not analgesia. J Pain 2005; 6(2):116–124.

78. Holtman JR Jr, Wala EP. Characterization of the antinociceptive effect of oxycodone in male and female rats. Pharmacol Biochem Behav 2006; 83(1):100–108.

79. Gear RW, Gordon NC, Miaskowski, et al. Sexual dimorphism in very low dose nalbuphine postoperative analgesia. Neurosci Lett 2003; 339(1):1–4.

80. Gear RW, Gordon NC, Miaskowski C, et al. Dose ratio is important in maximizing naloxone enhancement of nalbuphine analgesia in humans. Neurosci Lett 2003; 351(1):5–8.

81. Levine JD, Khasar SG, Green PG. Neurogenic inflammation and arthritis. Ann N Y Acad Sci 2006; 1069:155–167.

82. Federal Register, August 26, 2005; 70(165):50408–50409.

83. Kaufman M. New DEA statement has pain doctors more fearful. Washing Post, Washington, DC, Nov 30, 2004.

84. Satel S. Essay: Doctors behind bars: Treating Pain is now risky. New York, NY: New York Times, October 19, 2004.

85. The New York State Public Health Council. Breaking down the barriers to effective pain management. Recommendations to improve the assessment and treatment of pain in New York State. Report to the Commissioner of Health Barbara A. DeBuono, M.D., M.P.H. January, 1998.

86. Field MJ, Cassel CK, eds. Committee on Care at the End of Life, Institute of Medicine. Approaching death: Improving Care at the end of life. National Academies of Press 1997; 191:197.
87. Joranson D. State Medical Board Guidelines for treatment of intractable pain. Am Pain Soc Bull. 1995; 5(3):1–5.
88. Shapiro RS. Health care providers' liability exposure for inappropriate pain management. J Law Med & Ethics 1996; 24(4):360–363.
89. Tierney J. Handcuffs and Stethoscopes. Editorial. New York, NY: New York Times, July 23, 2005.
90. Libby RT. Treating doctors as drug dealers. The DEA's war on prescription painkillers. Cato Institute, Policy Analysis 545, June 6, 2005:1–22.
91. U.S. Department of Justice, Drug Enforcement Administration, Action plan to prevent the diversion and abuse of Oxycontin, 2001; U.S. Department of Justice, Drug Enforcement Administration, DEA-Industry Communicator: Oxy-Contin Special, Vol. 1.
92. Will new law frighten pain doctors or liberate them? Pain Medicine News: McMohan Publishing Group, NYC, September/October 2005; 3(5):1, 6, 7, 14.
93. www.legalsideofpain.com

Psychological Aspects of Chronic Non-Cancer Pain

"Pain, the barking watchdog of our health, is normally temporary. It immobilizes the damaged muscle, tendon, or ligament so that healing can occur. This acute or subacute pain usually passes quickly and is completely forgotten after it has (1)."

There are psychological aspects of all forms of pain, particularly when the pain becomes chronic. The neurochemical changes associated with chronic myofascial pain were discussed earlier in this work. The changes of serotonergic tonus, for example, do appear to play a role in depression, as well as other affective changes found in the chronic-pain patient. This may help explain why the chronic-pain patient may suffer from at least subclinical depression, and why serotonergic medications are helpful.

On the other hand, pain has *meaning* to some patients. Pain becomes as close as a lover to some chronic-pain patients. It directs and runs their lives. It takes on a life of its own, irrespective of its etiology. It can be an acceptable reason for a patient NOT to do things. It is a socially acceptable reason for obtaining opiates. It can be many things. Part of the job of the pain-management specialist is to determine exactly what it means to a specific patient.

Chronic pain can mean so much to a patient that the pain specialist, if he or she does not understand exactly what it entails, may do a significant disservice to a patient by quickly eradicating their pain.

CASE STUDY 1

A 36-year-old woman, RT, with a history of low-back pain for four and half years, had been injured at work. She had done a fair bit of rehabilitation without success. The man she lived with had accepted his role as her caretaker. She was on social security disability. She was no longer working. Her back pain kept her from making love to her significant other (SO), who did all the housework, shopping, and took care of two pets. She did not like going out of the house for anything, including going to a restaurant.

Her "diagnosis" was chronic low-back pain secondary to her injury. It was unresponsive to physical therapy, and she was kept on Valium® and sustained-release opiates. Her primary care physician sent her to a pain specialist who did an appropriate workup and found that her pain was treatable with a series of facet blocks. This led him to perform a radiofrequency (RF) neurolysis that ended her complaints of pain. She admitted that her pain was gone, but according to her SO she remained in bed, becoming more and more depressed. Three weeks after the RF treatment, she overdosed on the medication she had at home. Her SO returned home in time to call the paramedics and she was taken to the emergency room (ER) where she was resuscitated. She was found by the hospital social worker to be suicidal, and was placed on a psychiatric hold. When released, on her way home, she was the passenger in her SO's car and they were rear-ended when stopped at a red light. She was taken back to the same ER by ambulance and found to have an acceleration-deceleration injury and was placed back on medications. She did not want to see the pain specialist who had previously helped her and was referred to the author's center several weeks later.

The first thing stated by her boyfriend was that her mood had lifted significantly since the automobile accident. RT was very quiet at first and did not want to participate in the psychological aspects of her treatment program. Two weeks later, during a medical recheck, because she essentially refused to speak with the clinical psychologist, a very empathetic woman, as well as claiming that nothing was helping her neck pain, I had a team meeting with RT and her boyfriend. The plan was to get her involved in treatment or discharge her. As we had done before, we staged it so that the psychologist was seated next to her, between RT and her boyfriend. The author played "bad guy" and in a nice but firm way, began to question her as to the reasons that she was not interested in working to get better. One thing led to another and she was asked why she had tried to commit suicide. The two other times I had asked her, the only answer was "Because I couldn't take it anymore." This time I pushed her harder, and finally she stated that for the week before she overdosed, her boyfriend had been pushing her to get out of bed, to go out for dinner, and most importantly, to make love. She wanted no part of any of that; so, not knowing what else to do, she overdosed. It was like lancing a boil. All of her frustration and rage came out. She said that she liked her life the way it was. Her pain allowed her to "check out" and gave her an excuse not to do anything she did not want to do. Her boy friend was shattered.

Further questioning, in a much more supportive manner, enabled her to state that she had fallen out of love with her SO even before the workers compensation injury, but did not know how to end the relationship without hurting him, who she described as a "really wonderful man." Her pain enabled her to escape anything and everything she did not want to do, including work.

Questioning her boyfriend revealed that she had had the three neurovegetative signs of depression prior to her work-related injury: poor sleep, no appetite, and no libido. After that, RT was able to work well with the clinic's psychologist. We obtained a separate psychologist to perform couples therapy for the patient and her boyfriend. Three months later, she was pain free again, and she and her boy friend were continuing in therapy.

The bottom line here is clear. Without knowing more about the patient's pain, getting rid of it without investigating this patient's psychological status resulted in a major, almost catastrophic problem. The patient needed her pain. It was her friend, her protector, and her only lover. Just taking it away left her unable to deal with the other problems in her life, as she was totally unable to deal with being pain free. Her pain was the mechanism she used to cope with her everyday life and distance herself from her boy friend.

There is another important usage of clinical psychology in a pain center. Technology has certainly grown, faster, in some cases, than we know what to do with it, or how best to use it.

CASE STUDY 2

Back in the mid-1980s the use of implanted spinal cord stimulators was in its developmental stages. The process of a percutaneous test of the spinal cord stimulator was showing that the technology worked. Then the stimulator was implanted, a battery-powered tool about the size of a pacemaker, into the abdomen, close to the skin. Back then pain specialists were few and far between. The pain specialist who had done the implant for the patient, W.E., did it well. As the reader should know, a stimulator does not "eradicate the pain" and leave the patient feeling "normal." It works, possibly best explained, by producing an area of paresthesia, which "covers" the painful area. Having worked with other clinicians to bring this technology into the southern California area, I had been working closely with the anesthesiologist who had done the implantation, with the help of a neurosurgeon.

W.E. was sent to my center for two reasons. First, he had become more and more unsettled and agitated at the thought of having this foreign metal object in his belly, so one night he cut it out of himself with a steak knife. He was sutured back together in the hospital. Second, he had developed neuropathic pain in the region of his impromptu surgery secondary to cutting a number of sensory nerves. And, of course, his leg pain had come back.

We learned then, and it has become standard practice now to perform a psychological consult on people prior to placing foreign objects, even those used for treatment, into them.

Most insurance companies do not want to pay for this consult, usually with associated psychological testing, either.

It is imperative to perform a thorough psychological evaluation prior to any neuroaugmentative procedures, even if the insurance company does not wish to pay for it. Any "similar" problems, down the line postoperatively, belong to the pain specialist. Getting psychological testing done is needed for any clinician's insurance.

This chapter is specifically meant to refer to chronic noncancer pain secondary to chronic soft-tissue pain, but this can certainly be generalized. Please see the detailed clinical information regarding myofascial pain syndrome and other chronic soft-tissue disorders elsewhere in this text.

The specificity theory of pain still prevails in today's medical education. This theory suggests that pain is a specific sensation and that its intensity is initially proportional to the degree of peripheral tissue damage. This concept has been gradually modified in that the perception of pain, in addition to the degree of peripheral tissue damage, is influenced by attention, anxiety, suggestion, prior conditioning, learning, and other variables (2). This change in thinking in no way demeans the newer neurophysiologic, neurohormonal, pharmacologic, and mechanical aspects of soft-tissue injury, but does significantly influence the approaches to pain management.

Pain is not considered merely sensory, because it has motivational affective consequences (3).

Behavioral and physiological studies (4) have proposed the following sequence in appreciating pain:

1. A precise evolution of neurophysiologic aspect of the mechanism of pain (see Chapter 1).
2. Activation of the reticular and limbic systems through ascending neuropathways that involve emotional aspects of neurophysiology by studying these neurologic sites which are anatomically linked (Chapters 1 and 10).
3. Involvement of higher centers implicating powerful motivational drives such as suggestion, learned responses, anxiety, and fears that exert control over physiologic activities. (see "Limbically Activated Pain Syndrome" in Chapter 10.)

Acute pain is usually responsive to a specific treatment approach, but chronic pain is a totally different matter. The presence of pain with no discernible organic etiology presents a dichotomy. The "benign" aspect of pain (while there is nothing benign about chronic non-cancer pain) is a term that denotes the enigma of disabling pain proceeding from a relatively innocuous etiology. Individual treatments often fail to diminish such pain and may even enhance it. Disruptions of the nerve tracts that are recognized as mediators of pain may not relieve pain. Patients who fail to respond to a specific treatment may become depressed, resentful, and suffer further from being dismissed as malingerers, or neurotics, rather than fully diagnosed.

A major reason for this is the type of treatment that is utilized. Treating the chronic non-cancer pain patient without utilizing an inter/transdisciplinary approach that deals with the psychological aspects of a patient's pain, in addition to simultaneously treating the organic aspects, is typically doomed to failure. This, in turn, increases a patient's emotional and physical discomfort as well as their fears that the "system" is not out to help them. It also makes the physicians frustrated and less likely to be amenable to viewing the patient's problem as one entity with various parts. It is easier to label the patient as having a major psychological problem and ignore the reality of any concurrent physical/organic aspects of their pain.

Responses to placebo therapy have also further categorized patients in this manner (5). Placebo responses were initially discredited but now that study design flaws have been eliminated, it may be proven to be an effective tool in evaluating and controlling pain. Suggestion is one example of this enhancement (6), and it is now recognized that multiple approaches are more effective (7). Anywhere from 7% to 49% of placebo users muster a definite endogenous opiate system response. This is absolutely not to say that patients should receive "placebo" medications, versus "real" pain medications while in treatment. Nothing erodes trust in the physician faster than the patient feeling "tricked."

Chronic pain has frequently grown progressively worse when the inferred pathologic cause has been removed. It persists day after day and night after night leading to an endless circle of sleeplessness, depression, "agony," and social isolation. Pain, formerly, merely a symptom has now become a disease. Scientific attempts to explain chronic pain may be incomplete. Although many claims have been advanced regarding liability of specific personality traits and genetic hereditary factors, none have withstood the test of time and subsequent studies.

A recent hypothesis (8) is that muscular responses of an injured part persist due to a psychophysiologic mechanism. This learned cortical process (memory) responds to stressful events that trigger the latent increased state of muscular tension (9,10). Muscles that undergo prolonged muscular tension are those in the region of the initial tissue injury site.

Moderate levels of muscle tension may induce pain in both healthy subjects and patients with chronic pain (11). In people prone to reactive stress, these muscles fail to relax to baseline levels in a normal time, which causes them to become the site of pain (12,13). This implies a central mechanism, because both electrophysiologic and imaging studies have demonstrated (experimentally) that pain activates cortical and other central nervous system structures (14,15).

Psychophysiological reactivity is a major contributing and confounding problem in the persistence of chronic soft-tissue pain. The term itself indicates that the patient's physiologic etiology of pain (muscle spasm in the upper trapezius musculature, for example) may be increased and/or reinforced by psychologic aspects such as stress, anxiety, and depression.

A supporting study (16) has shown electromyographically that patients with carpal tunnel syndrome and low-back pain initiate co-contraction of the agonist and antagonist muscles simultaneously and that the antagonists fail to reciprocally relax. This may well explain the onset and persistence of low-back pain in individuals prone to it. This proneness, however, remains unclear in terms of neurophysiologic causes. Psychophysiologic aspects play an important role here.

Each individual appears to have (or have had) a breaking point under stress, after which his/her coping mechanisms have failed. Learned maladaptive coping mechanisms have emerged.

It is good to remember that early in the history of the subspecialty of pain medicine a major disagreement between its originators was whether pain was "peripheral" or "central." The peripheralists, if you will, perceived pain as originating specifically from the site of peripheral injury. When that area healed, the pain was terminated. The centralists felt that pain may have begun in the periphery, but was perceived and perseverated centrally. Some of us felt that acute and chronic pain has both peripheral and central components. A strong argument for this connection is frequently seen in the ER. Patients with acute pain from (soft-tissue) injury can perceive a reduction in their pain from the early use of an anxiolytic, a reminder that the fear and acute anxiety post injury occurs immediately.

Brena (17) postulated the five consequences of chronic pain in what he termed the Five D syndrome:

1. Drug misuse and abuse
2. Dysfunction
3. Dependency
4. Depression
5. Disability

The importance of psychosocial factors as determinants of low-back pain and resultant disability has become increasingly prominent in the literature (18) Frymoyer (19) developed a model based on the experience of numerous experts in determining the resulting disability from low-back pain. He concluded that the following factors had equal weight: physical requirements and job satisfaction were equal to stress, Minnesota Multiphasic Personality Inventory (MMPI) scores, and psychologic symptoms. The Boeing study made the relationship between job satisfaction and recovery after a soft-tissue low back injury equally clear (20).

In those patients with chronic low back problems who do not respond to rehabilitation efforts, there was evidence of depression, anxiety, distress, and pain behaviors (21–25). To rehabilitate work-injured patients, studies discerning pertinent factors needing correction have been produced (26). Physical work load reduction has been accepted, but recent studies emphasize avoidance of sick leaves of long duration and early initiation of rehabilitation measures in poorly educated injured people.

The old technique of allowing a day off after a simple, uncomplicated work-related soft-tissue injury has been rejected. Keeping and injured employee at work in a light-duty job has become a much more appropriate treatment strategy.

A qualitative study (27) emphasized the fact that people sustaining a low-back injury perceive their back problem as being a lifelong one to which they remain susceptible. This indication highlights the need to indoctrinate and educate the injured person, as early as possible, about the cause, significance, and prognosis of the given musculoskeletal problem using meaningful and easily understood terminology.

PANIC AND ANXIETY DISORDERS

Undoubtedly chronic pain is prevalent in patients who develop acute pain and panic secondary to the threatening symptoms. Anxiety disorders are among the most prevalent forms of psychiatric illness in the United States. They are more prevalent in women and in both genders in lower socioeconomic groups.

Differentiation must be made between significant anxiety and everyday normal episodic anxiety associated with upsetting life experiences ("daily hassles"). A clinically significant anxiety reaction literally interferes with a person's ability to function and thus can be considered an illness.

The biological basis of anxiety is an abnormality in chemical neurotransmission. Presynaptic neurons normally transmit impulses both electrically and chemically. These neurotransmitters are both fast and slow signals. Fast signals are mediated by glutamate ("on") and gamma-amino-butyric acid (GABA) ("off "). The slow signals are mediated by monoamines and peptides.

Effective chemical treatment of anxiety disorders, in recent decades, has clarified much of this chemical interplay. The discovery of benzodiazepine receptors and delineation of reciprocal relationships between benzodiazepines and GABA have evolved. Their effect on the locus coeruleus has been postulated.

Besides GABA and norepinephrine, current evidence shows that serotonin, which is significantly involved in pain perception, is also intrinsic to mood disorders and anxiety disorders, as well as in obsessive-compulsive disorders. Anxiety has been considered as a disorder caused by serotonin excess. At least one of the newer anti-anxiety medications is a specific serotonin (5HT-IB) receptor antagonist. Higher levels of serotonin have also been found in most obsessive-compulsive disorders, whereas aggressive impulsive patients may suffer from lower serotonin levels.

The uses of specific medications that help to obviate psychological problems with the help of psychotherapy are an integral part of an appropriate interdisciplinary treatment approach (28).

PAIN BEHAVIOR

Evaluation of pain behavior to indicate the presence and severity of pain has been the starting point for behavioral psychologists in their management of pain (29) Such patient behaviors have been verbal, nonverbal, related to medications, emotional attitudes and postures, and evidence in facial expressions (30). In an attempt to document behavior objectively, electromechanical devices are being developed to record activity and gait patterns (31).

Pain behaviors are most frequently observed directly and are then recorded. Observations can be modified depending on whether the action is being performed in a natural situation or a regulated one, which may simulate the natural production of pain and may be videotaped for further clinical evaluation (32).

Objectivity is a challenge to the trained observer. Most criteria are considered too simplistic and focus on behavior that denies the presence of pain and questions whether such behavior is an expression of pain or merely a mechanism for coping (33).

In the 1980s, Waddell described five nonorganic signs (34). These five types or categories of signs are tenderness, simulation, distraction, regional disturbances, and overreaction.

Tenderness is not related to a particular skeletal or neuromuscular structure. It is nonspecific and diffuse. Examples include superficial tenderness such as skin tenderness to light pinch over a large area not specifically associated with a specific dermatome. Also, there may be a nonanatomic sign of deep tenderness over a wide area not localized to one structure and which often extends to areas other than the lumbar spine.

Simulation tests give the patient the impression that a particular examination is being carried out when it really is not. These tests must be nonpainful. Then, if pain is reported, a nonorganic influence is suggested. These may include axial loading, where a patient is asked to sit straight and a quick downward pressure is applied to the top of the patient's head and the patient then reports low-back pain. Another, the rotational test, may be performed by passively rotating the shoulders and pelvis in the same plane in which the patient stands relaxed with their feet together and low-back pain may be described.

Distraction tests are used after a positive physical finding is demonstrated in a routine manner. This finding is then rechecked while the patient's attention is distracted. The testing should be nonpainful, nonemotional, and nonsurprising. A simple example is to perform the plantar reflex (Babinski) while the patient is in a sitting position. If the patient is able to fully extend the lower extremity, without significant pelvic tilting, and the patient complains of significant pain and a very positive straight leg-raising test when prone, an obvious lack of consistency is noted.

Regional disturbances are indicated by a divergence from neuroanatomically established motor and sensory distributions. First, however, multiple nerve root involvement must be ruled out, as well as a history of multiple spinal surgeries and spinal stenosis. An example would be "give-way" weakness of an extremity that involves multiple muscle groups.

Overreaction to stimulation includes disproportionate verbalization, facial grimacing, muscle tension and tremor, collapsing, or sweating during a nonpainful examination. This sign mandates that the clinician takes into consideration observations and judgements made over the entire patient contact, including how they were reacting to sitting and answering historical questions.

Waddell noted that the presence of three or more types of nonorganic signs correlated with abnormal psychologic profiles and was considered "positive."

Other techniques include performing a simple vibratory stimulation test, looking for changes in perception of vibration on similar areas, bilaterally. The examination ends when the tuning fork is placed in the middle of the sternum and the patient is asked if there is a sensory difference on either side. Neurophysiologically, the answer should be no. A positive answer also adds suspicion that the patient may not be fully forthcoming.

It is extremely important to note that patients with positive inorganic signs may also have true organic findings. There are many reasons for this, including the fact that patients in the Workers' Compensation system, or those who have experienced a motor vehicle accident, may have already seen numerous physicians who, they feel, discounted their complaints and did not find any organic pathology at all. This is not uncommon in contested cases where the patient is forced to attend any number of insurance company mandated Independent Medical Examinations from clinicians being paid by the insurance company.

The patients' may develop a somatoform disorder in which their complaints are magnified, at least in part, as a cry for help from a patient who feels helpless and feels that no one is listening to them or trying to help them. They feel that if they can "up the physical ante" someone, sometime, somewhere along their medical odyssey will listen to them and/or find some organic pathology.

Overexaggeration of pain/discomfort may exist because a patient has a real, albeit not necessarily medically serious, injury. For this reason, it is imperative that patients be fully examined for organic pathology, even simple muscle spasm, in spite of overexaggeration of pain or the finding of nonorganic signs.

Psychological Testing in Patients with Chronic Pain

Pain has traditionally been considered a stimulus-evoked response with the response being equivalent to the stimulus. Relief of pain should therefore follow removal of the noxious stimulus. Repeated stimuli over time, however, modifies, diminishes, or eliminates the relationship of time to stimulus and the response becomes dependent upon other factors (2).

Through generalized stimuli, sensations similar to the original noxious stimulus acquire the ability to elicit a pain response. These stimuli are then considered to be *conditioned* and *learned.* The pain response loses its correspondence with the original stimulus, which was *unconditioned* and becomes a response to a variety of stimuli (35) not necessarily similar to the original.

There is a large difference between pain and suffering. The former is secondary to nociception while the second is an emotional response. Many times, the clinician sees more evidence of suffering than pain in the chronic soft-tissue pain patient. This can be, in many cases, the only thing noted on an examination. It should be noted, but in the context of the patient as a whole.

In many patients, pain may have a specific meaning. That is, there may be a direct, transcendent relationship between a patient's pain and another experience. An example of this may include patients who see their pain as a result of something they have done wrong and feel that the pain is their punishment. Giving up that pain, or punishment, may create an even more untenable situation for the patient than continuing to have the pain. The pain may be, on an unconscious level, a reminder of something exceptionally potent in their consciousness.

The phenomenon of pain can be conceptualized as a *behavior* controlled by the initial unconditioned (pathologic) stimulus and the conditioned stimuli that follow (36). Tissue pathology initiates the noxious stimulus that is transmitted throughout all neural mechanisms, or the entire neuromatrix, following which a given pain behavior evolves.

Unfortunately, physical pain cannot be measured. A patient's verbal pain measurement may be subject to any number of contravening factors. While it is certainly important, if not mandatory, to obtain this patient data, it is best associated or correlated with the patient's level of function, before, during and at the end of treatment. Physical function is typically a much better measure of a patient's physical gain and possible diminution of pain.

CASE STUDY 3

D.R. was a 62-year-old right-handed Caucasian female with a 40-year history of constant headache. A local headache specialist who had treated her for four years without success had sent her for consultation and treatment. Multiple medications had been used, all to no effect. The patient, as she had been taught in the past, had created a diary of her pain levels on a three times a day basis, and, in our first meeting, she seemed pleased to show me how unremitting her headache had been. Examination revealed that she had a cervical myofascial pain syndrome, with active trigger points which referred pain to her head from both cervical and shoulder muscles, as well as decreased cervical and bilateral upper extremity range of motion.

The first task was to stop all of her medications, as she clearly had medication-overuse headache. This was done via an outpatient intravenous dihydroergotamine (DHE-45) and Reglan protocol. She was started in physical therapy and she was asked to meet with the clinic's clinical psychologist. She had great difficulty dealing with any discussions that dealt with her past, particularly her family and her relationship with various family members. She continued to maintain her pain diary, now with the addition of pictures that depicted her day. She chose to use simple pictures of her face. I asked her to continue to do this and add her daily activities. Over the next three weeks, her pain remained at an 8/10 or even 8.5/10. However, she had begun to perform a number of activities that she had not participated in for "a long time," according to her husband. He also reflected that she had discovered her "shopping gene." Aside from leaving the house and going to the mall to shop, she began to do other things such as swim 20 laps in an Olympic-sized pool. She was doing more and more functional activities, and appropriately writing them down. As she continued in physical therapy and psychotherapy, it became obvious that she was becoming more and more active, but her subjective pain level never changed. When she described her continued pain level of 8/10, which used to place her in bed, she continued, as she had from the beginning to talk about it with *la belle indifférence.*

When she had recorded that her pain level had decreased to seven or even 6/10, the same indifferent attitude was noted. She had never shown any pain behavior or even grimaced or frowned when describing her constant pain. As several more weeks passed, she began to do even more activities. When I would compliment her on how well she was doing, she always responded that her headache was terrible. She began to become more resistant, at first, to participating in psychotherapy as the psychologist continued to try to have her understand past experiences associated with her headache. When we had decided to do more work on positive reinforcement, she began to do much better. Finally, when she had continued for several more weeks to show markedly improved function, treatment was stopped. Her myofascial pain syndrome was gone—there were no trigger points, active or latent, to be found. The range of motion of her neck as well as her upper extremities had returned to normal. In spite of her regained physical status, as well as the markedly significant functional gains she had made and which had persisted, she continued to complain in an indifferent manner, of continued "severe" headache pain.

This patient is an excellent example of an important clinical outcome measure-function. In some patients, getting rid of their complaints of headache or pain can be very difficult. D.R. needed to maintain her complaints of headache pain for several reasons, including the secondary gain of having a very accommodating husband, who took very good care of her, especially when she was in pain. After a great number of years, it is difficult in the extreme to totally change a patient's life, which, in this case, had been predicated on headache pain for over 40 years. Her entire life had been predicated on her headaches—what she could and could not do, when and how, along with how much help was needed from her husband. In the end, both D.R. and her husband were pleased with the significant functional gains she had made. She was even driving by herself for the first time in many years. Essentially, we all made the implicit bargain that as long as she had regained and maintained her improved functionality, she could keep her complaints of headache.

A Pyrrhic victory? Not really. The patient was functional for the first time in years. She NEEDED to keep her complaints of pain. It is hard to let go of a close friend, even a "bad" one.

It is obvious that the chronic non-cancer pain patients have both physical as well as emotional aspects to their pain. While a good neurologic or musculo-skeletal examination can give a clinician a great deal of information, to treat the entire person additional information is needed. Psychological testing can be used to provide a good part of the remaining, necessary information needed to treat the chronic benign pain patient. Psychological testing can be used for a number of things. It is a good screening tool for determining the level of psychopathology a patient may have. It can determine specific psychiatric diagnoses. These aspects are mandatory in determining an appropriate, individualized interdisciplinary treatment protocol for a chronic benign pain patient.

Numerous tests for substantiating and quantifying pain have been reported in the literature. Only a few of these tests will be discussed here because most have validity, level of acceptance, and worth as outcome assessments. Any test must be used carefully to diagnose a patient with pain. The initial assumption of the existence of a psychological aspect, not necessarily a basis, which may then be therapeutically pursued, must be validated; treatment, as well as diagnosis, must not be based solely on the outcome of such a test. Patients, not test results, must be treated.

Treatment that ensues from the interpretation of any test must also be based on the age, sex, cultural background, educational level, and potential secondary gains, including economic (e.g., litigation), as well as acceptance by the patient. The competence of the therapist must be measured as well.

The Melzack or Melzack-McGill Pain Questionnaire consists of three major classes of word descriptors: sensory, affective, and evaluative. Reviewing the total score and the categories selected by the patient to describe their pain can give a good, initial indication of the presence or absence of a mild, moderate, or large affective component to the patient's pain complaints (37).

A test that has had acceptance for many years is the MMPI (38). This test has a self-administered true—and-false format. It consists of either a 550-question form or an abbreviated 399-question form. The test, in its original form, had statements requiring an answer of "true or false." The test is computer-scored and computer interpreted. It is a checklist of physical and emotional symptoms, both at the time of examination and in the past.

Scores vary in patients with acute pain and those with chronic pain. In the latter, patients score lower in hypochondriasis (Hs), depression (D), and hysteria (Hy), whereas patients in acute pain score higher in Hs and Hy. Because patients with both acute and chronic pain are preoccupied with the significance of their pain they may express agitation [i.e., elevated Ma (mania) score], which mitigates when the pain becomes chronic, and depression (D) rises.

Rejection of the MMPI test was based on the fact that the study group used to determine normal or average behaviors was not a good cross-section of the general public. The original group had 700 men and women, all white and all residents of Minnesota. The average members of the group interviewed were semi-skilled workers or farmers with an eighth grade education. The phrasing of the statements was considered awkward and unclear. Many topics such as drug abuse, alcoholism, and suicidal tendencies were not addressed. The revised MMPI-2 corrected these flaws and now consists of 567 items, which include a post-traumatic stress scale and a gender role scale; this revision has been evaluated to determine its efficacy.

In evaluating a MMPI-2 scale, the physician cannot determine whether the scores were elevated before or after onset of chronic pain (39). Another disadvantage is the length of time needed for the patient to take the test and the differing interpretation placed on its scores by psychologists.

The MMPI-2 results, or the actual configuration of the results, were looked at as a possible diagnostic indicator for specific pain types. The "Conversion V," with elevations of scales 1, 2, and 3, with 1 and 3 more elevated than scale 2 was felt to be diagnostic for tension-type headache (40). Other work showed that the configuration noted was seen in many other chronic benign pain syndromes (41).

The Eysenck Personality Test (EPT) measures mental stability versus neurosis and introversion versus extroversion (42). This test primarily indicates the stability of the patient's reaction to stress and the tendency for the patient to break down. A direct relationship of susceptibility to the N score exists. A high N score does not indicate neurosis but merely susceptibility; it indicates an introverted person. Extroverts allegedly complain more freely than introverts but have a higher threshold to pain. The EPI test is not as much help in therapy as it is in evaluating the patient's susceptibility to decompensate under stress.

The Beck Depression Inventory (43) test consists of 21 items, is self-administered, and can be taken in five minutes. Each item relates to a factor connected with depression but not to other psychological factors that may aggravate pain.

The Hospital Anxiety and Depression Scale (HADS) has been found to be a useful screening tool for the detection of comorbid depression and anxiety disorders in patients with musculoskeletal pain disorders, and cardiovascular disorders (44,45).

More specific tests, such as the Behavioral Assessment of Pain, have emerged and are useful in the evaluation of the chronic benign pain patient (46).

The Fibromyalgia Impact Questionnaire was developed by Bennett and first published in 1991. It has been modified twice since that time, and translated into eight languages (47). It measures physical functioning, work status, depression, anxiety, sleep, pain, stiffness, fatigue, and well being (47,48).

Hendler (49,50) proposed a test validating the complaint of chronic pain but it has been used mainly for low-back pain. Its value to substantiate other types of chronic pain, such as that likely to result from surgical intervention in low-back pain remains untested (51).

The strong emotional component of any significant pain and the proportion of the emotional component frequently remains obscure, often to the detriment of the patient and to the frustration of the clinician. Cultural and educational factors in today's society imply potential ominous sequelae of any pain with possible mitigating psychological involvement.

Considering these claims and implications, it is evident that many soft-tissue pains, as subjective complaints, with little, if any, confirmatory, objective findings, especially to those clinicians who do not know how to evaluate for these problems, tend to be labeled psychogenic. Failure of the patient to respond to what is considered appropriate treatment lends further support to a psychogenic basis for the pain, rather than an organic basis. Accusation, rather than diagnosis, ensues. Pain becomes chronic, resistant, and intractable. Inappropriate exotic treatments may be pursued by the patient in search of another solution that fails and thus further frustrates them.

Patient–physician rapport and communication are the cornerstones of appropriate examination, diagnosis, and treatment. "Listening" to the complaint and interpreting it properly is the basis for diagnosis and the beginning of effective treatment. The examiner should have knowledge of the presence of the underlying psychological aspect of any, if not all pain complaints, especially when evaluating soft-tissue pain.

CASE STUDY 4

When I first started to practice pain medicine, several decades ago, I was asked to see a 68-year-old woman who had complaints of chest pain. These complaints had occurred for seven years. Each time the pain would occur the patient was hospitalized for a total cardiac work up. Each time the workup was negative. This patient was in the coronary care unit of the hospital when I was asked to see her. Now, being a neurologist, I knew that there was nothing I was going to find regarding her cardiac status that her admitting cardiologist had not found. So, I did a full musculoskeletal examination. It was normal. Her neurologic examination was negative. As I had started my practice only months before, I did not want my consultation to be totally useless, however it appeared to be. Finally, after examining this very nice woman, I sat down with all of her old charts and started reading through them. Nothing came right out at me that would explain the patient's problems. So, I began to outline the charts, to see if there was possibly something I was missing. New in practice, I had the time to spend several hours doing this review. Nothing struck me as pertinent until I made a graph of WHEN she had been admitted to the hospital over the prior seven years. She had been admitted twice a year for six years, once the first year. Each admission, each year, was on the same date. I had no idea what this meant, so I went back to talk to the patient. Pulling up a chair, I asked her if she knew that she had been admitted to the hospital on the same dates each year. She looked at me and said, "Of course I do. The first time is the date my husband died and the second date is the date of the unveiling (of his tombstone)." I had one last question: How did her husband die? Of course, he died of a heart attack.

The information was there, but no one had ever either put it together or, more importantly, asked the patient. She had been left widowed, without family, staying in the apartment she and her husband had inhabited, full of pictures, and other reminders of her dead husband. Her anniversary reactions were really not all that unusual, just a bit extreme.

The use of understandable "words" in explaining the cause and effects of a patient's pain is mandatory. It can never be denied that a patient's cooperation in receiving benefit from any treatment begins with the patient's clear understanding of the problem. The presence of a psychological component to the acceptance of pain—either causative or as an aggravation—can and must be conveyed to the chronic noncancer pain patient. Its acceptance is the beginning of relief and even, in extremely rare situations, a "cure."

One relatively simple way of doing this in a manner that will not alienate a patient who may feel that the clinician thinks their pain is "all in their head", is to explain that many common psychologic problems such as depression and anxiety are (neuro) chemical in nature and are very common *effects* of chronic pain, and thus out of their control.

The validity of psychologic testing has not been demeaned but its proportion of etiology needs clarification before a treatment protocol is initiated and evaluated. In too many chronic pain centers, the psychological aspect is stressed even where it is not used to the exclusion of other modalities. The exact psychological test remains to be accepted and management of the psychological abnormality needs to be outcomes assessed. Use of a standardized test and conventional, one-size-fits-all treatment protocol, regardless of any specific diagnosis for the individual patient, inevitably will lead to failure.

SECONDARY GAIN

Nowhere is the term secondary gain so rampantly used as in therapy for pain and disability resulting from soft-tissue disorders. Fishbain (52) noted in 1994 that the term secondary gain was mentioned in 163 articles by authors of various specialties and disciplines.

The definition of secondary gain, however, remains unclear. Whether it is consciously or unconsciously motivated remains objectively undetermined; its relationship with malingering needs clarification.

Gain was first noted as a psychoanalytic concept by Freud in 1917 (53), who described two types of gain from illness: primary and secondary. He defined primary gain "as a decrease in anxiety brought about through a defensive operation that had resulted in the production of the symptom of the (an) illness." He termed this *intrapsychic*. Freud considered secondary gain as "an interpersonal (social) advantage attained by the patient as a consequence of the illness."

Barsky (54) also defined primary gain as "a reduction in intrapsychic conflict and the partial gratification accomplished by the defense operation." He defined secondary gain as "acceptable or legitimate interpersonal advantages that result when one has the symptoms of a physical disease."

Tertiary gains were described and defined by Dansak (55) as gains sought or attained by someone other than the patient from the patient's illness.

The operant conditioning concept claimed that "reinforcers" enhanced the concept of gain (30,56). Operant behaviors were considered as "rewards" that maintained and promoted chronic pain behavior. Some of these behaviors included: rest, excessive, and inappropriate; relief from pain including narcotic medications taken as needed; avoidance of responsibility; compensation, including financial compensation; avoidance of sexual activities; approval and justification from physician; pending litigation and its rewards; little job satisfaction before injury and consequent avoidance of work; and a poor relationship with an employer.

The relationship between the secondary gain concept and operant reinforcers has never been clearly defined. Fordyce (56) believed that although reinforcers can maintain pain behavior, they did not necessarily produce that behavior and he further believed that reinforcers did not necessitate real or imaginary pain. Fordyce's theory was that observed behavior is merely a response to reinforcers, whereas psychodynamic gains have an unconscious meaning and motivation. Cameron (57) claimed that secondary gains are the result of a neurotic process and not its cause. It is apparent that the relationship between secondary gains and reinforcers remains unclear.

If a patient responds because of secondary gains, the subsequent behavior generally results in secondary losses (58).

Some of these losses may include earnings, meaningful social relationships, recreational activities, community approval, guilt over disability, and the perception of social stigma.

The secondary gain concept unfortunately has been associated with malingering. According to recent definitions, the presence of unconscious secondary gain is a somatoform disorder and not an example of malingering. Also confusing the issue is the fact that financial rewards are often associated with disability (59). The mere presence of litigation or disability benefits can be considered by some as secondary gain.

Chronic-pain patients are usually only sick for a short time, after which they develop their subsequent impairment and disability, which becomes a disability role. The sick-role concept now differs from the disability concept. Studies have not been published to determine whether secondary gain necessarily has an etiologic or a reinforcing effect on the chronic pain.

The conscious–unconscious dichotomy regarding secondary gain is critical to establishing a clear definition. This is particularly true of patients involved in litigation (60,61)

Another form of secondary gain may be seen to have an acceptable etiology. Pain-fear is another problem, where in the patient does not want to do anything, or perform any task that will increase or re-establish his or her pain. The secondary gain seen by a patient's not working must also be evaluated in terms of pain-fear.

Secondary gain may help or harm the patient (62) because there are unanswered terms of insinuation such as unfulfilled dependency or unconscious motivation, which may be difficult to define.

CASE STUDY 5

While practicing in California during the 1980s I saw a patient, P.K., who was a 52-year-old right-handed male longshoreman. He had been injured at work and developed chronic low-back pain, by the time I saw him, two years after his injury. He did not have a history of surgery for the injury, just a number of failed trials of physical therapy and transcutaneous electrical nerve stimulation. He had been taking pain medications for most of the two-year period. He and his wife attended the consultation. They related that he had picked up a heavy box, with the help of another man, who had dropped his end, leaving the patient to try to hold the box alone. He complained of low-back pain immediately and left work for a medical evaluation. The initial examination revealed some lumbosacral paravertebral muscle spasm and pain. CAT scans of his low back were negative, as was a myelogram. Muscle relaxants did not help him, and the narcotic he took for his pain "just made me comfortable."

When seen, his examination was essentially clinically unrevealing, showing that P.K. was very deconditioned physically. He had minimal spasm of his low back. His wife, who had insisted she come into the examination room, a request he heartily agreed with, stood by the exam-room door, watching every move I made. The important examination point was that when he was seated on the exam table, I asked him to extend his legs, one at a time, so that I could check his Babinski reflex. He was able to extend his leg 90° bilaterally. Later, when I checked his straight-leg raising, he literally began to howl in pain when I had moved his legs upward to 30° to 35°. Now, as Waddell might say, this could be problematic. His wife responded to his verbal pain complaints by running over to him and cupping his head with her arms, telling me to leave him alone. Now, at least, I had a preliminary diagnosis to consider.

It took a month of treatment to get to the bottom of his pain problem. He was absolutely convinced that he was not crazy (and he was not) and should not have to see a psychologist. I made psychotherapy a condition of his care, however, and he relented, as long as his low back was being treated with physical therapy.

The story, when it finally became decipherable, was this: P.K. was a very good husband and provider. He had worked as a longshoreman for over 30 years, and had never missed a day of work. He and his wife had raised two children who had left home and gone out on their own. This made P.K.'s wife feel that her life was empty. It was less than a year after her youngest son moved out of their house that P.K. was injured. So, it was within days after the injury, when he was home lying on the couch, that she realized that she still had someone she could take care of: P.K. So, she took care of him very well indeed. P.K., on the other hand, had never been in the position of being taken care of before, hard working man and good provider that he was. Then, not so strangely, he began to like being taken care of by his wife. For the first time since he was a child someone was taking care of HIS needs. Things went swimmingly for several months, with P.K. and his wife essentially changing roles. Then P.K.'s wife found out that her girl friend received a new fur coat from her husband. She had always wanted a fur coat. So, she began to withdraw from P.K., essentially telling him, in so many words, that it was time for him to get off of the couch and get back to work. What did P.K. do when he realized that his wife was getting tired of taking care of him? He upped the ante—his complaints of pain increased. His wife, being a good woman, "felt his pain" and resumed taking care of him. Thus the pattern for the ensuing time between the injury and the next two years, when I saw him for the first time, had developed.

Yes, there was a great deal of secondary gain in play for both P.K. and his wife. At the end, neither one wanted to disappoint the other. Two months of psychotherapy for P.K. alone and with his wife, along with strengthening exercises helped get P.K. back to work. The fact that P.K. had not worked for two years and still went back to work was thought by the workers' compensation company to be amazing. What was really amazing was watching the dysfunctional relationship between P.K. and his wife straighten out so that both could get their needs met after P.K. had returned to work.

Observed reinforcers are suggested to represent "rewards for secondary gain behaviors or perceptions," (63) which seemingly rewrites the definition of operant psychology (30).

The relationship between a patient's emotional and physical difficulties must be determined and used, together, to determine an individualized treatment program. It is therefore imperative to have a psychologist experienced in working with chronic non-cancer pain patients as part of the interdisciplinary treatment team. Without this input and treatment, the ability to help the chronic benign pain patient is markedly, negatively impacted.

Another empirical clinical point is that, particularly in the lower socioeconomic classes, the concept of emotional or psychological distress is not considered pertinent or possibly even real. As the clinician's job is to help the patient, despite their feelings, it may best benefit the patient to utilize some physical treatment along with any necessary psychological care, with the patient therefore understanding that a primarily "physical" problem is being dealt with, in spite of the extreme importance of the work being done in the psychologist's office.

Unfortunately, the importance of individual and group psychotherapy has been discounted by the insurance companies who typically "authorize" an inappropriately small number of sessions to be used by the psychologist and the patient, if any are authorized at all. The majority of these companies will not "authorize" or pay for group psychological therapy. This is very unfortunate, as the chronic non-cancer pain patient may learn more about how to help themselves from their peers, who have moved along the road to improved health and decreased pain, than from the clinicians alone.

In considering the relationship between soft-tissue pain and disability, which may lack objective definition and acceptance, much abuse and argument has come from physicians, insurers, attorney, and claims adjusters. Only the patient, however, is experiencing pain and continues to suffer until all aspects of their diagnoses are made and treated.

REFERENCES

1. Brom B. Corticalization of chronic pain. APS Journal 1994; 3:131–135.
2. Melzack R. The Puzzle of Pain. New York: Basic Books, 1973.
3. Melzack R. Psychological Concepts and Methods for the Control of Pain. In: Advances in Neurology, vol. 4. New York: Raven Press, 1974:275–280.
4. Melzack R, Casey KL. In: Kenshalo D, ed. The Skin Senses, Vol. III, Springfield, IL: Charles C Thomas, 1968:423.
5. Beecher HK: Measurement of subjective response. New York: Oxford University Press, 1959.
6. Turk DC, Wack JT, Kerns RD. An empirical examination of the Pain Behavior construct. J Behav Med 1985; 8:119–130.
7. Sternbach RA. Acute versus chronic pain. In: Wall PD, Melzack, R, eds. Textbook of Pain. London: Churchill Livingstone, 1984:606.
8. Flor H, Birbaumer N. Acquisition of chronic pain: psychophysiological mechanisms. APS 1994; 3:119–127.
9. Flor H, Birbaumer N, Turk DC. A diathesis-stress model of chronic back pain: Empirical evaluation and therapeutic implications. In: Gerber WD, Miltner W, Mayer K, eds. Behavioral medicine: results and perspectives of empirical research. Weinheim: Edition Medizin, 1987.
10. Flor H, Turk DC, Birbaumer N. Assessment of stress-related psychophysiological reactions in chronic back pain patients. J Consult Clin Psychol 1985; 53:354–364.
11. Borgeat F, Hade B, Elie R, Larouche LM. Effects of voluntary muscle tension increases in tension headaches. Headache 1983; 24:199–202.
12. Christensen LV. Physiology and pathophysiology of skeletal muscle contraction. Part 1, Dynamic activity. J Oral Rehabil 1986; 13:451–461.
13. Christensen LV. Physiology and pathophysiology of skeletal muscle contraction. Part II, Static activity. J Oral Rehabil 1986; 13:463–477.
14. Backonja M, Miletic G. Somatosensory cortical neurons on mononeuropathy model. Soc Neurosci Abst 1983; 19:1074.
15. Kenshalo DR Jr, Willis WD Jr. The role of the cerebral cortex in pain sensations. In: Jones PA, ed. EG: Cerebral Cortex. New York: Plenum Press, 1991:153–212.
16. Donaldson CCS, Romney D, Donaldson M, Skubick D. Randomized study of the application of single motor unit biofeedback training to chronic low back pain. J Occup Rehabil 1994; 4(1):23–37.
17. Brena SF. Chronic pain: America's Hidden Epidemic. New York: Atheneum, 1978.
18. Linton SJ, Althoff B, Melin L, et al. Psychological factors related to health, back pain, and dysfunction. J Occup Rehabil 1994; 4:1–10.
19. Frymoyer JW. Predicting disability from low back pain. Clin Orthop Rel Res 1992; 279:101–109.
20. Bigos SJ, Spengler DM, Martin NA, et al. Back injuries in Industry: A retrospective study III. Employee-related factors. Spine 1986; 11:252–256.
21. Jensen MP, Karoly P. Pain-specific beliefs, perceived symptoms severity, and adjustment to chronic pain 1992; 8:123–130.
22. Keefe FJ, Williams DA. Assessment of pain behaviors. In: Turk DC, Melzack R, eds. Handbook of Pain Assessment. New York: Guilford Press, 1992:275–294.
23. Truner JA, Robinson J, McCreary CP. Chronic low back pain: Predicting response to nonsurgical treatment. Arch Phys Med Rehabil 1983; 64:560–563.

24. Jensen MP, Turner JA, Romano JM, Karoly P. Coping with chronic pain: A critical review of the literature. Pain 1991; 47:249–283.
25. Feuerstein M, Thebarge RW. Perceptions of disability and occupational stress as discriminators of work disability in patients with chronic pain. J Occup Rehabil 1991; 1:185–195.
26. Kemmlert K, Lundholm L. Factors influencing ergonomic conditions and employment rate after an occupational musculoskeletal injury. J Occup Rehabil 1994; 4:11–21.
27. Tarasuk V, Eakin JM. Back problems are for life: Perceived vulnerability and its implications for chronic disability. J Occup Rehabil 1994; 4:55–64.
28. Keltner NL, Folks DG. Psychotropic Drugs, 2nd edn. St. Louis: Mosby-Year Book, 1997.
29. Keefe FJ, Dunsmore J. Pain behavior: concepts and controversies. APS Journal 1992; 1:92–100.
30. Fordyce WE. Behavioral methods for chronic pain and Illness. St. Louis, CV Mosby: 1976.
31. Keefe FJ, Hill RW. An objective approach to quantifying pain behavior and gait patterns in low back pain patients. Pain 1985; 21:153–161.
32. Follick MJ, Ahern DK, Aberger EW. Development of an audio-visual taxonomy of pain behavior: Reliability discriminate validity. Health Psych 1985; 4:555–568.
33. Turk DC, Wack JT, Kerns RD. An empirical examination of the pain behavior construct. J Behav Med 1985; 8:119–130.
34. Waddell G. Low back pain: A framework for clinical decision making. Drug Therap 1983; 8(3):92–96.
35. Fordyce WE, Fowler RS, Lehman JF, Delateur BJ. Some implications of learning in problems of chronic pain. J Chron Dis 1968; 21:179.
36. Brena SF, Koch DL. A pain estimate model for quantification and classification of chronic pain states. Anesthesia Review 1975; 2:8–13.
37. Melzack R. The McGill pain questionnaire: major properties and scoring methods. Pain 1975; 1:277–299.
38. Dahlstrom WG, Welsh GS, Dahlstrom LE. An MMPI handbook, Vol. 1. Minneapolis: University of Minnesota Press, 1960.
39. Naliboff BD, Cohen MJ, Yellen AN. Does the MMPI differentiate chronic illness from chronic pain? Pain 1982; 13:333–341.
40. Kudrow L. Muscle contraction headaches. In: Rose FC ed. Handbook of Clinical Neurology. Vol. 48. Amsterdam: Elsevier Science Publishing, 1986:343–352.
41. Jay GW, Grove RN, Grove KS. Differentiation of chronic headache from non-headache pain patients using the millon clinical multiaxial inventory (MCMI). Headache 1987; 27:124–129.
42. Bond MR. Personality and Pain. Edinburgh: Churchill Livingstone, 1984:45–50.
43. Beck AT, Ward CH, Mendelson M, et al. An inventory for measuring depression. Arch Gen Psychiatry 1961; 4:561–571.
44. Bambauer KZ, Locke SE, Aupont O, et al. Using the hospital anxiety and depression scale to screen for depression in cardiac patients. Gen Hosp Psychiatry 2005; 27(4):275–284.
45. Bennett R. The fibromyalgia impact questionnaire (FIQ): a review of its development, current version, operating characteristics and uses. Clin Exp Rheumatol 2005; 23(5 suppl 39):S154–S162.
46. Jay GW. Headache handbook: diagnosis and treatment. Boca Raton: CRC Press, 1999:89.
47. Harter M, Reuter K, Gross-Hardt K, Bengel J. Screening for anxiety, depressive and somatoform disorders in rehabilitation—validity of HADS and GHQ-12 in patients with musculoskeletal disease. Disabil Rehabil 2001; 23(16):737–744.
48. Buskila D, Neumann L. Assessing functional disability and health status of women with fibromyalgia: validation of a hebrew version of the fibromyalgia impact questionnaire. J Rheumatol 1996; 23(5):903–906.
49. Hendler NH. The four stages of pain. In: Hendler NH, Long DM, Wise TN, eds. Diagnosis and treatment of chronic pain. Boston: John Wright, PSG Publishing, 1982:1–8.
50. Hendler N, Viernstein M, Gucer P, Long D. The hendler ten minute screen test for chronic back pain patients. The chronic pain treatment Center, Baltimore: The Johns Hopkins Hospital, 1978.
51. Mersky H. Classification of chronic pain descriptions of chronic pain syndromes and definitions of pain terms. Pain 1986; 3(suppl):S1–S225.

52. Fishbain DA. Secondary gain concept: Definition problems and its abuse in medical practice. APS J 1994; 3:264–277.
53. Freud S. Introductory Lectures on Psychoanalysis (1917). London: Hogarth Press, 1959:378–391.
54. Barsky AJ, Klerman GL. Overview: hypochondriasis bodily complaints and somatic styles. Am J Psychiatry 1983; 140:273–282.
55. Dansak D. On the tertiary gain of illness. Compr Psychiatry 1973; 14:523–534.
56. Fordyce WE, Fowler RS, Lehmann JF, DeLateur BJ. Some implications of learning in problems of chronic pain. J Chron Dis 1968; 21:179–190.
57. Cameron N. Personality development and psychopathology. Boston: Houghton Mifflin, 1963:273–274.
58. Bienoff J. Traumatic neurosis of industry. Industr Med Surg 1946; 15:109–112.
59. Finneson BE. Modulating effect of secondary gain on the low back pain syndrome. Adv Pain Res Ther 1976; 1:949–952.
60. Thompson DL. Secondary gain, a second look: Issues in counseling the industrially injured worker. NARPPS J News 1991; 6:59–63.
61. Weissman FIN. Distortions and deceptions in self-presentation: Effects of protracted litigation in personal injury cases. Behav Sci Law 1990; 8:67–74.
62. Gallagher RM. Secondary gain in pain medicine. APS J 1994; 3:274–278.
63. Whitehead W, Kuhn WF. Chronic pain: an overview. In: Miller TW, ed. Chronic Pain. Vol. 1, Madison, WI: International Universities Press, 1990:5–48.

16 Interventional Pain Medicine in the Treatment of Chronic Non-Cancer Pain

At this time, the majority of pain medicine specialists are interventional anesthesiologists; a decade or so ago, this was not the case.

Many of these anesthesiologists have done a fellowship for additional certification in interventional pain medicine. Increasing numbers of psychiatrists and neurologists earn pain fellowships, so that they can perform interventional procedures. Much or most of this treatment, according to many interventional anesthesiologists, is based on finding an abnormality on a CAT scan or MRI.

This appears to ignore the literature demonstrating that in spite of having abnormalities of the spine found on an MRI or CAT scan, many people remain pain-free (1,45–47). This is also true clinically. The author has reviewed hundreds of patient charts after international procedures that show only brief neurological exams and a paucity of pertinent pain history. The issue here is that these patients may have abnormal test results but pain from another problem, such as MPS.

Boden et al. (1) found that out of 67 pain-free individuals with no history of low-back pain, sciatica, or neurogenic claudication, about one-third had substantial abnormalities on lumbosacral MRIs. Of the patients under 60 years old, 20% had a herniated nucleus pulposis, and one had spinal stenosis. In the patients who were over 60, 57% had abnormal MRIs, with 36% of these having herniated nucleus pulposus (HNP), and 21% having spinal stenosis. Thirty-five percent of the subjects between 20 and 39 years of age had degeneration or bulging of a disk at at least one level.

Jensen's study in the *New England Journal of Medicine* (45) looked at the MRI of the lumbar spine in 98 asymptomatic subjects. Fifty-two percent had a disk bulge at at least one level, and 27% of these had a disk protrusion and 1% an extrusion. Thirty-eight percent had abnormalities in more than one intervertebral disk. Annular defects were found in 14% of patients, facet arthropathy in 8% of patients. No substantial differences were seen between men and women. The authors commented that the discovery by MRI of bulges or disk protrusions in people with low-back pain may "frequently be coincidental."

Stadnik et al. (46) found that annular tears and focal-disk protrusions on MRI images were frequently found in an asymptomatic population. Savage et al. (47) found that 32% of asymptomatic subjects had "abnormal" lumbar spines and 47% of subjects with complaints of low-back pain (LBP) had "normal" lumbar MRIs (n = 149 subjects; 78 of these were between 20 and 30 years of age and 71 were between 31 and 58 years).

The majority of physicians with a patient in pain will gladly send their patients to the interventionalist, many of whom will also use pain medications, too often, while giving injections. Patients who show improvements may do so secondary to pain medications. This solves the referring physician's problems—they do not want to prescribe pain medications in today's fear-ridden atmosphere regarding opioid use.

Another issue is that the proliferation of interventionalists, along with insurance companies that do not want to pay for anything else (except possibly two to three physical therapy treatments prior to a two-week stop to get more treatments approved), makes other types of treatment difficult to access.

Also, pain medication, for the most part, is far cheaper than neuro-rehabilitative treatment.

EVIDENCE-BASED MEDICINE

An evaluation of interventional pain medicine literature, using an evidence-based medicine (EBM) approach, is extremely interesting. There are four basic levels (some consider five) of EBM.

Level I: Strong research-based evidence—Several high-quality randomized controlled trials (RCTs), high-quality scientific studies with homogeneous results, one or more meta-analyses

Level II: Moderate research-based evidence—At least one relevant RCT or several adequate studies

Level III: Limited research-based evidence—No RCT, at least one adequate scientific study

Level IV: No scientific evidence—Expert panel evaluations, other published case studies

There is a lack of scientific evidence regarding the value of interventional procedures secondary, at least in part, to significant and unnecessary variation in the provision of interventional pain procedures (2,3). Further, revue of the literature shows that in spite of unclear criteria and "uncertain long-term value" (2) regarding facet injections, Medicare was billed $60 million for these procedures in 2001. The Medpac (3) study shows different rates of usage of the various interventional procedures, which were geographically based. This poses the question: if these therapies are the most up-to-date and efficacious procedures for pain in the hands of physicians of adequate and equivalent training, why should such geographic barriers/variations occur?

In 2001, Medicare paid physician charges of over $370 million for interventional pain procedures, not including facility fees (4). The national bill in 2001 for physician charges alone for interventional pain procedures for acute, chronic, and cancer-related pain would be higher than $1.8 billion (as Medicare pays on average 21% of the total national bill for physician charges) (2).

The question of the efficacy of interventional pain procedures and the EBM used to determine such efficacy is therefore markedly important, as an enormous amount of medical fees, on a yearly basis, is paid for interventional pain procedures by such national programs.

There are multiple treatment guidelines for the same clinical problem. The question is which guideline should/must be used, and why?

Such treatment guidelines are based on expert opinion, systematic reviews, and meta-analyses. Ioannidis et al (5) noted that significant problems may exist between the findings of large trials and meta-analyses including significant discrepancies, secondary to heterogeneity of study populations, treatment protocols, and bias. Another group (6) noted that at least 90% of meta-analyses of interventional pain management studies had serious flaws in methodology. This would create an amplification of the negative effect of a poor-quality RCT by its inclusion in a meta-analysis, inducing a 30–50% overestimation of the value of the intervention being evaluated (2,7,8).

Merrill (2) , an anesthesiologist, noted that interventional pain medicine is based on the belief in the "value of acute, invasive interventions in chronic disease." He further noted that "EBM has befallen interventional pain therapy early in the development of both and has found that the scientific underpinnings of these invasive therapies are as yet unprepared for scrutiny."

EPIDURAL STERIOD INJECTIONS

One of the questions here is whether acute invasive intervention can effectively intervene in a chronic disease process. Many consider chronic pain as a chronic disease that should be treated as one, and are doubtful that a few epidural steroid injections (ESIs) (i.e., between one and three series of three ESIs) will stop a chronic biological-psychological-social disease process. Proponents of interventional pain medicine appear to disagree with this issue.

There is apparent chaos in the ranks. A recent study found that there is no clear consensus as to the best or ideal method to use in the performance of an ESI: fluoroscopy should or should not be used; a transforaminal approach should be taken or not (9).

The answer to the question, "What is the most effective treatment for acute LBP?" asked in the Journal of Family Practice in February 2002, included the statement, "There is no consistent evidence that epidural steroid injections are effective for acute low-back pain (evidence grade: D)" (48).

Sciatica, or sciatic pain, is a common sequelae of an HNP. Watts and Silagy (10) did a meta-analysis on the efficacy of ESIs in the treatment of sciatica and described "quantitative evidence from meta-analysis of pooled data from randomized trials that epidural administration of corticosteroids is effective in the management of lumbosacral radicular pain." Then, Carette et al. (11) performed an RCT to evaluate the efficacy of up to three ESIs in the treatment of sciatic pain secondary to an HNP. They found that while ESIs with methylprednisolone could afford short-term decrements in leg pain and sensory changes in the lower extremities, they offered no significant functional benefit and did not reduce the need for surgery.

Out of twelve controlled trials, ESIs were found to be effective in six (12–17), and in six (18–23) they were found to be no different than placebo or reference treatment. As these trials go back to the early 1970s, there are certainly better ways to perform these trials today. Koes et al. (24) noted that many, if not most, of these trials had significant methodological problems. They found that the best studies showed inconsistent results of ESIs and they concluded that the efficacy of ESIs has not been established. They felt that the benefits of ESIs, if any, appeared to be only of short duration.

There are studies favorable to interventional procedures. Nimgade et al. (25) found that steroid injections for lateral epicondylosis are the most successful short-term intervention for pain relief. Active physical therapy was efficacious no matter what the time frame.

Delport et al. (26) treated patients with lumbar spinal stenosis with ESIs under fluoroscopy. Of 140 patients, 32% noted greater than two months of pain relief; 39% reported less than two months pain relief; and 29% noted no relief from the injections. Twenty percent had surgery. Of note, 53% noted better functioning, and 74% were at least somewhat satisfied with their treatment.

Rosen et al. (27) found that 50% of patients with LBP and sciatica with radicular symptoms who received ESIs received temporary relief. Long-term relief was seen in fewer than 25% of patients.

In Butterman's study (28), he found that ESIs were not as effective as discectomy in their ability to reduce symptoms and disability associated with HNPs in the lumbar region. He noted that ESIs did have a role: they were found to be effective for up to three years by almost 50% of patients who had not had improvement with six or more weeks of noninvasive care.

In a more ambitious study, looking at the place of minimally invasive procedures in the treatment of chronic LBP, Cahana et al. (29) noted the contradictory interventional literature. They found that there was moderate evidence (via small randomized, nonrandomized, single group, or matched case controlled studies) for medial branch neurotomy and limited evidence (nonexperimental one or more center studies) for intradiscal treatments in mechanical LBP. They found moderate evidence for the use of transforaminal ESIs, lumbar percutaneous adhesiolysis, and spinal endoscopy for lumbar radiculopathy. They found no "gold standard treatment" for chronic LBP.

It was noted that the conflicting information from various reviews of ESIs made it difficult for general practitioners to determine how or if they should be used. Hopayian and Mugford (49) indicated that the choice of methods used for systematic reviews may alter views about the medical evidence.

McLain et al. (50) noted that clinical studies have alternatively either supported or refuted the efficacy of ESIs in the treatment of patients with back and leg pain. They noted that steroid medications did benefit some patients with radicular pain, but the benefits were limited in duration, therefore making efficacy over time difficult to prove. They also indicated the need for good randomized, controlled trials to identify those patients most likely to benefit from ESIs and when and for how long.

A more recent study found only moderate evidence for the use of transforaminal ESIs, along with lumbar percutaneous adhesiolysis and spinal endoscopy for pain resulting from lumbar radiculopathy (51).

Tong et al. (52) called into question the practice of giving ESIs to patients who were on SSDI/workers' compensation and/or had work requiring heavy lifting.

Slipman et al. (53) did an EBM analysis of the current literature and indicated that current studies gave only sparse evidence to support the use of interventional techniques in the treatment of lumbar zygapophysial joint-mediated LBP.

Other data showed similar findings. Nelemans et al. (30) found, in their Cochrane Database EBM evaluation of RCTs of injection therapy for pain relief in patients with LBP, that convincing evidence for the effects of injection therapies for LBP is lacking, and that there was a need for more and better designed trials.

Bogduk (31) found that while literature endorses the use of ESIs, there is little compelling data on rationale and efficacy for the procedure. In a more recent paper, Bogduk (54) stated that "The apparent efficacy of lumbar intra-articular steroids is no greater than that of a sham injection. There is no justification for the continued use of this intervention. Better outcomes can be achieved with deliberate placebo therapy."

Valat et al. (32) looked at the efficacy of ESIs in RCT comparing prednisolone to saline administered to patients with sciatica. They found that the efficacy of saline could not be excluded, but ESIs provided no additional improvement.

Rozenberg et al. (33) did a review of 13 trials published between 1966 and 1997. They concluded that they could not determine if ESIs were effective in common LBP and sciatica.

A study by Lafuma et al. (34) looking at the cost-effectiveness of ESIs requiring in-hospital management for lumbosciatic syndrome found that adding an epidural injection as a first-line treatment to rest and the use of nonsteroidal anti-inflammatory medication resulted in additional costs and no gain in efficacy.

An editorial in the *British Medical Journal* (35) noted that evidence for the efficacy of ESIs for LBP is equivocal; they may be useful as adjunctive treatment in some patients with symptoms lasting longer than three months in the absence of indicators of "chronic pain", and in patients who may have radicular symptoms.

A review by the Institute for Clinical Systems Improvement looked at fluoroscopically guided transforaminal ESIs for lumbar radicular pain and found that they are generally safe, but there was insufficient evidence to comment on the efficacy of ESIs (36).

Zhou et al. (55) looked at quality assurance for interventional pain management procedures and noted a good QA program was helpful. They did a survey of 566 patients and found that the majority had immediate pain relief after a procedure. No follow-up was done, however, to determine if the decrement in pain persisted, or for how long. A number of different interventional pain management procedures were involved.

In an effort to look at the costs of interventional procedures in the United States, Straus (37) noted that the costs of interventional treatment for spinal pain were minimally $13 billion in 1990, with costs growing 7% per year. Cost minimization analysis suggested that ESIs under fluoroscopy "may not be justified by the current literature."

The findings noted above are also found in the German literature where Hildebrandt (38) found that intra-articular injections of steroids offered no greater benefit than normal saline and that long-lasting success from this procedure was lacking.

Vad et al. (39) stated that they did a randomized study to evaluate the efficacy of transforaminal ESIs. However, the study was not blinded or randomized—patients were "randomized by choice." The data, secondary to these significant methodologic problems, are not objective.

Patients, in a retrospective study done by Lin et al. (56), who had failed conservative treatment for cervical pain and were otherwise surgical candidates were given a trial of cervical ESIs, which were found to be a reasonable choice for nonoperative treatment of patients with symptomatic cervical disk herniations. Cervical ESIs are less studied than lumbar ESIs and have "less support" than lumbar and caudal ESIs (57).

An RCT looking at intradiscal steroid therapy for lumbar spinal discogenic pain found that intradiscal steroid injections did not improve clinical outcome in patients with discogenic back pain compared to placebo (40).

OTHER PROCEDURES

A systematic review of spinal cord stimulation identified one RCT, one cohort study, and 72 case studies. Taylor et al. (41) found that the level of evidence for the efficacy of spinal cord stimulation in chronic back and leg pain was only "moderate."

Two studies of percutaneous vertebroplasty done in the same time period found in one case that the procedure was safe and useful (58), while the other noted that there were no data from controlled clinical trials or from studies with long-term follow-up and that the procedure was still investigational, but may be appropriate for patients with no other treatment options (59).

Finally, Abram (42) noted that it is difficult to determine whether interventional procedures are truly effective and, further, there is almost no data on whether or not they are cost-effective. He made a number of conclusions, which bear further evaluation:

1. Some patients do obtain excellent and lasting pain relief with all interventional techniques, but the same can be found in placebo studies.
2. ESIs are widely used, but there is little good data regarding efficacy and to recruit patients for a blinded, definitive outcome study would be very difficult.
3. There is minimal evidence, if any, suggesting that fluoroscopic translaminar, transforaminal, caudal, or epiduroscopic ESIs are safer or more effective than the older "blind" translaminar approach—no comparison studies have been done.
4. Steroid facet injections can give temporary and on occasion, prolonged relief for some patients with axial back pain, but no evidence is noted that they are more effective or longer lasting than placebo.
5. Radiofrequency ablation of lumbar facet nerves is more effective than sham procedures and gives longer lasting relief than facet injections.
6. Intradiscal electrotherapy studies have not shown good evidence for efficacy.

PRACTICE GUIDELINES

Boswell (43) noted that new practice guidelines were presented in 2005 (44). The conclusions of this publication are based on much the same published information, yet are very different. Note that these recommendations were developed from "all types of evidence." Furthermore, "if an evidence-based approach failed to provide adequate levels of evidence, consensus and expert opinions were utilized." This would unfortunately fail the EBM established tests for the highest reliability of evidence, or at the very least make them a low level IV or V.

1. Transforaminal ESIs—moderate-level evidence found for this procedure or selective nerve roots in preoperative evaluation of patients with negative imaging studies and clinical findings of nerve root irritation.
2. Evidence for interlaminar ESIs in managing lumbar radiculopathy was strong for short-term relief and limited for long-term relief. The evidence is presented as moderate for both short and long-term pain reliefs for cervical radiculopathy.
3. Evidence for transforaminal ESIs for lumbar nerve root pain was felt to be strong for short-term and moderate for long-term improvement. Moderate evidence for managing cervical nerve root pain was found. Evidence was limited in lumbar postlaminectomy syndrome, and lumbar spinal stenosis. The effectiveness of transforaminal ESIs in axial LBP, lumbar disc extrusions, and axial neck pain was indeterminate.
4. Evidence of lumbar and cervical medial branch blocks in decreasing chronic LBP and cervical pain was moderate.

5. Medial branch neurotomy via radiofrequency neurotomy was moderate to strong for short- and long-term reliefs of lumbar and cervical facet joint pain.
6. There was moderate evidence for efficacy of short-term and limited evidence for long-term improvement in managing LBP via intra-articular blocks, and evidence was negative for this procedure in managing neck pain.
7. Evidence for intra-articular sacroiliac joint injections was moderate for short-term relief (< six weeks) and limited for long-term relief.
8. Evidence for spinal cord stimulation in failed back surgery patients as well as complex regional pain syndrome patients was strong for short-term relief (< one year) and moderate for long-term relief.

CONCLUSIONS

It is interesting that so many different conclusions can be taken from essentially the same data. It would therefore seem that there is not yet enough evidence to give fully credible EBM unequivocal statements of efficacy to interventional procedures at this time.

Clinically speaking, the adjunctive use of interventional procedures has been found to be useful when the procedures are done by a well-trained interventional anesthesiologist. However, there are several issues here:

1. Adjunctive treatment should be the operational term.
2. Proper diagnosis should be established by a specialist in neurology, physiatry, or orthopedics prior to patients undergoing invasive treatments.
3. These procedures are possibly limited to moderate evaluative and analgesic appropriateness. Patients should be given ALL of the information—both the positive and negative aspects as well as information on all alternative treatments prior to undergoing invasive procedures.
4. The insurance companies favor interventional pain medicine to the exclusion of interdisciplinary pain medicine treatment for chronic non-cancer pain patients. This has eliminated many outstanding programs, which have closed for lack of insurance reimbursement.
5. Finally, in today's cost-conscious medical environment, the minority of inter-ventionalists who utilize the procedures as a form of lottery—performing as many procedures as possible on patients who are not showing responsiveness—needs to stop. This is a waste of our valuable but limited medical resources.

The author knows and holds in high regard many interventionalists from around the world. The EBM statements above are based on just what is reported: reports of EBM evaluations of interventional procedures, mostly by interventional-ists. The truly expert clinicians known to the author who practice state-of-the-art interventional pain medicine do the best possible clinical treatments known at this time. More work certainly needs to be done to establish a greater in-depth knowl-edge of such work, when EBM hopefully catches up to better investigated interven-tional tretment.

REFERENCES

1. Boden SD, David DO, Dina TS, et al. Abnormal magnetic-resonance scans of the lumbar spine in asymptomatic subjects. A prospective investigation. J Bone Joint Surg Am 1990; 72(3):403–408.

2. Merrill DG. Hoffman's Glasses: evidence-Based medicine and the search for quality in the literature of interventional pain medicine. Reg Anesth Pain Med 2003; 28(6):547–560.
3. Medpac. Medicare Payment Advisory Commission Report to the Congress: Paying for Interventional Pain Services in the Ambulatory Settings. Dec. 2001. www.medpac.gov/publications/contressional_reports/dec2001Pain Management.pdf.
4. HHS.CMS. 2001 Medicare physician/supplier procedure summary master file (formerly Part B Procedure File). June 30, 2002. Electronic file.
5. Ioannidis JPA, Cappelleri JC, Lau J. Issues in comparisons between meta-analyses and large trials. JAMA 1998; 279:1089–1093.
6. Jadad AR, McQuay HJ. Meta-analyses to evaluate analgesic interventions: a systemic qualitative review of their methodology. J Clin Epidemiol 1996; 49:235–243.
7. Moher D, Cook DJ, Jadad AR, Tugwell, et al. Assessing the quality of reports of randomized trials: implications for the conduct of meta-analyses. Heath Technol Assess 1999; 3:1–100.
8. Moher D, Pham B, Jones A, et al. Does the quality of reports of randomized trials affect estimates of intervention efficacy reported in meta-analyses? Lancet 1998; 352:609–613.
9. Cluff R, Abdel-Kader M, Cohen SP, et al. The technical aspects of epidural steroid injections: a national survey. Anesth Analg 2002; 95:403–408.
10. Watts RW, Silagy CA. A meta-analysis on the effacy of epidural corticosteroids in the treatment of sciatica. Anaesth Intensive Care 1995; 23(5):564–569.
11. Carette S, LeClaire R, Marcoux S, et al. Epidural corticosteroid injections for sciatica due to herniated nucleus pulposus. N Engl J Med 1997; 336:1634–1640.
12. Dilke TFW, Burry HC, Grahame R. Extradural corticosteroid injection in management of lumbar nerve root compression. BMJ 1973; 2:635–637.
13. Breivik H, Helsa PE, Molnar I, Lind B. Treatment of chronic low back pain and sciatica: comparison of caudal epidural injections of bupivacaine and methylprenisolone with bupivacaine followed by saline. In: Bonica, JJ, Albe-Fessard, DG, eds. Advances in pain research and therapy. Vol. 1. New York: Raven Press, 1976:927–932.
14. Yates DW. A comparison of the types of epidural injection commonly used in the treatment of low back pain and sciatica. Rheumatoid Rehabil 1978; 17:181–186.
15. Mathews JA, Mills SB, Jenkins VM, et al. Back pain and sciatica: controlled trials of manipulation, traction, sclerosant and epidural injections. Br J Rheumatol 1987; 26:416–423.
16. Ridley MG, Kingsley GH, Gibson T, Grahame R. Outpatient lumbar epidural co4rticosteroid injection in the management of sciatica. Br J Rheumatol 1988; 27:295–299.
17. Bush K, Hillier S. A controlled study of caudal epidural injections of triamcinolone plus procaine for the management of intractable sciatica. Spine 1991; 16:572–575.
18. Beliveau P. A comparison between epidural anaesthesia with and without corticosteroid in the treatment of sciatica. Rheumatol Phys Med 1971; 11:40–43.
19. Snoek W, Weber H, Jorgensen B. Double blind evaluation of extradural methylprednisolone for herniated lumbar discs. Acta Orthop Scand 1977; 48:635–641.
20. Klenerman L, Greenwood R, Davenport HT, et al. Lumbar epidural injections in the treatment of sciatica. Br J Rheumatol 1984; 23:35–38.
21. Cuckler JM, Bernini PA, Wiesel SW, et al. The use of epidural steroids in the treatment of lumbar radicular pain: a prospective, randomized, double-blind study. J Bone Joint Surg Am 1985; 67:63–66.
22. Rocco AG, Frank E, Kaul AF, et al. Epidural steroids, epidural morphine and epidural morphine and epidural steroids combined with morphine in the treatment of post-laminectomy syndrome. Pain 1989; 36:297–303.
23. Serrao JM, Marks RL, Morley SJ, Goodchild CS. Intrathecal midazolam for the treatment of chronic mechanical low back pain: a controlled comparison with epidural steroid in a pilot study. Pain 1992; 48:5–12.
24. Koes BW, Scholten RJ, Mens JMA, Bouter LM. Efficacy of epidural stoerid injections for low-back pain and sciatica: a systematic review of randomized clinical trials. Pain 1995; 63:279–288.
25. Nimgade AS, Sullivan M, Goldman R. Physiotherapy, steroid injections or rest for lateral epicondylosis? What the evidence suggests. Pain Practice 2005; 5(3):203.
26. Delport EG, Cucuzzella AR, Marley JK, et al. Treatment of lumbar spinal stenosis with epidural steroid injections: a retrospective outcome study. Arch Phys Med Rehab 2004; 85(3):479–484.

27. Rosen CD, Kahanovitz N, Bernstein R, Viola K. A retrospective analysis of the efficacy of epidural steroid injections. Clin Orthop Relat Res 1988; 228:270–272.
28. Butterman GR. Treatment of lumbar disc herniation: epidural steroid injection compared with discectomy. A prospective, randomized study. J Bone Joint Surg Am 2004; 86-A(4):670–679.
29. Cahana A, Mavrocordatos P, Geurts JW, Groen GJ. Do minimally invasive procedures have a place in the treatment of chronic low back pain? Expert Rev Neurother 2004; 4(3):479–490.
30. Nelemans PJ, Bie RA de, Bet HCW de, Sturmans F. Injection therapy for subacute and chronic benign low back pain. In: Cochrane Database Syst Rev 2000 (2): CD001824, ISSN:1469–493X.
31. Bogduk N. Epidural Steroids. Spine 1995; 20(7):845–848.
32. Valat JP, Giraudeau B, Rozenberg S, et al. Epidural corticosteroid injections for sciatica: a randomised, double blind, controlled clinical trial. Ann Rheum Dis 2003; 62(7): 639–643.
33. Rozenberg S, Dubourg G, Khalifa P, et al. Efficacy of epidural steroid in low back pain and sciatica. A critical appraisal by a French task force of randomized trials. Critical Analysis Group of the French Society for Rheumatology. Rev Rhum Engl Ed 1999; 66(2):79–85.
34. Lafuma A, Bouvenot G, Cohen C, et al. A pragmatic cost-effectiveness study of routine epidural corticosteroid injections for lumbosciatic syndrome requiring inhospital management. Rev Rhum Engl Ed 1997; 64(10):549–555.
35. Samanta A, Samanta J. Editorial: is epidural injection of steroids effective for low back pain? BMJ 2004; 328:1509–1510.
36. Institute for Clinical Systems Improvement. Fluoroscipically guided transforaminal epidural steroid injections for lumbar radicular pain. Bloomington, MN. Institute for Clinical Systems Improvement, August 2004.
37. Straus BN. Chronic pain of spinal origin: the costs of intervention. Spine 2002; 27(22): 2614–2619.
38. Hildebrandt J. Relevance of nerve blocks in treating and diagnosis low back pain—is the quality decisive? Schmerz 2001; 15(6):474–483.
39. Vad VB, Bhat A, Lutz GE, Cammisa F. Transforaminal epidural steroid injections in lumbosacral radiculopathy: a prospective randomized study. Spine 2002; 27:11–15.
40. Khot A, Bowditch M, Powell J, Sharp D. The use of intradiscal steroid therapy for lumbar spinal discogenic pain. Spine 2004; 29(8):833–837.
41. Taylor RS, Van Buyten JP, Buchser E. Spinal cord stimulation for chronic back and leg pain and failed back surgery syndrome: a systemic review and analysis of prognostic factors. Spine 2005; 30:152–160.
42. Abram S. Efficacy of interventional therapies for low back and neck pain. In: Justins, DM. ed. Pain 2005-An updated Review: Refresher Course syllabus. Seattle: IASP Press, 2005:123–129.
43. Boswell MV. Evidence-Based use of interventional techniques for chronic spinal pain. Lecture, American Academy of Pain Management, 16th Annual Clinical Meeting, San Diego, CA, September 24, 2005.
44. Boswell MV, Shah RV, Everett CR, et al. Interventional techniques in the management of chronic spinal pain: evidence-based practice guidelines. Pain Phys 2005;8(1):1–47.
45. Jensen MC, Brant-Zawadzki MN, et al. Magnetic resonance imaging of the lumbar spine in people without back pain. N Engl J Med 1994; 331(2):69–73.
46. Stadnik TW, Lee RR, Coen HL, et al. Annular tears and disk herniation: Prevalence and contrast enhancement on MR images in the absence of low back pain or sciatica. Radiology 1998; 206(1):49–55.
47. Savage RA, Whitehouse GH, Roberts N. The relationship between the magnetic resonance imaging appearance of the lumbar spine and low back pain, age and occupation in males. Eur Spine J 1997; 6(2):106–114.
48. Harwood MI. What is the most effective treatment for acute low back pain? J Family Practice. 2002; 51(2): www.jfponline.com/pages.asp?AID=1106.
49. Hopayian K, Mugford M. Conflicting conclusions from two systematic reviews of epidural steroid injections for sciatica: which evidence should general practitioners heed? Br J Gen Pract 1999; 49(438):57–61.

50. McLain RF, Kapural L, Mekhail NA. Epidural steroid therapy for back and leg pain: mechanisms of action and efficacy. Spine J 2005; 5(2):191–201.
51. Macrocordatos P, Cahana A. Minimally invasive procedures for the treatment of failed back surgery syndrome. Adv Tech Stand Neurosurg 2006; 31:221–252.
52. Tong HC, Williams JC, Haig AJ, et al. Predicting outcomes of transforaminal epidural injections for sciatica. Spine J 2003; 3(6):430–434.
53. Slipman CW, Bhat AL, Gilchrist RV, et al. A critical review of the evidence for the use of zygapophysial injections and radiofrequency denervation in the treatment of low back pain. Spine J 2003; 3(4):310–316.
54. Bogduk N. A narrative review of intra-articular corticosteroid injections for low back pain. Pain Med 2005; 6(4):287–296.
55. Grados F, Depriester C, Cayrolle G, et al. Long-term observations of vertebral osteoporotic fractures treated by percutaneous vertebroplasty. Rheumatology (Oxford) 2000; 39(12):1410–1414.
56. Lin EL, Lieu V, Halevi L, et al. Cervical epidural steroid injections for symptomatic disc herniations. J Disord Tech 2006; 19(3):183–186.
57. Hession WG, Stanczak JD, David KW, Choi JJ. Epidural steroid injections. Semin Roentgenol 2004; 39(1):7–23.
58. Levine SA, Perin LA, Hayes D, Hayes WS. An evidence based evaluation of percutaneous vertebroplasty. Manag Care 2000; 9(3):56–60, 63.
59. Zhou Y, Furgang FA, Zhang Y. Quality assurance for interventional pain management procedures. Pain Physician 2006; 9:107–114.

17 Interdisciplinary Treatment of Chronic Non-Cancer Pain

Acute pain may last days to weeks, even two to three months or so. Chronic pain, in existence for three to six months or more, is in itself a disease. It is the cause of a great deal of financial distress to patients from increased medical system utilization and loss of work, and familial disintegration. It is also leads tosignificant cost increases to insurers and patients for medical services and medications.

The treatment of pain is relatively uncomplicated in the acute pain patient. Once the cause of the pain is identified, it may be treated in a rather straightforward manner. The problems involved in the treatment of the chronic-pain patient increase substantially, as chronic pain is biological (organic), psychological and sociological in nature, making treatment far more complex and of necessity more significantly encompassing.

While medication and possibly a modality (such as a short course of physical therapy) may be all that is necessary to treat an acute-pain patient (who is not suffering from a significant primary problem such as cancer or a specific disk herniation), 15% of acute-pain patients who go on to become chronic-pain patients need an integrated treatment paradigm.

The pain treatment armamentarium includes medication, physical therapy, occupational therapy, interventional anesthesiological procedures ("nerve blocks"), psychiatric treatment, neuropharmacological treatment, work hardening, and much more.

What has been learned over the past several decades is that "shot-gunning" a patient with various treatments given by different providers at different places or overreliance on narcotic pain medication will not help the patient to obtain more than temporary relief.

To treat only one aspect of a chronic-pain patient's problem may do more harm than good. For example, prescribing pain medication and physical therapy for a chronic soft-tissue injury, while ignoring the patient's depression, anxiety, loss of self-esteem, and their inability to return to work may well potentiate the problem and makes the patient's chronic pain harder to treat. It becomes more costly in time, services, and funds to remedy these problems, so the patient can return to a normal life.

The International Association for the Study of Pain has defined four levels of pain-treatment facilities (1). At the first level are single- or dual-modality–oriented facilities. These organizations provide treatment limited to a specific intervention, such as nerve blocks, physical therapy, or biofeedback. These are the most common types of pain treatment facilities, mostly run by interventional anesthesiologists, who utilize nerve blocks and pain medications, sometimes with physical therapy. These healthcare facilities do not manage the pain condition or evaluate the patient with a comprehensive interdisciplinary approach.

The second level includes so-called syndrome-oriented facilities, such as headache clinics or a low-back pain centers. These entities specialize in a particular diagnosis or pain associated with a specific area of the body.

The third level, the interdisciplinary pain clinic, is a facility containing a diverse group of health care specialists that offers evaluation and treatment of both acute and chronic pain disorders. Multiple therapeutic assessments and interventions/treatments are available, with the healthcare providers working as a team.

The fourth and "highest" level, the interdisciplinary pain center, is similar to the interdisciplinary pain clinics. These centers treat both acute and chronic pain disorders using a variety of healthcare specialists led by a physician pain specialist; they have the added components of research and teaching as an operating feature. Unlike a "multidisciplinary pain clinic," where members of various disciplines may work in different locations, a key feature of the interdisciplinary pain center is that all members of the pain-treatment team work "under one roof." This enhances the ability to communicate and work as a true team to help patients.

INEFFICIENCIES IN CURRENT TREATMENT METHODS

Generally speaking, pain is first encountered by the family physician who will attempt to treat it within their frame of expertise. If they need to, they may send the patient to a mono- or bi-modality facility or a syndrome-oriented clinic, which treats only one form of pain problem, that is, a "back pain" clinic, or uses one modality, such as nerve blocks. Over the course of years, the chronic pain patient may have been seen at three to six such facilities.

In terms of chronic pain patients (patients with pain for three to six months or longer) these forms of pain treatment may initially help up to 60% to 80% of them, leaving, in the rest, a continuous drain on health resources—insurance, workers' compensation insurance, and personal finances, which will typically go on for years.

Only 6% of chronic-pain patients find a way to obtain treatment at a tertiary care center for pain—a comprehensive, interdisciplinary pain management/neuro-rehabilitation center. As noted earlier, such a center is constructed around the ability to diagnose and treat all aspects of all forms of acute and chronic pain under one roof. These centers have at least one physician who is the "Captain of the Medical Ship." This individual is able to obtain the correct diagnosis, treat with appropriate neuropharmacological medications (not typically narcotic analgesics), and design a specific treatment plan for a specific patient. The other members of the center's treatment team are typically a psychologist (PhD or Psy.D) or psychiatrist (MD), physical therapists, occupational therapists, and nurse specialists, all on a fulltime basis, and any other necessary clinicians on a full- or part-time basis. The center typically begins treatment by detoxifying or weaning patients off of unnecessary medications and obtaining a complete and correct diagnosis.

In the large comprehensive interdisciplinary pain management/neuro-rehab center overseen by the author, patient outcome data was kept for seven years, where it was placed on the center's Web site. The average patient had suffered from pain for over 5.6 years before arriving at the center; 63% of the patients seen were incorrectly and/or incompletely diagnosed; and 85% needed to be taken off unnecessary medications, including narcotics and barbiturates. These were significant factors in the patients coming to the center. Essentially, all previous treating clinicians had given up on these patients.

Aside from pain reduction and decreasing or eliminating inappropriate/unnecessary opioid medications, the major outcome data from this form of treatment should also include increased physical activity, return to work where possible, closure of disability claims, and reduction in health care (over) utilization.

Patients, all too commonly, when they initially develop pain—low-back pain for example (low-back pain is a description, not a real diagnosis, but is frequently seen as a patient diagnosis)—become labeled with the diagnosis; physicians may rarely reevaluate such patients to ascertain if the initial diagnosis was correct. With the development of chronicity, the initial pain-related diagnosis becomes only one of several diagnoses—including, possibly, depression, anxiety disorder, and iatrogenic substance abuse—all of which must be identified and treated for the patient to achieve some return to wellness/work or reduction in symptomatology.

A study performed in 1995 (2) found that only 6% of all patients treated by "pain specialists" (6% = 176,850 patients) were treated at an interdisciplinary pain center. These patients were sent to these facilities almost as a "last resort," as they had already had a mean seven-year history of pain and pain treatments. An average $13,284 was spent per patient each year on nonsurgical pain-related healthcare costs. These patients also had an average of 1.7 surgeries performed at an average cost of $15,000 per surgery (1994 USD).

The total cost of health care for these patients (only 6% of the pain patients seen in that year) was greater than $20 billion.

The cost for treatment at the interdisciplinary centers was greater than $1.4 billion (1995 average cost of $8,100 × 176,850). The medical cost savings after one year (post-treatment at the interdisciplinary centers) was greater than $1.87 billion, an 86% reduction in healthcare costs (3).

Chronic pain is a biological–psychological–sociological phenomenon. If all aspects of a patient's pain are not dealt with appropriately, and simultaneously, the overall effectiveness of treatment is poor. A number of published studies go further, stating that it is the inclusion of treatment of the chronic-pain patients' psychological and sociological (including economic factors, i.e. return to work) problems that enables the interdisciplinary pain centers to successfully treat these patients (4–6).

The full focus of the biological–psychological–sociological aspects of chronic pain (as well as return to work) is not dealt with in the mono- or bi-modality pain treatment facilities, or in typical "syndrome-oriented" pain treatment facilities.

CHRONIC NON-CANCER PAIN SYNDROME TREATMENT

The fact that the interdisciplinary pain center is clinically effective, cost-effective, and provides clinical relief that lasts during the first year post-treatment has been well documented (2,7–9).

In one systematic review, it was concluded that patients could be returned to work with nonsurgical, interdisciplinary pain center treatment (37 controlled and noncontrolled studies were evaluated) (7). In another systematic review (8), 65 controlled and noncontrolled studies were evaluated. The reviewed studies supported the effectiveness of interdisciplinary treatment but noted methodological problems existed in some of these studies.

The costs of chronic pain, particularly in the Workers' Compensation environment have been well documented. In 1994, the direct costs (medical costs, disability payments) and indirect costs (training substitute workers, paying them, legal costs) for injured workers totalled $171 billion. In 1999, the total financial impact of

Workers' Compensation injuries (direct and indirect) equaled more than $240 billion. A day lost from work equals one day's salary times 3.75, a significant cost when one looks at over 20 million days a year lost from work, just from headache.

Another study found that treatment at an interdisciplinary center was more clinically effective and more cost-effective than the traditional treatment methods, including medication, surgery, interventional procedures (nerve blocks), noninvasive treatment modalities such as physical therapy, and implantable devices such as spinal cord stimulators and medication pumps (10).

It was also found that the cost to return one injured worker after treatment at an interdisciplinary pain center was $11,913, while the cost to return one patient to work after back surgery was $75,000. The cost to return patients to work indicates that treatment at an interdisciplinary pain center is 6.3 times more cost-effective than surgery (3).

As medicine is starting to be driven by cost and outcome data, such information is extremely important. Also, as noted earlier, MPS may be the single most common cause of chronic non-cancer pain syndrome patients. Research has noted that there is "overwhelming, consistent meta-analytic evidence that pain facilities provide effective treatment for a wide range of outcome variables for such patients (11)." The same study noted that referring physicians should be aware of the type of pain treatment facility to which they send their patients, as not all facilities use the same treatment methods.

As indicated in great detail in Chapter 6, in the section on "Evidence-Based Medicine," an EBM review (from the Cochrane Database) entitled "Multidisciplinary rehabilitation for fibromyalgia syndrome (FMG) and musculoskeletal pain in working age results," which used a different definition of multidisciplinary pain management than pain specialists use, found all poor studies and stated the level of scientific evidence regarding multidisciplinary pain rehabilitation for "this diagnosis (sic) is limited" (12).

When utilizing more commonly accepted criteria, another systematic review (from the Cochrane Database) entitled "Multidisciplinary Bio-psycho-social rehabilitation for chronic low-back pain" (13) concluded that evidence showed intensive (> 100 hours of therapy) interdisciplinary bio-psycho-social pain rehabilitation programs with a functional restoration approach engendered greater improvements in pain and function for patients with "disabling chronic low-back pain," than did nonmultidisciplinary rehabilitation or "usual care."

Please note that some utilize the terms "interdisciplinary" and "multidisciplinary" synonymously—as is done here, while other use them differently. Of interest, the term "multidisciplinary" predated and, in some ways has been updated to, "interdisciplinary."

Finally, dual diagnosis multidisciplinary pain programs that deal with chronic non-cancer pain and substance-abusing patients are also found to work well (14).

Turk and Burwinkle (15) noted an "epidemic of 'Mural Dyslexia," the "inability to read the handwriting on the wall." They noted that outcome data are necessary and important to have for the sake of the payers as well as the patients. They reiterate that there is a large cohort of published information indicating that the interdisciplinary pain centers are clinically effective, cost-effective, and, via their treatment paradigm, able to provide significant savings in health care and disability payments.

In an important study, Robbins et al. (16) noted that patients in their interdisciplinary pain management programs who were forced by insurance company "carve outs" to have physical therapy elsewhere experienced negative treatment outcomes at one year, in comparison with those patients who were able to participate in the full, intact program.

As previously discussed in this book, the restoration of function must be a primary goal of all interdisciplinary treatment programs. Rehabilitation, while it focuses on function and not specifically pain, is associated with decreased pain and improvements in psychological status as function improves (17).

A recent study looking at a more abbreviated "comprehensive pain management programme" including education, cognitive, and behavioral interventions for patients experiencing neuropathic pain status post– spinal cord injury were considered an important and valuable complement to the patients' treatment (18).

FIBROMYALGIA TREATMENT STUDIES

A half-day treatment program for FMS was done by Kaiser Permanente and evaluated by patient questionnaires (19). It was found to be helpful in both mental health and functional measures.

Another FMS study (20) found that when interdisciplinary treatment was customized, based on patients' individualized psychosocial needs, outcomes are enhanced.

Davidson (21) indicated that a multidisciplinary treatment approach to FMS patients offers the best method to achieving effective pain relief.

Other studies also showed the efficacy of interdisciplinary pain management programs for FMS patients (22,23).

TECHNIQUE

Over the last 26 years, the author has found that neurological and musculoskeletal examination and diagnosis come first—then, if the patient has chronic pain and needs an interdisciplinary treatment program, the physical therapist, the psychologist, and the occupational therapist perform evaluations. The entire team then meets and discusses diagnoses and examination findings.

An individualized interdisciplinary treatment program is then determined, if found to be appropriate.

The team meets weekly to discuss the patient's progress or lack of progress in each individual treatment modality. In many cases, the patient may join the staff to discuss how treatment is progressing. During the weekly team staff meeting, each clinician who is treating a specific patient gives a report of the patient's progress or lack of progress during the past week.

The interdisciplinary team is the most important treatment tool available to the chronic-pain patient. Each member of the team should be "cross-trained" regarding the basics of each other's discipline. It is not unusual for a patient to tell the physical therapist, rather than the physician or the psychologist, their feelings of suicidality. The physical therapist would need to understand how to deal with this information without ab-reacting, and should be trained in how to handle the situation while waiting for the physician, whom they would immediately notify, to come to talk to the patient.

The clinic's nurse specialists should be the patients' internal case managers, who make certain that all orders from the physician and/or the rest of the treatment team have been carried out. The nurse also serves as each patient's primary liaison with the physician and the team. The nurse's role is of extreme importance. They must have a good degree of knowledge about pain medicine and medication. For one thing, some physicians never give medication refills—patients must call each month for refills, and the nurse is responsible for determining if the patient has been taking their medications in a timely fashion, and discussing any problems with the physician. Training is well worth the time and effort for the nurse and the entire team.

The weekly team staff briefings are also the best time to have appropriate third-party visitors come to the clinic. This would include outside nurse case managers or, if they can get away, adjustors. The patient's attorney may desire to attend such a staff meeting.

Interdisciplinary pain management programs have been the most medically efficacious, time, and cost-effective treatment paradigm for the chronic non-cancer pain patients with a chronic MPS or FMS. Unfortunately, a very limited number of this type of treatment facility exist. Many excellent programs at prestigious medical institutions have been forced to close as a result of poor insurance reimbursement.

The dwindling numbers of these programs bodes poorly for the chronic-pain patient and their insurers, for the reasons—both clinical and financial—noted earlier.

REFERENCES

1. Loeser JD. Desirable characteristics for pain treatment facilities: report of the IASP taskforce. In: Bond MR, Charleon JE, Woolf CJ eds. Proceedings of the Sixth World Congress on Pain. Seattle, International Association for the Study of Pain, 1991:411–415.
2. Marketdata Enterprises: Chronic pain management programs: A Market analysis. Tampa, FL, 1995.
3. Turk DC, Loeser JD, Monarch ES. Chronic pain: purposes and costs of interdisciplinary pain rehabilitation programs. TEN 2002; 4(2):64–69.
4. Roy R. Pain clinics: reassessment of objectives and outcomes. Arch Phys Med Rehabil 1984; 65(8):448–451.
5. Rosomoff HL, Rosomoff RS. Comprehensive multidisciplinary pain center approach to the treatment of low back pain. Neurosurg Clin N Am 1991; 2:877–890.
6. Becker N, Hojsted J, Sjogren P, Eriksen J. Sociodemographic predictors of treatment outcome in chronic non-malignant pain patients. Do patients receiving or applying for disability pension benefit from multidisciplinary pain treatment? Pain 1998; 77:279–287.
7. Cutler RB, Fishbain DA, Rosomoff HL, et al. Does nonsurgical pain center treatment of chronic pain return patients to work? A review and meta-analysis of the literature. Spine 1994; 19(6):643–652.
8. Flor H, Fydich T, Turk DC. Efficacy of multidisciplinary pain treatment centers: a meta-analytic review. Pain 1992; 49:221–230.
9. Chapman SL, Brena SF, Bradford LA. Treatment outcome in a chronic pain rehabilitation problem. Pain 1981; 11:155–268.
10. Turk DC, Okifuji A. Treatment of chronic pain patients: clinical outcomes, cost-effectiveness and cost-benefits of multidisciplinary pain centers. Crit Rev Phys Med Rehabil 1998; 10:181–208.
11. Fishbain DA, Cutler R, Rosomoff H, Rosomoff RS. Pain facilities: a review of their effectiveness and referral selection criteria. Curr Headache Pain Rep 1997; 1(2):107–115.
12. Karjalainen K, Malmivaara A, van Tulder M, et al. Multidisciplinary rehabilitation for fibromyalgia an musculoskeletal pain in working age adults (Cochrane Review). IN: the Cochrane Library, Issue 4, 2002. Oxford: Update Software.
13. Guzman J, Esmail R, Karjalainen KI, et al. Multidisciplinary Bio-Psycho-Social Rehabilitation for chronic low back pain (Cochrane Review). In: the 3 Cochrane Library, Issue 4, 2002. Oxford: Update Software.

14. Mahoney ND, Devine JE, Angres D. Multidisciplinary treatment of benign chronic pain syndrome in substance abusing patients. Curr Rev Pain 1999; 3:321–331.
15. Turk D, Burwinkle T. Treatment of chronic pain sufferers- an antidote to mural dyslexia. The Pain Practitioner (American Academy of Pain Management) 2004; 14(3):20–25.
16. Robbins H, Gatchel RJ, Noe C, et al. A prospective one-year outcome study of interdisciplinary chronic pain management: compromising its efficacy by managed care policies. Anesth Analg 2003; 97(1):156–162.
17. Schofferman J. Restoration of function: the missing link in pain medicine? Pain Med 2006; 7(Suppl 1):S159–S165.
18. Norrbrink Budh C, Kowalski J, Lundeberg T. A comprehensive pain management programme comprising educational, cognitive and behavioural interventions for neuropathic pain following spinal cord injury. J Rehabil Med 2006; 38(3):172–180.
19. Beck A, Breth G, Ellis J, et al. Multidisciplinary group intervention for fibromyalgia: a study of psychiatric symptom and functional disability outcomes. Permanente J 2002; 6(2): www.kaiserpermanente.org/medicine/permjournal/spring02/fibromyaglia.html
20. Turk DC, Okifuji A, Sinclair JD, Starz TW. Differential responses by psychosocial subgroups of fibromyalgia syndrome patients to an interdisciplinary treatment. Arthritis Care Res 1998; 11(5):397–404.
21. Davidson P. Fibromyalgia: A painful and treatable illness. San Francisco Medical Society: www.sfms.org/sfm/sfm202b.htm. (Accessed on Feb 2002.)
22. Bennett RM, Burckhardt CS, Clark SR, et al. Group treatment of fibromyalgia: a 6 month outpatient program. J Rheumatol 23(3):521–528.
23. Bennett RM. Multidisciplinary group programs to treat fibromyalgia patients. Rheum Dis Clin North Am 1996; 22(2):351–367.

Index